HEALING AUTISM IN THE KITCHEN

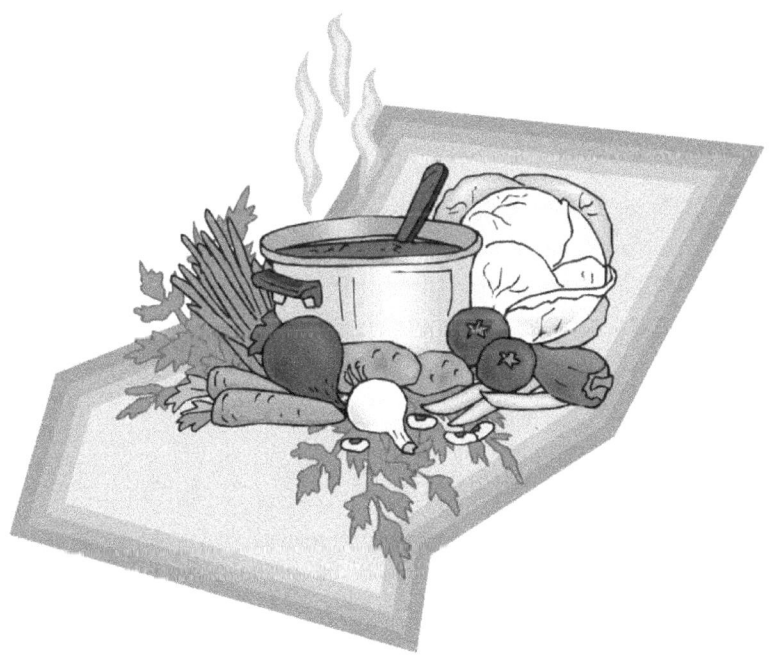

Healing with Healthy Nutrition

Healing aspects of a healthy diet, with specific emphasis on oral motor difficulties in children with autism spectrum and developmental disorders.

By Annette Cartaxo MD and Garima Jain ND

The information in this book is presented to assist parents of children with special needs. This book is not intended to diagnose or treat any medical condition. Readers should use common sense in applying the information in this book and consult with their medical doctor if there are questions about whether specific foods or diets are appropriate for their child. Since each child is different, specific reactions to foods recommended in these diets cannot be accounted for; therefore, the use of caution is advised. The book is solely intended to share information based on the experience and research of the authors. Neither the author nor publisher will assume any liability for inappropriate use of the information in this book.

Copyright ©2010 by GN Publishing LLC

All rights reserved. Printed in the United States of America. No part of this publication may be reproduced, stored in a retrieval system, or transmitted, in any form or by any means electronic, mechanical, photocopying, recording, or otherwise, without the prior written permission of the author.

ISBN: 978-0-615-23917-0
LCCN: 2008907249

Published by GN Publishing LLC
New Jersey, USA

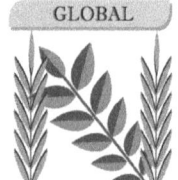

DEDICATION

Dr. Annette Cartaxo

This book is dedicated to the core of my emotional life — my family, those closest to me who have always loved and supported me.

My parents, **Richard and Antoinette Rossetti**

My husband, **Kenneth Cartaxo**

My daughter, **Danielle Cartaxo**

My son, **Joseph Cartaxo**

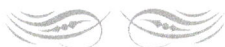

Dr. Garima Jain

This book is dedicated to my family and all the parents who go far above and beyond in helping their children achieve a fulfilling life.

My parents, **D.K Jain & Saroj Rani Jain**

My husband, **Vinod Jain**
My special dedication goes to my husband, whose enormous efforts have made this book come to reality.

My son, **Harshil Jain**
He came to me as a blessing and taught me how to love unconditionally.

ACKNOWLEDGMENT

This book has been a dream that was years in the making. Never before has such an intensive need to find answers to the Autism puzzle been apparent in our country and in the world. We wish to thank all the children and their parents who taught us so much; some who are our patients and some who are our own children. As we see the unique aspects of every individual who is diagnosed with Autistic Spectrum Disorder (ASD) and developmental delay, we also see the similarities that run as a common thread of this complex disorder. It must be realized that in helping treat those with ASD and developmental delay one must consider the natural laws of the function of the human body. It has been a great challenge to combine sound overall nutritional advice while paying close attention to addressing the unique problems and aspects of those with ASD and developmental delay.

We thank those researchers and clinicians who are brave enough to find answers for these individuals with complex and multifaceted developmental problems.

Special thanks to Hope Fernicola and the members of TeamHope Speech and Pediatric Center (www.teamhope.com), whose input on the oral motor aspects of children with ASD and assistance in rating the recipes in terms of level of oral motor difficulty, is an invaluable portion of this book. We would like to acknowledge Maurice Johnson for the design and artwork of the cover of this book.

Our deepest gratitude goes to the team at Body Bio Corporation who helped so much with their efforts, time and expertise, especially Dr. Tom Wnorowski, Reggie Scott and Judy Schneider, and most of all to Dr. Patricia Kane, a friend, a mentor and a healer who truly cares about making a difference in the lives of patients who are suffering from illness. Finally to Ed Kane, a brilliant mind, innovator and "Renaissance Man".

TABLE OF CONTENTS

PREFACE i

INTRODUCTION iii

CHAPTER 1 – NUTRITIONAL WELLNESS 1
    Nutrients and Nutrient-Dense Foods 3
    Carbohydrates: Main Source of Energy 4
    Proteins and Amino Acids..5
    Fats and Essential Fatty Acids...7
    Introduction to Vitamins...9
    Fat Soluble Vitamins 11
    Introduction to Minerals 18
    Macro Minerals 20
    Trace Minerals 23

CHAPTER 2 – GETTING STARTED WITH NUTRITION 27
    Guide to Food Selection 28
    Nuts and Seeds: Nutrient-Dense Foods..29
    Health Benefits of Nuts..30
    Seeds That Nourish Growth 32
    Guide to Natural Oils and Their Health Benefits 34
    Guidelines for Using Natural Oils..36
    Sea Weeds: Health Treasure 37
    Types of Sea Weed and Health Benefits 39
    Lesser-Known Healthy Foods and Their Health Benefits 42
    Fermented Foods: Fruits and Vegetables.....................................45
    Beneficial Fermented Foods and Recipes 46
    Beans, Lentils, and Legumes Guide 51
    Pressure-Cooking Beans 52

CHAPTER 3 – THE PRACTICAL GUIDE TO HEALTHY LIVING 55
- Preventing Cross-Contamination in the Kitchen....................................56
- Tips and Hints to Avoid Cross-Contamination 57
- Healthy Eating Habits – Tips & Hints 58
- Hidden Food Allergens – Tips & Hints 60
- Unhealthy Hidden Ingredients in Food 61
- Guide to Natural Sweeteners 63
- Refined Sugar vs. Natural Sweeteners 64
- Impact of a High-Sugar Diet 67
- Tips for Limiting Children's Sugar Intake 67
- Planning Lunch Box Meals That Kids Enjoy..69

CHAPTER 4 – KITCHEN SAVVY AND COOKING AIDS – TIPS & HINTS..........73
- Suggested List of Cookware for Healthy Cooking................................74
- Suggested List of Cookware to Avoid 76
- Cooking Pans 77
- Kitchen Accessories Guide 78
- Small Kitchen Appliance Suggestions..79
- Tips for Using Food Storage Containers 80
- General Kitchen Tips & Hints 81
- Cooking Efficiently 82
- Ideas for Baking 84
- Kitchen Safety Tips & Hints 85

CHAPTER 5 – DIET AND DIETARY PLANNING – INTRODUCTION TO DIETS................87
- Gluten and Casein-Free Diet (GFCF)...89
- Gluten and Casein-Free Diet: Guidelines for Parents..........................93
- Low Oxalate Diet (LOD) 94
- Low Oxalate Diet: Guidelines for Parents 96
- Phenol-Free Diet 97
- Phenol-and Additives-Free Diet: Guidelines for Parents 100
- Specific Carbohydrate Diet (SCD) Diet..101
- Specific Carbohydrate Diet: Guidelines for Parents...........................104

Chapter 6 – Other Diet Options 107
Raw Food Diet 108
Food Rotation Diet 109
Food Elimination Diet 110

Chapter 7 – Special Diet: Food List and Resources 111
Gluten-Free & Casein-Free (GFCF Diet) Food List 112
Gluten-Free Casein-Free Resources Shopping List 113
Dairy Substitutes & Sources 115
Low Oxalate Diet Food List 117
Phenol-Free Diet Food List 118
Specific Carbohydrate Diet Food List (Foods "Legal" and "Illegal") 119

Chapter 8 – Aspects of Oral Motor Development 157
Understanding Your Child's Eating Problems 160
Setting Up the Eating Environment and Behavior Guidelines 162

Chapter 9 – Getting Started in Meal Planning 165
Gluten-Free Cooking Flour Options 166
Quick Recipes to Speed Cooking 170
Homemade Specialties 172

Oral Motor Rating Chart 177

Chapter 10 – Breakfast Recipes 179
The Importance of a Good Breakfast

Chapter 11 – The Main Course 221
Lunch and Dinner Recipes

Chapter 12 – Tasty Meal Companions 269
Soups and Salads Recipes

CHAPTER 13 – DELICIOUS ACCOMPANIMENTS 315
    Recipes for Sauces, Dips, Dressings and Condiments

CHAPTER 14 – HEALTHY BETWEEN-MEAL TREATS..331
    Hunger-Satisfying Snacks Recipes

CHAPTER 15 – SWEETS 'N' DESSERTS...347
    Cookies, Pies, Cakes, Brownies and Biscotti Recipes, and More

CHAPTER 16 – SMOOTHIES AND POWER SHAKES
    "Power Shakes" 379

CONVERSION TABLES AND MEASUREMENT CHARTS 393

INDEX OF RECIPES..394

RESOURCES 402

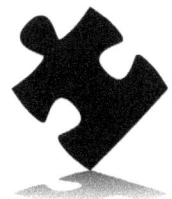

PREFACE

Healing Autism in the Kitchen is devoted to children with Autism Spectrum and other development disorders, as well as to children who are overfed, yet undernourished. This book is not a nutritional manual. Rather, it is a cookbook that focuses on how to nourish children, with a special focus on children with ASD. Food has healing power that can stabilize one both physically and mentally.

This book is written with the intention of making a person healthy. Diet is the key and not necessarily dietary supplements, which are not a replacement for a healthy diet. Eating whole foods is first and foremost where one should start as the basis of sound nutrition.

Everyone appreciates a great meal, and many of us would love to be able to prepare one. With busy lives and other family commitments, however, sometimes the ability to prepare a healthy meal eludes us. Cooking, for some parents who are cooking for children with special needs, is a complex process in itself. This book was written to create healthy meals for children with special needs a simple process. The recipes are easy, and once you understand the basics, you will be able to make many fabulous meals in a matter of minutes.

This book also provides the necessary tools and guidelines for parents, and introduces them to the fundamentals of cooking. Parents will learn how to shop for healthy foods, to identify and select healthy ingredients, to learn to read labels, and to identify (parallel) unhealthy hidden ingredients, all of which are steps towards a fabulous culinary experience. Parents will also learn how to increase their chances of success in the kitchen by selecting proper equipment and kitchen accessories, and by learning healthy tips on how to cook. Included are individualized recipes suited to children's specific needs.

All efforts have been taken to make preparation of the recipes easy and fun. The ingredients selected are nutritious and can easily be found in local supermarkets, health foods stores, or online. Each recipe includes an informative box with tips or other helpful information. This book will give you the background to step into your kitchen with confidence in the knowledge that you're truly equipped with all that you need to serve a nutritious meal to your child and entire family.

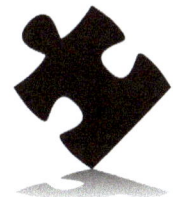

INTRODUCTION

Autism is one of the five pervasive development disorders (PDDs). Children with autism spectrum disorders (ASD) exhibit a broad range of behaviors and levels of severity. These are defined as severe deficits in social interactions, language, communication and play, with stereotypic and repetitive behaviors with a narrow range of interests. Children with autism spectrum disorder also have gross-motor, fine motor and oral motor problems, which impact their overall function and development.

This book focuses on a healthy diet while addressing the feeding-related oral motor problems of children with ASD. Feeding and speech problems can also result from sensitivity in and around the mouth. These problems are related to hyper (over) or hypo (under) reactions to sensory input. Many children with ASD demonstrate delayed, primitive and/or abnormal oral motor development that impacts their expressive language and eating development. We recommend that some children will need an oral motor skills evaluation by a licensed speech-language pathologist or a feeding specialist.

It is our observation that many children with ASD and other developmental disorders have a limited diet and prefer crunchy foods such as pretzels, crackers and cookies that are quick and easy to chew. They reject meats, most fruits and vegetables, and are usually messy eaters, often over-stuffing food into their mouths and frequently rejecting having their teeth brushed. They have difficulty accepting new foods and have an aversion to tactile input in the mouth.

Some of the problems parents face in feeding a wholesome diet to their children with ASD and other developmental disorders relate to their specific oral motor problems, which are commonly seen and observed. These include excessive food loss while eating, mouthing inedible objects after the age of two, presence of immature oral reflexes, sensitivities to food textures and temperature, excessive drooling, and unintelligent speech after the age of three.

This book will help you simplify how to start and maintain a wholesome diet, with specific attention to the problems parents face with their children diagnosed with ASD and other developmental disorders. It focuses on biochemical issues, behavioral issues, and oral motor function.

CHAPTER ONE

Nutritional Wellness

NUTRITIOUS FOODS ARE THE EASIEST WAY to start your child on a wholesome diet and lifestyle. Most foods, especially "whole foods," are those that have not been radically changed. They are in their natural state and contain a variety of nutrients, such as vitamins, minerals, carbohydrates, proteins and fats. Some foods have better quantity and quality of these components, and those that contain the highest are considered "nutrient dense" foods.

Everyone needs good food to obtain proper nutrition. For some individuals, especially some diagnosed with ASD, getting proper nutrition is difficult due to many obstacles inherent in their unique biochemistry and physiology. The easiest way to help these children is to offer them a choice of healthy foods to eat. Just taking vitamins and minerals in supplements is not enough. For example, often if a child is deficient in good fats the requirement for vitamins and minerals is increased. When adequate EFA nourishment is supplied in the diet, the need for vitamins and mineral quantities is diminished. As your child gets the essential components in a healthy diet, he or she gets healthier overall.

New Nutritional Wellness Model: It is our philosophy that if a child is healthy — really healthy — eats a truly good diet, and is not exposed to environmental toxins, then one may not need supplements. However, in our world today, one needs nutritional support along with diet to be healthy because we are exposed to toxins both in the environment and in foods, so our bodies are in a constant state of detoxification.

The New Wellness Model incorporates a nutrient dense diet with nutritional supplements. Positive attitude is the key and nature's healthy foods are what we need to maintain our health.

Nutrient and Nutrient-Dense Foods

As mentioned a **nutrient** is described as a substance contained in a food used by the body to promote growth, maintenance and repair of tissues, or simply a substance that provides nourishment.

Nutrients are categorized into two groups

Macro-nutrients: These are present in our diets in large amounts, and make up the foundation of our diet and include:

- Carbohydrates
- Proteins
- Fats

Micro-nutrients: Found in various quantities in nutrient dense foods, micronutrients are essential to ensure that metabolism, growth and development, along with our cellular processes function properly. Even though their presence is in minute amounts, it should in no way diminish their importance to nutrition.

Most micro-nutrients are known to be essential nutrients — as they are indispensable to life processes as the body cannot manufacture them. In other words, micro-nutrients can only be obtained from the food in which we eat. Micronutrients:

- Vitamins
- Minerals

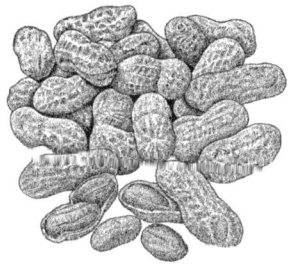

Carbohydrates: Main Source of Energy

Carbohydrates are your body's main source of energy. Carbohydrates are actually built of sugar molecules, called saccharides. The body requires around 45 to 65 percent of total calories in the form of carbohydrates. However, these need to be nutrient dense carbohydrates found in fruits and vegetables, not donuts and candy. These saccharides are arranged together like beads on a necklace.

Carbohydrates include sugars, starches, and fiber. Both sugars and starches are broken down by the body into the simple sugar, glucose. Glucose molecules then circulate in the bloodstream, supplying cells with fuel on an as-needed basis. Extra glucose is converted into glycogen, which is stored in muscles and the liver. If the body is already storing enough glycogen, glucose gets changed into fat. Your body prefers to burn glucose or glycogen for energy, but when these reserves are depleted it draws on fat, the reserve fuel. Carbohydrates are an important part of the diet, since your body needs energy to grow, to work, and to repair itself.

Effects of Carbohydrates on Children with ASD: Foods high in refined carbohydrates, like white sugar and white flour, provide quick breakdown and easy assimilation of simple sugars that provide the energy to the cells with very little digestive work. Many children with developmental delay and ASD who eat this type of diet tend to snack all day. This is the case because carbohydrates are not digested in the stomach; they exit quickly, leaving an empty feeling that elicits a hunger response. As these carbohydrates leave the stomach, they make their way into the small intestine where they are quickly broken down into simple sugars that are released into the blood stream. This causes an increase in insulin which in turn causes a drop in blood sugar level as sugar now enters the cells to be used as energy. This low blood sugar will in turn elicit the drive to restore adequate levels by causing the individual to seek these foods again.

It has been observed by many parents that behavior in children with ASD is affected by this rise and fall in sugar levels. When sugar levels are rapidly increasing and decreasing it can cause hyperactivity, aggression, tantrums, self-stimulatory behaviors, and melt downs.

Proteins and Amino Acids

Proteins: Proteins are large, complex molecules that play many critical roles in the body. They do most of the work in cells and are required for the structure, function, and regulation of the body's tissues and organs. Proteins are the building blocks of the body. The human body on average assembles about 50,000 different proteins to form organs, nerves, and muscles essential for growth and development. Proteins also provide the body with energy, and are needed in the manufacture of hormones, antibodies, enzymes, and tissues.

Amino Acids: When protein is consumed, it is broken down into its smallest components, amino acids, the building blocks of proteins. Humans can produce eleven of the twenty amino acids called "non-essential." The others (the "essentials") must be supplied in the foods we eat. Normally we obtain amino acids from our food sources, particularly those high in protein. The body breaks these proteins down into their constituent parts and our cells use these to build the specific types of protein each of them needs.

Types of Amino Acids

Essential Amino Acids: These are called essential amino acids because the body cannot synthesize them; instead they have to be obtained by the diet. The nine essential amino acids are Histidine, Isoleucine, Leucine, Lysine, Methionine, Phenylalanine, Threonine, Tryptophan and Valine.

Non-Essential Amino Acids: These are called non-essential, not because they are not needed, but because they do not have to be obtained as part of one's diet. Instead the body makes non-essential amino acids from other amino acids already in the body. The eleven non-essential amino acids are Alanine, Arginine, Asparagine, Aspartic Acid, Cysteine, Glutamic Acid, Glutamine, Glycine and Proline.

Failure to obtain enough of even one of the nine essential amino acids results in degradation of the body's muscle proteins. Unlike fat and starch, the human body does not store excess amino acids for later use; they must be in the diet every day.

The National Academy of Sciences says people need to get 10 to 35 percent of their daily calories from protein. Lack of consumption of good protein is commonly found in children with ASD, as these children tend to eat less protein in their diets.

This may be due in part to a child's oral motor and sensitivity problems or pancreatic insufficiencies in the release of digestive enzymes, which could have been created by a low protein diet in the first place, since approximately half of the dietary protein consumed daily goes into making enzymes.

When protein is lacking in the diet, the brain and other organs cannot function or develop properly, and the child may have failure to thrive. **Poor diets which exclude protein foods, such as a, vegetarian diet, need to be monitored carefully to include wide range of complementary plant proteins such as seeds, nuts, legumes, and perhaps egg.**

Common Symptoms of Protein Deficiency include wasting and shrinkage of muscle tissue, edema (swelling, including the brain), anemia (the blood's inability to deliver sufficient oxygen to the cells), and diminished growth in children, neurotransmitter imbalances (which can lead to depression & behavior disorders) etc. may result.

For children with ASD the diet needs to be balanced with a variety of healthy foods in the form of proteins, complex carbohydrates, fats and essential fatty acids.

Fats and Essential Fatty Acids

Fats are a concentrated form of energy available to the body just as carbohydrates are. Much attention has been focused on reducing dietary fat, but the body does need fats to function properly. It is the man-made fats — margarine and hydrogenated oil — that cause a health challenge. Fatty acids provide building blocks for cell membranes and a variety of hormones and hormone-like substances and make up 60% of the brain. Fats, as part of a healthy meal, slow down the digestive process, which prolongs the phase of nutrient absorption and give a feeling of fullness. This is crucial for children with ASD, as they need to snack frequently for biochemical stability.

Trans Fats: Children tend to eat poor quality foods which often contain "trans" fats found commonly in fast foods and commercial baked goods. Trans fats act as plastic deposited in the cell membranes, where they interrupt normal cell function. Margarine, hydrogenated vegetable oil, shortening and all foods containing trans fat must be avoided as much as possible.

Unsaturated Essential Fatty Acids: EFAs (Essential Fatty Acids) are specialized fats the body cannot manufacture. They make up the membrane barrier that surrounds every cells and intracellular organelles in our bodies. EFAs determine fluidity and chemical reactivity of membranes. They also regulate oxygen use, help form red blood pigment (hemoglobin), the immune system fight infections, prevent the development of allergies, and increase metabolic rate, and energy levels. EFAs also play a role in every life process in the body. *Life without EFAis impossible.*

Saturated Fatty Acids: Are highly stable, can withstand high cooking temperatures, and do not go rancid at room temperature. These fats are solid or semi-solid at room temperature. They are found in animal fats and tropical oils. The body can also make them from carbohydrates. Saturated fat sources include meat fat, poultry fat and butter cream. Saturated fats have tremendous benefits to the body as supportive architecture for cell membranes and the formation of hormones.

Unsaturated Fatty Acids:

Monounsaturated Fatty Acids: Tend to be liquid at room temperature, solid when cooled. They are relatively heat-stable, do not become rancid, and therefore can be used for cooking. The body can make monounsaturated fatty acids and uses them as energy. They are found in olive oil as well as in fats from almonds, cashews, pecans and avocados.

Polyunsaturated Fatty Acids or PuFAs: Highly reactive and become rancid easily, particularly omega-3 fatty acids. They are always in the liquid state, even when frozen. These fatty acids should never be heated or used generally in cooking, and should be handled with care. PuFAs are found in seeds, walnuts, egg yolk and cold water fish.

Deficiency Symptoms of EFAs in Autism Spectrum Disorder: EFA deficiency in children with developmental delay and autism may experience excessive thirst, frequent urination, asthma, depression, anxiety, dry skin/hair, hyperactivity, mood changes, learning difficulties, and problems with attention and focus. Many children have a very low intake of essential fatty acids. Omega-6 fatty acids and omega-3 fatty acids are equally important, but it is important to take these fats in the proper ratio. The ratio of omega-6 to omega-3 should be about 4:1. This means that we need four times as much omega-6 as omega-3.

Signs and Symptoms in Children with ASD Where EFAs Can Help

- Dry, flaky skin
- Asthma
- Bedwetting
- Behavior difficulties
- Recurrent illness
- Dry, straw-like hair
- Excessive thirst
- Cognitive problems
- Dandruff
- Eczema

Introduction to Vitamins

Vitamins are a group of nutrients found only in living things, plants and animals. Vitamins are divided into two classes based on their solubility:

- **The fat-soluble vitamins**, which include vitamin A, D, E, and K.

- **The water-soluble vitamins**, which include folate (folic acid), vitamin B12, biotin, vitamin B6, vitamin B3 (niacin), vitamin B1 (thiamin), vitamin B2 (riboflavin), vitamin B5 (pantothenic acid), and vitamin C (ascorbic acid).

Fat-soluble vitamins can be stored in appreciable amounts in the body, and so caution should be used not to overdose them. Water-soluble vitamins cannot be stored in the body; however, when water soluble vitamins are used for children with ASD (such as the B vitamins and vitamin C), it is important to consider that dosages should be individualized, as each child may react to the same dose differently.

Functions of Vitamins in the Human Body: Vitamins are sometimes referred to as the "spark plugs" of our human machine. They promote normal growth, ensure good health, and protect against certain diseases. Vitamins are required by the body in small amounts to help regulate metabolism, to protect health, and for proper growth in children. They assist in the formation of hormones, blood cells, nervous-system chemicals, and genetic material. They are responsible for keeping cells & connective tissue strong, and fighting infections.

Vitamins also help convert fat and carbohydrates into energy, and assist in forming bone and tissues. Vitamins and minerals have no calories and are not an energy source, but they assist in making it possible for other nutrients to be digested, absorbed and metabolized by the body. Without vitamins our cells would not function properly and thus our organs would fail and eventually we would no longer be able to survive.

Modern Methods and Vitamins' Value in Food: Fifty years ago, commercial farmers started using chemical fertilizers to grow the crops. Now, today's methods of food handling, food processing, cooking on high heat, and oxidation are greatly impacting the nutritional contents of food. Deep-frying foods and long periods of high heat used in canning are destructive to some vitamins, but not all. Vitamin content in food varies enormously with farming methods too, as nitrogen fertilizers produce initial high yields, in part by pulling minerals from the soil. In time, commercially fertilized soils become depleted, and foods grown on them suffer greatly. Many commercial foods contain vitamins, but if they also contain additives and sugar, the detrimental effects of these preservatives will do more harm than the vitamins can offset.

Vitamins and Children with ASD: Children with ASD can be deficient in many nutrients including vitamins and minerals, since they have absorption problems and a limited diet, which may not provide proper nutrition. It thus becomes important for children with ASD to have a good multivitamin and to eat a healthy diet with foods that are organically grown and in their whole state. Processed foods should be limited. For optimum health, the American Medical Association now encourages that a multivitamin accompanies a healthy diet.

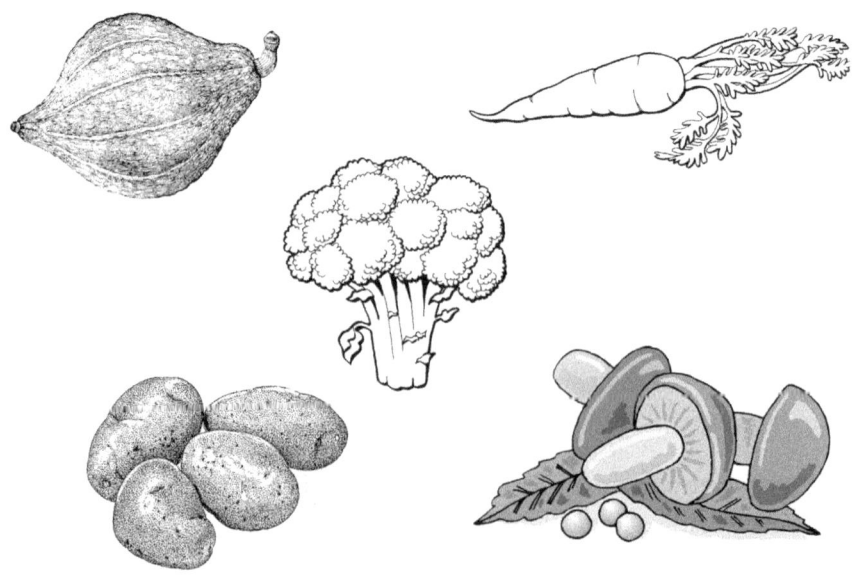

Fat Soluble Vitamins

Vitamin	Function	Common signs of Deficiency in ASD	Overdose Symptoms	Food Sources
Vitamin A (Retinol)	Strengthens mucous membranes, immune system, adrenal glands, and eyes Promotes skin health, hair, bones and teeth Anti-cancer for breast, bladder, cervical	Increased susceptibility to infections Poor appetite Dry and rough skin Hearing, taste, smell and nerve damage Night blindness, eye problems Impaired growth Reduced hair growth in children	Fatigue Diarrhea Dry, cracked Lips Rashes Headache Blurred or double vision Irregular menstrual periods Joint & bone pain Loss of hair Liver damage Birth defects Bone loss	Cod liver oil Crab Red pepper Dandelion Greens Carrot Nori Kale Parsley Spinach Swiss Chard Chives Watercress Broccoli Pumpkin Kombu Onion Cantaloupe Apricot <u>**Other Sources:**</u> Dark green leafy vegetables Yellow fruits & vegetables Vitamin A fortified milk Butter - summer Egg yolks
Vitamin D (Cholecalciferol)	Supports bone, tooth and muscle function Aids calcium, phosphorus, magnesium and zinc absorption Supports healthy function of thyroid gland Anti-cancer and anti-inflammatory properties	Rickets in children Bone softening in adults Osteoporosis Weak muscles Pain with brushing teeth	Nausea Vomiting Headaches Constipation Diarrhea Fatigue Appetite Loss Excessive Thirst and urination Protein in urine Liver and kidney damage	Cod liver oil Shiitake Mushroom Kippers Mackerel Sardines Tuna Cod Fish Liver Oil Fortified milk Butter Egg yolks

Fat Soluble Vitamins

Vitamin	Function	Common signs of Deficiency in ASD	Overdose Symptoms	Food Sources
Vitamin E (Tocopherols) and (TocoTrienols)	Antioxidant – (This property of this nutrient may be a factor in reducing the risk of certain forms of cancer.) Helps form red blood cells, muscles and other tissues; preserves fatty acids Anti-clotting properties; helps to keep blood platelets from sticking together	Anemia Edema Dry Skin Nerve abnormality Red blood cells fragility Weak muscles Impaired reflexes	Can cause stomach upset, diarrhea, and dizziness Nausea Overdose of Vitamin E can interfere with the body's ability to clot (especially dangerous if taking the blood thinning drugs Warfarin or Coumadin).	Wheat germ oil Corn oil Safflower oil Soybean oil Cod liver oil Sesame oil / Seeds Hazelnuts Pecans Sunflower oil / Seeds Kale Brazil nuts Turnip greens Spinach Peas Herring Millet Mackerel Brown rice Swiss chard Mangos Lettuce Apples Bananas Strawberries
Vitamin K	Allows your blood to clot normally Help protect against osteoporosis Prevents oxidative cell damage Helps in absorption of calcium, so contributes in forming bone cells	Excessive bruising and bleeding Digestive system problems, especially malabsorption Liver or gallbladder problems Defective blood coagulation	Generally non-toxic; elevated levels of vitamin K can interfere with the effects of anti-coagulants	Broccoli Brussels sprouts Cabbage Cauliflower Kale/Kombu (seaweeds) Spinach Soybeans Dark green vegetables

Water Soluble Vitamins

Vitamin	Function	Common signs of Deficiency in ASD	Overdose Symptoms	Food Sources
Vitamin B1 (Thiamine)	Key role in metabolism of carbohydrates, fat and protein Assists production of energy within the body Essential for normal function of muscles, heart and nervous system Stabilizes the appetite Promotes growth and good muscle tone	Vitamin B1 deficiency affects the functioning of gastrointestinal, cardiovascular, and peripheral nervous systems Anxiety Depression Hysteria Muscle weakness Nausea Vomiting Fatigue Memory loss Muscle cramps Loss of appetite Irritability Extreme cases causes beriberi, Edema, enlarged heart	Generally non-toxic alone, but excess of one B vitamin may cause deficiency of others	Brewer's Yeast Sunflower seeds Peanuts Chestnuts Brazil nuts Sesame seeds Soybeans Millet Aduki beans Rye Lentils Brown rice
Vitamin B2 (Riboflavin)	Key role in metabolism of carbohydrates, fat and proteins Assists production of energy within the body Aids in the formation of antibodies and red blood cells Helps maintain good vision, skin, nails and hair Alleviates eye fatigue May prevent cataracts May help combat migraine Promotes general health	Cracks and sores around the mouth and nose Visual problems (red eyes, light sensitivity) Depression Dry skin and hair loss Insomnia Poor digestion Anemia Dizziness	Generally non-toxic alone, but excess of one B vitamin may cause deficiency of others	Brewer's Yeast Sunflower seeds Walnuts Salmon Rainbow trout Nori (seaweeds) Kelp/Kombu (seaweeds) Tempeh Soybeans Mackerel Buckwheat Brown rice Banana Beans Avocado Chestnuts Kale Spinach Brussels sprouts

Water Soluble Vitamins

Vitamin	Function	Common signs of Deficiency in ASD	Overdose Symptoms	Food Sources
Vitamin B3 (Niacinamide) **Niacin is converted to niacinamide in the body.**	Needed in many enzymes that convert food to energy Helps maintain a healthy digestive tract and nervous system Involved in production of sex hormones; helps maintain healthy skin Improves circulation and reduces the cholesterol level in the blood	Fatigue Irritability Insomnia Emotional instability Blood sugar fluctuations In extreme cases, pellagra (disease characterized by dermatitis, diarrhea and mouth sores)	Flushing into niacin Nausea Vomiting Abdominal cramps Diarrhea Ulcers Severe overdose — liver disorders Gouty arthritis Irregular heart rate	Brewer's yeast Almonds Sunflower seeds Sesame seeds Mackerel Trout Salmon kelp Sardines Nori (seaweeds) Wakame (seaweeds) Brown rice Buckwheat Dried peas Green peas Tempeh Aduki beans Millet Soybeans Kale Parsley
Vitamin B5 (Pantothenic Acid)	Converts food to molecular forms; involved in the breakdown of carbohydrates, proteins and fats Supports normal growth and development Needed to manufacture adrenal and sex hormones chemicals that regulate nerve function Helps body use other vitamins Gene expression, RBC and neurotransmitter formation.	Nausea, vomiting Depression, anxiety Restlessness Eczema Palpitation Edema Allergy Insomnia Hives Burning feet Irritable bowel Adrenal fatigue Loss of hair pigment Growth retardation	Generally non-toxic alone, but excess of one B vitamin may cause deficiency of others	Brewer's yeast Almonds Chestnuts Cashews Walnuts Sunflower seeds Dates Blackcurrants Lobster Salmon Trout Mushrooms Cabbage Avocado Cauliflower Kale; Parsley Peas; Parsnips Corn (cooked) Squash Pinto beans Black-eyed beans Brown rice

Water Soluble Vitamins

Vitamin	Function	Common signs of Deficiency in ASD	Overdose Symptoms	Food Sources
Vitamin B6 (Pyridoxine)	Key role in metabolism of carbohydrates, fat and protein Assists production of energy within the body Aids in the formation of antibodies Maintains health of the central nervous system Aids removal of excess fluid in premenstrual women and reduces muscle spasms and cramps Promotes healthy skin Reduces hand numbness and stiffness Helps maintain balance of sodium and phosphorous	Seizures Headaches Nausea Vomiting Dry, flaky and scaly skin Irritability Cracks on mouth Sore tongue Anemia	Problems with sense of position and vibration; reduced tendon reflexes; numbness in hands and feet; problems walking; problems with memory; depression, headache and tiredness Imbalances in nervous system activity have been shown to result from high levels of supplemental vitamin B6 intake. *(These imbalances do not seem to occur until supplementation exceeds one gram per day.)*	Brewer's yeast Sunflower seeds Walnuts Chestnuts Salmon Rainbow trout Mackerel Nori (seaweeds) Kelp/Kombu (seaweeds) Tempeh Soybeans Pinto beans Buckwheat Brown rice Pearled barley Avocado Kale Spinach Brussels sprouts Lima beans Bananas
Vitamin B12 (Cobalamin)	Plays key role in metabolism of carbohydrates, fat and protein, assisting in production of energy within the body; helps formation and regeneration of red blood cells, thus helping prevent anemia; maintains a healthy nervous system; promotes growth in children; needed for calcium absorption; improves memory; Helps body use folic acid, and supports healthy functioning of nervous system.	Irritability Memory loss Constipation Tactile hyper sensitivity Megaloblastic anemia Loss of coordination Development delays; slow growth	Generally non-toxic; (be careful when supplementing vitamin B12 with other B vitamins)	Beef liver Oysters Crab Herring Mackerel Haddock Salmon Tempeh Kelp/Kombu (seaweeds) Nori (seaweeds) Hiziki Gruyer cheese Low fat milk Eggs Yogurt

Water Soluble Vitamins

Vitamin	Function	Common signs of Deficiency in ASD	Overdose Symptoms	Food Sources
Biotin	Involved in metabolism of fatty acids, carbohydrates, and protein Involved in maintaining health of skin, hair, sweat glands, nerves and bone marrow Essential for proper body chemistry Aids utilization of protein, folic acid, Pantothenic acid, and vitamin B12	Nausea, vomiting Dry scaly skin Seborrhic dermatitis in infants (rare in adults, but can be induced by consuming large amounts of egg whites) Anorexia High cholesterol Muscle cramps Cracks in the corner of the mouth	Biotin supplements are rarely seen on their own, and biotin is usually included instead as part of a quality B-complex multivitamin. Biotin combines well with other B-vitamins, especially vitamin B5 and vitamin B9. The recommended daily intake of biotin is 300 mcg.	Chard Tomatoes Romaine lettuce Carrots Onions Cabbage Cucumber Cauliflower Almonds Walnuts Eggs Goat's milk Raspberries Strawberries Halibut
Folic Acid (Folinic Acid)	Essential for the manufacture of genetic material as well as protein metabolism and red blood cell formation Supports hair and skin health Involved in growth, development and reproduction Supports healthy functioning of nervous system, brain development, RNA, DNA, Hemoglobin Methionine metabolism; Amino acid and neurotransmitter production	Diarrhea Digestive problems Fatigue Sleep problems Irritability Weakness Pallor Anemia Mental retardation Neural tube defects Homocystoincmia Low WBC (White Blood Cells) Neuropathy Gingivitis Glossitis	Kidney damage, abdominal bloating / distention Nausea Loss of appetite Increased cholesterol LDL / HDL ratio Increased zinc and potassium requirements may mask pernicious anemia from Vitamin B12 deficiency	Liver Fenugreek Chick peas Pinto beans Spinach Parsley Soybeans Black-eyed beans Brussels sprouts Broccoli Cauliflower Watercress Avocado Hiziki (seaweeds) Brown rice Nori (seaweeds) Dates Pears Oranges Pumpkin seeds Almonds Hazelnuts

Water Soluble Vitamins

Vitamin	Function	Common signs of Deficiency in ASD	Overdose Symptoms	Food Sources
Vitamin C (Ascorbic Acid)	Antioxidant; helps bind cells together and strengthens blood vessel walls Aids in absorption of iron from GI tract Helps maintain normal enzyme function Important for healthy growth of teeth, bones, gums, ligaments, and blood vessels Involved in production of neurotransmitters and adrenal gland hormones Plays an important role in immune response to infections and in supporting wound healing	Muscle weakness Infections Allergies Depression Anxiety Immune dysfunction Slow wound healing Recurrent bleeding gums Easy bruising In extreme cases: scurvy, cataracts, periodontitis	Diarrhea symptoms, which go away once supplement is stopped	Cherry Strawberries Guava Orange Blackcurrant Red pepper Kale Parsley Turnip tops Broccoli Brussels sprouts Watercress Cauliflower Lotus root Chives Spinach Cabbage Onions Bean sprouts

Introduction to Minerals

Minerals are naturally occurring elements found in earth. They are equally important for the body as vitamins. Vitamins cannot be assimilated without the aid of minerals. Although the body can manufacture a few vitamins, it cannot manufacture a single mineral. All tissues and internal fluids contain varying quantities of minerals. Minerals are constituents of the bones, teeth, soft tissue, muscle, blood, and nerve cells. They are vital to overall mental and physical well-being.

Function of Minerals: Minerals act as catalysts for many biological reactions within the body. The regulation of mineral balance in the body is essential for survival. **Minerals have two general functions — building and regulating.** Their building functions affect your bones, teeth, and all soft tissues. Their regulating functions include a wide variety of systems, such as the beating of your heart, the clotting of your blood, maintaining nerve responses, and transporting oxygen from your lungs to the tissues.

Minerals belong to two-groups:

Macrominerals

- a) Calcium
- b) Magnesium
- c) Sodium
- d) Potassium
- e) Phosphorus
- f) Sulfur
- g) Chloride

Microminerals or Trace Minerals

- a) Boron
- b) Chromium
- c) Copper
- d) Germanium
- e) Iodine
- f) Iron
- g) Manganese
- h) Molybdenum
- i) Selenium
- j) Zinc

Minerals and Children with ASD: Symptoms of mineral deficiency common in ASD children include:

- **Zinc:** Acne, apathy, brittle nails, delayed sexual maturity, depression, diarrhea, eczema, fatigue, growth impairment, hair loss, immune impairment, irritability, lethargy, loss of appetite, loss of sense of taste, low stomach acid, memory impairment, night blindness, paranoia, white spots on nails, poor wound healing.

- **Magnesium:** Anxiety, confusion, cardiac problems, hyperactivity, insomnia, nervousness, muscular irritability, restlessness, weakness.

- **Calcium:** Eye pain, brittle nails, cramps, delusions, depression, insomnia, irritability, osteoporosis, palpitations, periodontal disease, tooth decay.

Points to Remember:

- Calcium competes with other minerals for absorption.

- There is a direct relationship in the body with zinc and copper ratio. Many children with ASD have high copper and low zinc levels. Eating foods that are rich in zinc and even zinc supplementation can be helpful. Zinc should always be taken with a balance of all trace minerals.

- Calcium needs magnesium and vitamin D for optimal absorption.

- Calcium carbonate is the least absorbable (citrate/chelate/glycinate forms are preferred).

- Zinc should be given separately from calcium.

The following tables will help you understand the function of minerals in the body, signs of deficiency, overdose symptoms, and in which foods they are contained.

Macro Minerals

Vitamin	Function	Common signs of Deficiency in ASD	Overdose Symptoms	Food Sources
Calcium (Ca)	Bone and tooth structure Muscle function Clotting Heart rhythm Nerve function and regulation of blood vessel Hormone and enzyme secretion Cell membrane permeability Nerve transmission Helps activate enzymes needed to convert food into energy	Seizures Insomnia Irritability Anxiety Brittle nails Rickets Osteoporosis Osteopenia Cramps Periodontitis Tremors Hypertension	Constipation Alkalosis Joint pain Soft tissue Calcification Kidney stones Hinders absorption of iron in body and other minerals	Hiziki (seaweeds) Wakame (seaweeds) Arame (seaweeds) Kelp/Kombu (seaweeds) Soybeans Parsley Carrot tops Watercress Chickpeas Buckwheat Broccoli Milk Brown rice Hazelnuts Sesame seeds Sardines
Phosphorus (P)	Along with calcium, is needed to build bones and teeth Needed for metabolism, nerve and muscle function Needed for body's utilization of carbohydrates and fats Required for synthesis of protein for growth, maintenance and repair of cells and tissues Crucial for the production of ATP, a molecule body uses to store energy Helps regulate acid base balance Kidney function Helps body use other vitamins	Dizziness Neurological problems Muscle cramps Bone problems Ataxia Muscle myopathy Paresthesia Rickets Cardiac myopathy	Hypocalcemia Hinders body's absorption of calcium	Pumpkin seeds Sunflower seeds Sesame seeds Arame (seaweeds) Nori (seaweeds) Brown rice Lentils Rye Adzuki beans Oats Dulse (seaweed) Snapper Cod Sardines Chicken Beef

Macro Minerals

Vitamin	Function	Common signs of Deficiency in ASD	Overdose Symptoms	Food Sources
Magnesium (Mg)	Activates enzymes to release energy in body (ATP) Needed by cells for genetic material and bone growth Hormone and neurotransmitter metabolism Blood pressure regulation Blood sugar metabolism Metabolism of Calcium and Vitamin C Involved in structuring basis genetic material (DNA & RNA)	Insomnia Irritability Depression Constipation ADHD Nervousness Fatigue Hyperactive Nausea Confusion Sleep seizures GI upset Cramps Arrhythmia Osteoporosis PMS Muscle tension Twitching Rapid heartbeat	Diarrhea Stomach cramps Nervous Disorders Vomiting Fatigue **Others** Low Ca, Phosphorus. Low BP Flushing	Kelp/Kombu (seaweeds) Almonds Dulse Sesame seeds Soybeans Lima beans Died peas Lentils Millet Wheat Rye Brown rice Spinach Swiss chard Avocado Parsley Kale Carrots Onions Blackberries Dried banana
Potassium (K)	Helps regulate neuromuscular function Stabilizes heart rhythm Maintains the proper electrolyte and acid-base balance in the body Helps lower risk of high blood pressure Supports kidney function Supports the function of the nervous system	Muscle weakness and cramping Lethargy Nervousness General fatigue Dry skin Diarrhea Impaired cognitive function Heart arrhythmias Acne Chills Edema Thirst Glucose intolerance Decreased reflex response Elevated cholesterol	Hyperkalemia (high potassium levels in the blood) Cardiac arrhythmia Cardiac arrest	Aduki beans Pinto beans Soybeans Chickpeas Almonds Sunflower seeds Sesame seeds Prunes Tangerines Oranges Watermelon Green, leafy vegetables Cantaloupe Berries Orange Juice Potato

Macro Minerals

Vitamin	Function	Common signs of Deficiency in ASD	Overdose Symptoms	Food Sources
Sodium (Na)	The body needs a small amount of sodium to help maintain normal blood pressure and normal function of muscles and nerves Sodium helps keep the fluid inside and outside the body's cells, thus it serves as important factor in maintaining an electrolyte balance of the body Helps regulate body pH	Abdominal pain Flatulence Impaired taste senses Lethargy Memory impairments Muscle weakness Nausea/vomiting Seizures Poor coordination Recurrent infections Headaches Anorexia Hallucinations Heart palpitation Low BP Weight loss	Edema High BP Potassium deficiency Liver and kidney diseases	Kelp/Kombu (seaweeds) Irish moss Sardines Oysters Cod Daikon raddish Kale Beet greens Celery Olives Sesame seeds Sunflower seeds Lentils Aduki beans Oats Brown rice Beef

Trace Minerals

Vitamin	Function	Common signs of Deficiency in ASD	Overdose Symptoms	Food Sources
Iron (Fe)	Helps in the formation of Hemoglobin and Myoglobin Helps oxygen transport Helps promote growth Aid in energy production and cell diffusion and cell differentiation Helps the immune and central nervous systems Electron transport	Glossitis (tongue inflammation) Stomatitis Dysphagia Intestinal malabsorption Fatigue Infections, spoon nails Pale eye membranes Anemia Palpitation Microcytosis Shortness of breath Pale eye membranes	Haemochromatosis (Thick blood) Constipation Liver damage Copper skin color Skin pigmentation Diabetes Enlargement of the spleen and liver Heart failure General weakness	Dulse Nori Kelp/ Kombu (seaweeds) Hiziki Brewer's yeast Pumpkin seeds Sesame seeds Chickpeas Lentils Millet Soybeans Parsley Red pepper Dried apricots Beet greens Chard Buckwheat Spinach
Copper (Cu)	Component of several enzymes in the body Stimulates iron absorption Needed to make RBC, connective tissue and nerve fibers Needed for synthesis of hemoglobin, proper iron metabolism, and maintenance of blood vessels Crucial for development of immunity Important for thyroid and Neurotransmitter functioning	Hypo chromia of RBCs Low WBC Immune dysfunction Depression Schizophrenia Abnormal development of nerve tissues Iron resistant anemia Hypo-pigmentation Cardio pulmonary dysfunction	Burning sensation in the body Chills Convulsions Diarrhea Metallic taste Muscular aches Nausea & vomiting Pain throughout the body; weakness Yellow eyes and skin Lack of urine	Lobster Crab Sunflower seeds Sesame seeds Walnuts Almonds Mushrooms Kidney beans Lima beans Soybeans Spinach Beets Squash Onions Carrots Avocado Brown rice

Trace Minerals

Vitamin	Function	Common signs of Deficiency in ASD	Overdose Symptoms	Food Sources
Chromium (Cr)	A mineral that acts directly on cell membrane Involved in amino acid transport and breakdown of glycogen and lipids Crucial for liver function Vital in synthesis of cholesterol, fats and proteins Helps to increase energy Suppresses the desire for sugar and flours, since it causes the existing insulin to work efficiently, which is good for those people suffering with diabetes	Blood sugar fluctuation Anxiety Fatigue Inadequate amino acids metabolism High triglycerides Arteriosclerosis Insulin resistance Neuropathy Poor collagen formation Weight loss Diabetes	Dermatitis Gastro intestinal ulcers Kidney and liver impairment Industrial exposure linked to lung cancer	Brewer's Yeast Blackstrap molasses Organ meats Calves liver Ham Chicken Grape juice Prunes Brown rice Potatoes Broccoli Mushrooms Dried beans Dairy products Eggs
Manganese (Mn)	Crucial in the reproduction and growth of bone and cartilage Assists in glucose control Assists thyroid function Helps in brain and CNS functioning Assists in lipid metabolism Componont of some enzymes important in metabolism	Impaired vision and hearing Skin rashes Irritability Mental impairment Teeth grinding Arthrosclerosis Confusion Tremors, increase in heart rate Elevated cholesterol levels Increased BP Pancreatic damage Sweating	Generally results from inhalation of manganese containing dust or fumes (not dietary ingestion) Has been linked to psychiatric and nervous disorders	Ginger Blackberries Blackcurrants Hazelnuts Chestnuts Brown rice Buckwheat Avocado Beets Leeks Turnip greens Onions Parsley Kale Greens Carrots Eggs Oysters Escargot

Trace Minerals

Vitamin	Function	Common signs of Deficiency in ASD	Overdose Symptoms	Food Sources
Selenium (Se)	Powerful antioxidant Interacts with vitamin E to prevent breakdown of fats and body chemicals Healthy function of cell membranes Increase resistance to cancer Supports pancreatic functioning Assists glutathione peroxidaseas; is a selenium-dependent enzyme with antioxidant properties Useful for cardiac function	Immune dysfunction Susceptibility to infections Cardiomyopathy Joint degeneration Pancreatic insufficiency Hair pigment loss Muscle wasting Calf tenderness Thyroid problems Cell fragility Growth retardation Elevated cholesterol levels Sterility	Dermatitis Irritability Fatigue Brittle hair and nails Paresthesia (pins & needles) Metallic mouth Liver and kidney damage Jaundice	Organ Meats Meat Poultry Seafood Lobster Shellfish Salmon Tuna Brazil nuts Brown rice Broccoli Onions Dairy products Torula yeast Wheat germ
Zinc	Involved in more than 200 enzyme activities Energy metabolism Helps develop immunity Needed for proper insulin function Protein metabolism	Hypersensitivity to taste and smell Thin and peeling nails White spots on nails Increased infection Acne Delayed sexual maturation Hair loss Elevated cholesterol Night vision problems Growth retardation	Nausea Vomiting Abdominal pain Impaired coordination Fatigue	Wheat germ Basil Caraway seeds Brazil nuts Hazelnuts Cashews Milk Brown rice Lentils Sprouted lentils Mushrooms Chickpeas Corn Black eyed beans Spinach Sauerkraut Cabbage Carrots Avocado Peaches

NOTES:

Chapter Two

Getting Started With Nutrition

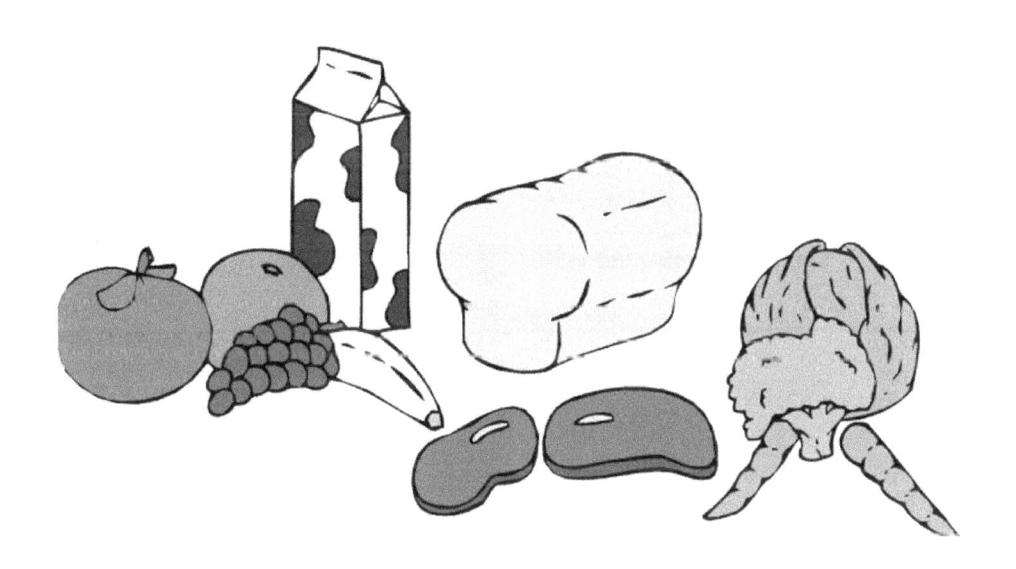

Guide to Food Selection

The National Institutes of Health recommends eating a variety of fruits, vegetables, and dark green, orange and starchy vegetables. The diet should also be rich in fiber. The table below shows the foods that are a part of a unhealthy fast food diet (unacceptable column). To achieve a state of health and well being, efforts should be made to slowly move from the direction of unhealthy fast food diet (unacceptable) to a wholesome, ideal nourishing diet (Optimum column).

Components	Optimum	Acceptable	Unacceptable
Proteins	Fresh, pasture raised meat including buffalo, beef, lamb, poultry, wild game, chicken, turkey, duck, organ meats from pasture fed animals, seafood cold water, fresh shellfish in season, organic eggs from free range poultry, and organic fermented soy such as tempeh, and natto.	Commercially raised beef, lamb, turkey and chicken. BBQ or smoked meat. Additive-free sausages and bacon. Free range non-organic eggs, tofu and soy milk (GMO) in very small amounts.	Processed meat containing additives and preservatives, such as luncheon meat, salami and bacon, hydrolyzed protein and protein isolates. Eggs from commercially raised hens (hormone treated, non-organic foods fed hens) Hg laden fish – swordfish, shark, sea bass.
Fats	Fresh raw and cultured butter ghee and cream from pasture-fed cows. Organic cocunt butter, sardines, wild salmon. Extra virgin olive oil, unrefined cold pressed flax seed, safflower oil, sunflower oil. Balanced 4:1 oil Omega 6 to Omega 3. Use coconut butter to cook french fries.	Olive oil that is not extra virgin. Butter that is not organic. Low fat food.	All processed vegetable oils, margarine, vegetable shortenings, fat substitutes, peanut oil, canola oil and fried food.
Beverages	Filtered high-mineral water, meat stocks and vegetable broths. Natural homemade fruit juices. Organic casein-free milk sources like hazelnut, hemp seed, almond, and coconut milk. Homemade milks (nut, seeds). **Note: See Beverages in recipes section.**	Filtered tap water, Sparkling Bottled Water. Natural organic fruits juices with non- added sugars and additives. Non-dairy commercial milks which are from non-organic sources. Fresh juice fruit smoothies **Note: See Beverages in recipes section.**	Unfiltered tap water, soft drinks, fruit juice with added sugars and additives / colors. Powered drink mix.
Carbs	Fruit, potato, sweet potato, beans, starchy vegetables, stevia, whole grains.	Honey, maple syrup, xylitol, unrefined sugar, sorghum syrup.	Refined sugar, white rice, white bread, refined flour, corn syrup, high fructose corn syrup.

Nuts and Seeds: Nutrient-Dense Foods

Nuts and Seeds are our favorite super nutrient-dense foods. Incorporating nuts and seeds in your diet is one of the best ways to replace saturated fats with heart-friendly polyunsaturated and monounsaturated fats that render a cardio-protective effect.

Nuts in general are very nutritious, providing abundant proteins, while seeds are also high in carbohydrate and oils. Nuts and seeds have a variety of nutrients like the vitamins and minerals in which children with ASD are deficient. Both nuts and seeds are abundant in magnesium, zinc, manganese, copper, calcium, iron, phosphorus and B vitamins. They are high in healthy vitamins like niacin and folic-acid, which make them an excellent nutritional package. All nuts and seeds are also good sources of vitamin E, an important antioxidant.

Health Benefits of Soaking Nuts and Seeds: Soaking nuts and seeds is important as they contain enzyme inhibitors. The purpose of these enzyme inhibitors is to protect the nut or seed itself. Soaking nuts and seeds in warm water will neutralize these enzyme inhibitors, and also help encourage the production of beneficial enzymes. When neutralized, these enzymes in turn increase the power of many vitamins, especially B vitamins. Soaking also makes these nuts and seeds much easier to digest and the nutrients more easily absorbed.

Nuts and Seeds and Children with ASD: In some individuals, nuts can cause some allergic reactions. Seeds as compared to nuts are less allergenic. If your child has digestive issues, soaking nuts and seeds will ensure that they are better digested. It is also beneficial if you start with seeds and later add nuts in the diet of these children.

Peanut Problems in a Nutshell: Although peanuts are grouped with nuts, they actually are part of the bean (legumes) family. There are some individuals who are allergic to peanuts, but not allergic to nuts and seeds. However, there are individuals who are allergic to peanuts, nuts and seeds. Peanut butter is many parents' first choice when it comes to making sandwiches for their children, but it is still important to note that more people die from allergenic reactions to peanuts than any other food. The vast majority of people who are allergic to peanuts do not outgrow this allergy. Peanuts are also a leading cause of childhood choking accidents. Aflatoxins are naturally occurring poisons produced by the molds apergillus flavus, which grow on peanuts and grains, and contribute to many health conditions.

Listed on the next page are other healthy nuts/nut butter choices that can offer both variety and high nutritional value.

Health Benefits of Nuts

Nuts	Health Benefits
Coconut	Although its name suggests that it is a nut, and it is often thought of as a fruit, the coconut it is actually a seed. Its cavity is filled with coconut water which contains sugar, fiber, proteins, antioxidants, vitamins and minerals. Coconut water provides an isotonic electrolyte balance, and is a highly nutritious food. **Coconut butter or coconut oil** is a tasty, healthy, naturally saturated vegetable product. It is also very stable, making it ideal for sauté cooking and baking.
Pistachios	Pistachios are an excellent source of protein. They're also high in potassium and low in sodium, which helps to regulate blood pressure, maintain water balance in the body, and strengthen muscle tissue. Their vitamin E content boosts the immune system and alleviates fatigue. They contain high levels of monounsaturated fats which help reduce the risk of heart disease. **Pistachio Nut Butter** tastes great with raw cultured vegetables in a bowl or on your sandwich. Make pistachio dressing in a blender by mixing with any of the following: avocados, a little water, garlic, tomatoes, or raw cultured vegetables.
Almonds	Almonds contain generous amounts of vitamin E, magnesium, phosphorus, potassium, iron, zinc, copper, manganese, and trace amounts of the B vitamins thiamin and riboflavin. **Almond Butter** is mildly sweet and one of the most popular alternatives to peanut butter. It is easily spreadable on bread or crackers, and can be thinned with liquid to make sauces or dips.
Cashews	Cashews provide more of the essential trace elements like iron, copper and zinc than all other nuts. Protein is present in abundance and that too is of a good quality. Cashews are also rich in sodium, potassium, calcium, phosphorus, magnesium and Vitamin B. **Cashew Butter** has a "rich" flavor, is a popular sandwich spread, and can be used to make soups, sauces, and dips. It can be eaten as snacks or used in combination with other foods such as salads and desserts.
Chestnuts	Chestnuts are an excellent source of vitamin B6, vitamin C, vitamin A, sodium, potassium and folate. They have an anti-inflammatory effect and also improve the tone of the veins. **Chestnut butter** is very mild in taste with a hint of sweetness. It is versatile and can be used to make dips, sauces, dressings, soups and baked goods.
Hazelnuts	Hazelnuts contain the highest level of folic acid of any tree nut, as well as fiber, vitamins E, B6 and A, potassium and calcium. Hazelnuts are rich in B vitamins, C and E. **Hazelnut Butter** has a sweet and rich taste and is a popular addition to entrees and side dishes. It is easily spreadable on sandwiches and snacks/appetizers. It is also a wonderful complement to jams, chocolate and crackers. It is especially known for calcium, folic acid, folate and protein content.

Nuts	Health Benefits
Macadamia Nuts	This tasty, upscale nut contains no cholesterol and is low in sodium and saturated fats. Macadamias are rich in vitamin A, Omega 3, riboflavin, iron, thiamine, niacin and Palmitoleic acid. They aid fat metabolism and lower blood cholesterol. **Macadamia Butter** is another great alternative to peanut butter and a good addition to ice cream. It is easily spreadable for sandwiches, snacks/appetizers and is an excellent addition to recipes. It is the most preferred nut butter choice for children with oral motor issues. It is also a wonderful complement to jams, chocolate and crackers. *(See note below).*
Pecans	Pecans contain an abundance of vitamin A, vitamin E, folic acid, calcium, magnesium, phosphorus, potassium, several B vitamins and zinc. Pecans are a good low fat source of vitamin E and also have anti-cancer effect. **Pecan Nut Butter** has a creamy butter taste, can be used as spread on breads or made in dips and sauces. It contributes great taste to recipes.
Pine Nuts	These nuts are also rich in vitamin D, vitamin C and vitamin A. They also strengthen bones and teeth and improve the cardiovascular system. **Pine Nut Butter,** is a creamy butter that can be used as dips and made in sauces.
Walnuts	Walnuts are rich in iron, thaimine, copper, potassium, folate, zinc, magnesium and phosphorus. Walnuts contain important vitamins, minerals, antioxidants and protein, and they contain a significant amount of essential omega-3 fatty acids. **Walnut butter** is great with breakfast foods, in that it add a tasty punch to grains, granolas and protein.

<u>NOTE</u>: Oral Motor Issues of Children with ASD and Nut Butter

For children with oral motor issues, the macademia nut butter is the preferred choice over other nut butters. It is easily spreadable and preferred over other nut butters, as it does not stick to the roof of the mouth.

Seeds That Nourish Growth

Seeds are the "eggs" that contain the nutrients needed to nourish the growth of a new plant. They are a gold mine of healthy vitamins and minerals, which makes them an excellent nutrition package. Seeds also provide more fiber per ounce than nuts.

Seeds	Health Benefits
Flax Seed	Flaxseeds are a good source of omega-3 essential fatty acids. They are a very good source of dietary fiber and manganese, folate and vitamin B6 as well as the minerals magnesium, phosphorus, and copper. In addition, flax seeds are concentrated in lignan phytonutrients.
Sesame Seeds	They are good source of manganese, copper, calcium, magnesium, iron, phosphorus, vitamin B1, zinc and dietary fibers.
Hemp Seeds	The hemp seed is 35 percent oil, the richest source of EFAs in the plant kingdom. It is also the king of protein. Of all plant-based sources, its 25 percent protein content — comprised of all eight essential amino acids — is second only to that of the soybean. The protein in hemp seed is readily digestible. In addition to its ideal balance of Omega 6 and 3, it has a huge trace mineral content. Hemp seeds and oils have EFAs a desirable omega-6/omega-3 ratio range of 3.6:1 which is the closest natural source of the optimal 4:1 ratio..
Sunflower Seeds	In addition to linoleic acid (an Omega 6 essential fatty acid), sunflower seeds are also an excellent source of dietary fiber, protein, vitamin E, B vitamins, and minerals such as magnesium, iron, phosphorus, selenium and zinc. They are also a good source of calories. These seeds are more readily available than safflower seeds.
Pumpkin Seeds	Pumpkin seeds are a very good source of the minerals phosphorus, magnesium and manganese. They are also a good source of other minerals including zinc, iron and copper. In addition, pumpkin seeds are a good source of protein and vitamin K. They are also an excellent source of carbohydrates and dietary fibers.

Nuts and Seeds, Copper Contents, and Children with ASD: Nuts and seeds are high in copper, and this is a concern for many children with ASD, as many children have high copper and low zinc levels. Copper is a component of, or a cofactor for, approximately 50 different enzymes. Copper is a strong antioxidant that works with an enzyme, superoxide dismutase (SOD), to protect cell membranes from destruction by free radicals. Copper is needed to make adenosine triphosphate (ATP), the energy source the body requires.

Nuts and seeds are nutrient-dense foods. They should be incorporated in the diet. If copper is found to be elevated, it should be noted that foods containing copper, like nuts and seeds, are also high in zinc. Zinc helps balance the levels of copper in the body.

Directions to Make Nut Butters: Soak nuts in water for 7 to 12 hrs. Drain and refrigerate, use to make nut milk or nut butter. Soaking increases digestibility. To make nut butter, combine nuts with a healthy oil in a food processor.

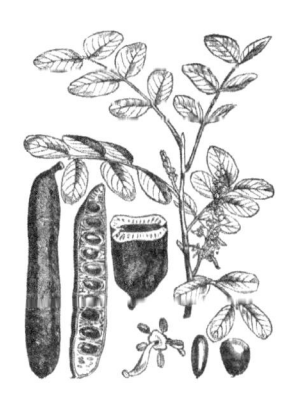

Guide to Natural Oils and Their Health Benefits

Vegetable fats and oils are lipid materials derived from plants. Physically, oils are liquid at room temperature, and fats are solid.

Edible Oil	Health Benefits
Flax Seed Oil	Flax seed oil contains omega-3 essential fatty acid, alpha linolenic acid.
Coconut Oil	Coconut oil is a "functional food," defined as a food that "provides a health benefit over and beyond the basic nutrients". Nearly two-thirds of the saturated fat in coconut oil consists of medium-chain fatty acids, which are are easily absorbed and converted into quick energy.
Safflower Oil and Sunflower Oil	These oils are similar, in nutrient content as they are both high in linoleic acid (omega 6 essential fatty acid). These oils are low in saturates and high in unsaturates. They both are essential fats, and have an abundance of antioxidants that are needed to keep our bodies healthy.
Sesame Oil	Sesame oil contains several important antioxidants, believed to promote cell integrity and the healthy function of body tissues.
Rice Bran Oil	Rice bran oil is a source of the vitamin E, antioxidants and other micronutrients to help fight free radicals and combat the effects of aging.
Olive Oil	The beneficial health effects of olive oil are due to both its high content of monounsaturated fatty acids and its high content of antioxidant substances. It contains a high amount of oleic acid and is a heat stable monounsaturated fat.
Grape Seed Oil	A good frying and salad oil. It is available commercially as a tasty mayonnaise.

Edible Oil	Health Benefits
Walnut Oil	Walnut oil is not cooking oil; high heat destroys its delicate flavor. Along with its EFA content, it is as an ingredient in a salad dressing or a fresh pasta sauce or to give a final fillip to a finished dish. It can also give class to a piece of freshly poached salmon or chicken breast. A mix of walnut oil, apple cider vinegar, a touch of garlic, prepared mustard, and salt makes an excellent salad dressing. Walnut oil contains the lower order omega 3 alpha linolenic acid.
Almond Oil	Almond oil primary contains oleic acid as is found in olive oil
Avocado Oil	Avocado oil is also similar in fatty acid content to olive oil, as it is high in oleic acid

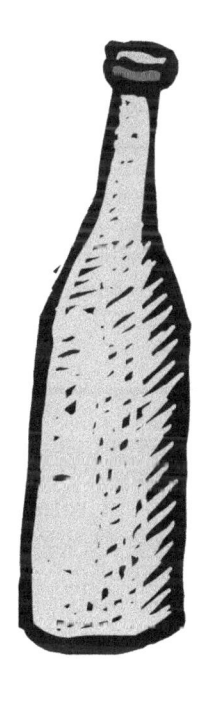

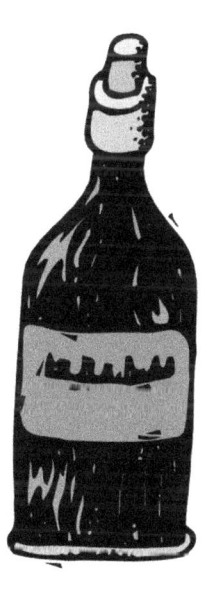

Guidelines for Using Natural Oils

Eliminate canola oil, corn oil, peanut oil and vegetable oil, all hydrogenated oils, margarines, commercial salad dressings, and mayo.

Purpose	Oils to Choose
High Heat Oils **Smoke Point:** Up to 510 degree F **Uses:** Oils can be used sautéing, frying and other high heat applications	Palm oil Grape seed oil Almond oil Avocado oil Coconut oil
Medium High Heat Oils **Smoke Point:** Up to 425 degrees F **Uses:** Oils with medium high smoke point are best for sautéing at medium high heat, also because of neutral flavor used for baking.	Grape seed oil Coconut oil Olive oil, virgin or extra light Rice bran oil
Low Heat Oils **Smoke Point:** Up to 350 degrees F **Uses:** Medium heat oils have flavors, making them ideal for sauces and dressings or for sautéing at medium heat where the oils flavor is intended as an integral part of the finished dish.	Sesame oil Peanut oil Toasted sesame oil Olive oil, extra virgin Corn oil Coconut oil
No Heat Oils **Smoke Oil:** No direct heat oils **Uses:** Oils with low smoke points have such rich, robust flavor and fragile structure that they're best poured directly onto a finished dish, or blended into dressing, simple sauce or taken directly.	Flax seed oil Borage oil Hemp oil Evening primrose oil Enriched flax oil BodyBio balance (4:1 ratio) oil

Seaweed: Health Treasures

Seaweed: Since ancient times, seaweeds have been appreciated as one of nature's most valuable food sources by coastal peoples from around the globe. Although their taste is distinctive and an acquired one for those with an uninitiated palate, sea vegetables are incredibly versatile and may be added to just about any dish.

Guidelines for Seaweed

- Soak before cooking, as dried seaweeds will expand considerably upon soaking. Save the soaking water, strain it, and use for soup broth and vegetable stock.

- Storage: Dried seaweed, if stored in a cool, dry place in an airtight container, will keep for several years. If seaweed becomes damp, simply dry briefly in a low oven and use.

Seaweed and Health Benefits

- Seaweed contain a whole spectrum of nutrients including calcium, iron, potassium, zinc, vitamins A, B complex, C, D, E, K, and trace minerals. They are one of nature's richest sources of vegetable protein and vitamin B12.

- Seaweed contains a substance (ergosterol) that converts to vitamin D in the body. Vitamin D has other roles in human health, including modulation of neuromuscular and immune function and reduction of inflammation.

- In addition to key nutrients, seaweeds provide us with carotene, chlorophyll, enzymes, and fiber. Seaweed's saltiness comes from a balanced, chelated combination of sodium, potassium, calcium, phosphorus, magnesium, iron, and a myriad of trace minerals found in the ocean.

- Seaweed have a balancing, alkalizing effect on the blood.

- Seaweed are known for their ability to reduce cholesterol, and remove radioactive elements from the body, and to prevent goiter

- The polysaccharide alginic acid, found in brown sea vegetables such as kombu, arame, hiziki and wakame, has been found to bind with heavy metals found in the intestines, rendering them indigestible, and causing them to be eliminated from the body.

- Seaweed has putative antibiotic properties that have shown to be effective against penicillin- resistant bacteria.

- Scientists have concluded that antioxidants in seaweed may promote immune system health.

- Some seaweed are treated with pesticides and fungicides while drying. So look for a safe source.

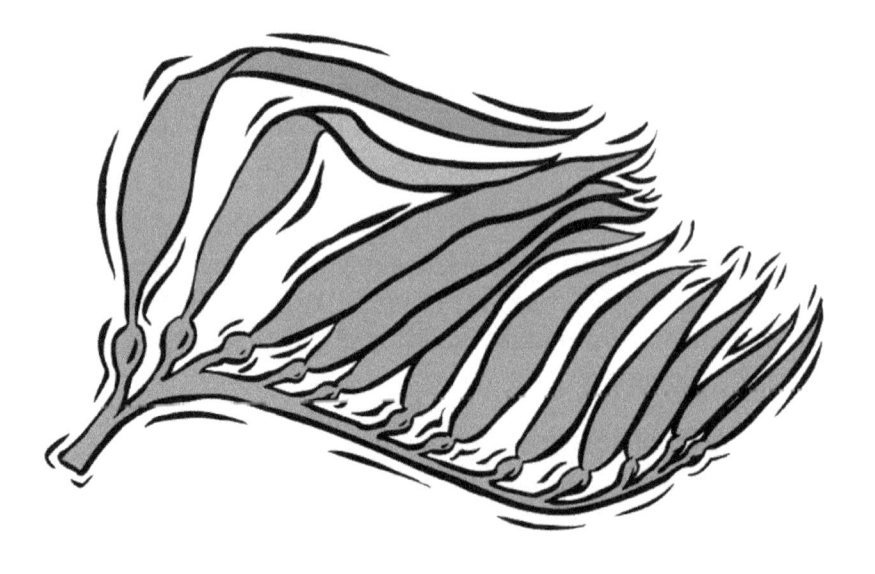

Types of Seaweed and Health Benefits

- **Arame:** Arame is a good introduction to seaweed because of its mild taste. It blends well with other flavors and is a rich source of iron. Arame can be steamed, sautéed, added to soup, or eaten in salads.

  Health Benefits: Arame and all other seaweeds are a rich source of calcium, zinc, potassium and iodine. Arame is also a good source of protein and lignans, which help fight cancer. Because it comes from the ocean, seaweed contains sodium. It should be avoided by anyone on a sodium-restricted diet.

- **Agar Agar (Kanten):** It is a vegan-quality odorless, tasteless, gelatin made from a variety of red sea vegetables that are simply boiled and naturally freeze dried in the cold of winter. The commercial uses are the same as animal gelatin: vegetable and fruit aspics, custard, pie fillings and more. Agar is high in dietary fiber. It acts as a mild laxative, adding bulk without the calories. Use agar agar to replace gelatin, as well as eggs and other thickening agents, in baking.

  Health Benefits: Agar agar is a fine source of iodine, calcium, iron, phosphorus and vitamins.

- **Hijiki (Hijicki, Hizicki):** It is an elegant, strong-tasting seaweed particularly good with onions and tofu, as well as carrots and other root vegetables. It may also be added to stir-fries and noodle dishes. Hijiki sweetens considerably when cooked. To cook, first rinse and soak for 20 minutes. Then, rinse again before simmering for 30 minutes to one hour. Try dressing with cider vinegar, tamari and roasted sesame oil. For a cold salad, combine with tamari, sunflower seeds, cooked onions, celery and carrots.

  Health Benefits: Among all the sea vegetables, hijiki is the richest in minerals and it has an abundance of trace elements. It is extremely high in calcium, iron and protein.

- **Irish moss:** Carrageen, the thickening agent used in food products from cottage cheese to salad dressing, comes from this seaweed.

  Health Benefits: Carrageen is rich in minerals, especially iodine, and contains a good supply of vitamin A.

- **Kombu (Kelp):** It is rich in minerals, vitamins and trace elements. Its natural mineral salts have long been valued as a flavor enhancer and tenderizer, especially for cooking dry beans. Kombu is always used to make the delicious Japanese noodle broth called "dashi," seasoned with shoyu soy sauce. It is a versatile sea vegetable that imparts delicious flavor and healthful nutrients to soup stock, soup, stew, sauces and vegetable dishes.

    Health Benefits: Kombu is low in sodium, and a good source of iodine, as are all sea vegetables. For those who cook with sea salt, which does not contain iodine, cooking with kombu and eating sea vegetables can be a valuable source of iodine in one's diet.

- **Nori (Sea Lettuce, Green Laver):** Nori has a mild, nutty, salty-sweet taste. It is best when roasted before using (pre-toasted nori is sold as "sushi nori"). Wild nori is excellent crumbled into soups, grains, salads, pasta, and popcorn. Nori is also great as a table condiment, either alone or with ginger. Nori, when sold in paper thin flat sheets, is used for wrapping sushi rolls or for cutting into strips to use in soup. Sea lettuce, "green nori" that resembles lettuce, is excellent in soups, salads, and in rice and noodle dishes.

    Health Benefits: Nori is nearly as rich in protein as eggs and meats, and has a tiny proportion of fats. It is also an excellent source of calcium, iron, manganese, fluoride, copper, and zinc. Of the sea vegetables, nori is one of the highest in vitamins B1, B2, B3, B6, B12, as well as vitamins A, C and E.

- **Wakame:** A traditional addition to miso soup, this sweet-flavored and tender sea vegetable may be softened in water for only about 5-10 minutes before slivering into a green salad. Wakame goes well with land vegetables, especially cooked greens. It is particularly delicious when sautéed with onions. Lightly bake and crumble wakame for a mineral-rich condiment for brown rice and other grain dishes. These wakame flakes can be used in place of salt, to enhance flavor.

    Health Benefits: Wakame has many of the same nutritional benefits as its close relative, kombu. It is especially rich in calcium and contains high levels of vitamins B and C.

- **Dulse:** Dulse is delicious as a raw snack with its distinctive, strong sea flavor, as well as its rich taste and salty, spicy flair. It is great in soups, stews, chowders, salads and sandwiches. It pairs well with corn and potatoes. Dulse is a favorite with children and first-time eaters of sea vegetables. Dulse is great sprinkled over grain dishes, and it combines well with onions.

Health Benefits: Dulse is approximately 22 percent protein, higher than chickpeas (garbanzo beans), almonds, or whole sesame seeds. A handful (about 30 g) offers more than 100 percent RDA of vitamin B6, iron and fluoride, as well as 66 percent RDA of vitamin B12. Dulse is relatively low in sodium, yet quite high in potassium, phosphorus, manganese, and iodine and vitamin A. It also a highly alkaline vegetable.

Seaweed and Children with ASD: Children with ASD are low in many vitamins, minerals, and especially trace minerals. Seaweeds like kombu (kelp), dulse and wakame all come in flake form, available in a shaker that can be used instead of salt to enhance the flavor of food.

Seaweed are not SCD (Specific Carbohydrate Diet) legal, but have very high nutritional value. So if parents are planning to consider the SCD Diet *(see Chapter 4)*, they have to avoid sea weeds in their child's diet.

Lesser-Known Healthy Foods and Their Health Benefits

- **Tahini:** Think peanut butter, only made with sesame seeds. To make tahini, sesame seeds are soaked in water for a day and then crushed to separate the bran from the kernels. The crushed seeds are put into salted water, where the bran sinks, but the kernels float and are skimmed off the surface. They are toasted, and then ground to produce an oily paste. There are two types of tahini, light and dark. The light, ivory version is considered to have both the best flavor and texture. Tahini is most closely associated with the Middle East, where it is eaten as is, and is often used to make hummus (mashed chickpeas, flavored with lemon juice and garlic), baba ghanoush (a purée of eggplant, lemon juice, garlic, and oil), halvah (a confection that includes honey or cane syrup), and other traditional dishes.

    Health Benefits: Tahini is a source of calcium, protein and B vitamins. It is also a good source of essential fatty acids (EFA), which are used to help maintain healthy skin. Tahini is a source of vitamin E, which helps to reduce the rate of aging in body cells. Sesame seeds are also a good source of the amino acid methionine, which is an important contributor to liver detoxification and helps with the absorption of other amino acids.

- **Tempeh:** Tempeh is made by a natural culturing and controlled fermentation process that binds soybeans into a cake form. It has a full body, meaty texture and can be used as a main course and substitute for animal foods in stews, soups, bread and sauces and sandwiches. Many varieties of Tempeh are readily available in the U.S., including Organic Soy Tempeh, Organic Flax Tempeh, Organic Wild Rice Tempeh, and Garden Veggie Tempeh., all of which are available at www.lightlife.com) or in many Whole Foods health food stores.

    Health Benefits: Tempeh is a good source of manganese, protein, copper, phosphorus, and magnesium. It supplies monounsaturated fats and some B vitamins. With these properties, tempeh is a good food choice for children with ASD..

- **Natto:** Natto is fermented soybean that has been a traditional Japanese staple for more than 1,000 years. Natto is fermented with bacillus natto, which produces various enzymes, vitamins, amino acids and other nutrients unique to natto during its fermentation. It is these unique elements that give natto its distinctive health and medical benefits.

  Health Benefits: Natto is a good source of protein and vitamin B2, which helps keep the skin young.

- **Umeboshi:** Umeboshi are pickled ume fruits. Ume is a species of fruit-bearing tree in the genus Prunus, which is often called a plum but is actually more closely related to the apricot.

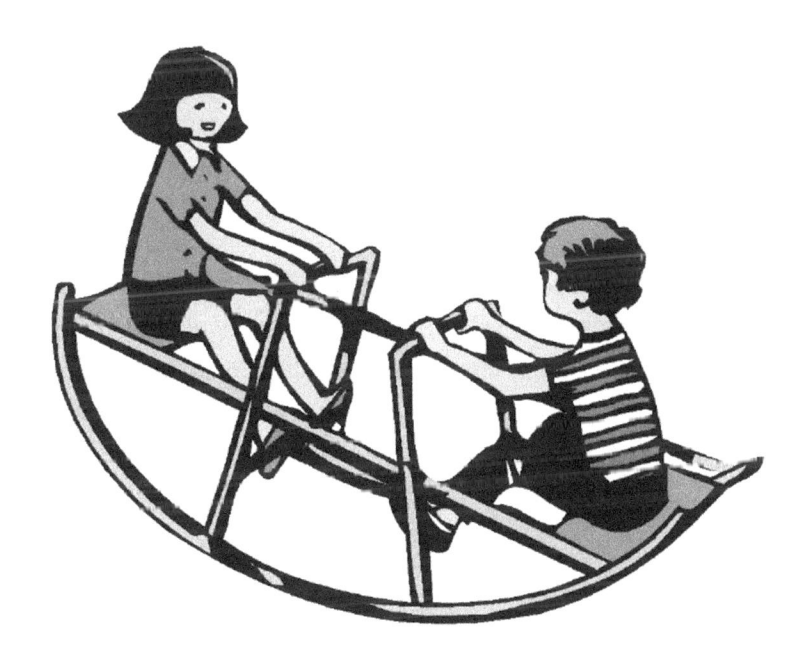

Health Benefits: Their powerful acidity has a paradoxical alkalinizing effect on the body, neutralizing fatigue, stimulating the digestion, and promoting the elimination of toxins. This is the far eastern equivalent to both aspirin and apple; not only is it a potent hangover remedy for mornings after, but also is regarded as one of the best preventive medicines available.

- **Mochi:** It is delicious pounded sweet rice. The sweet rice is soaked, steamed, and pounded; then it is allowed to dry until it is firm enough to slice.

  Health Benefits: Mochi warms the body and increases energy. Its sweet taste nourishes the pancreas, spleen, and stomach. It is physically strengthening and an easy-to-digest food which makes it an excellent food for people who are in a weakened condition. Mochi is recommended for such health problems as anemia, blood-sugar imbalances, and weak intestines. Pregnant and lactating women benefit because it strengthens both mother and child and encourages a plentiful supply of milk. Mochi is high in calcium and iron and is traditionally given to women after childbirth.

- **Miso:** Miso is a versatile condiment that originated in Japan. It is usually made from fermented soybeans and then ground into a buttery textured paste. There are many varieties of Miso like red miso, white miso, barley miso and soybean miso. For children with ASD on the SCD diet, however, miso is "not legal."

  Health Benefits: Miso is high in the minerals iron, copper and manganese. Miso is often recommended for vegans to eat regularly because it is naturally high in protein, vitamin K, and vitamin B12. Miso is rich in the immune boosting mineral zinc and great for the digestive tract because it is high in fiber and probiotics.

Fermented Foods: Fruits and Vegetables

Fermentation is one of the oldest forms of food preservation technologies in the world. Indigenous fermented foods such as bread, cheese and wine, have been prepared and consumed for thousands of years and are strongly linked to culture and tradition.

Benefits of Eating Fermented Foods

- **Fermentation allows the bacteria, yeasts and molds to "predigest"** and therefore break down the carbohydrates, fats, and proteins to create "probiotics," which offer friendly bacteria to the digestive tract. This helps to keep the immune system strong, and to support overall digestive health. The healthier drinks made from grains and nuts qualify as foods.

- **Fermented foods are enzyme-rich foods** that are alive with micro-organisms. These foods allow beneficial microflora to "colonize" in our intestines to keep us healthy. Our "inner ecosystem" helps to support our health, and to fight infection. A healthy gastrointestinal tract (GI) is critical to a strong immune system.

- **Fermented foods aid in digestion**, promote healthy flora in our digestive tract, produce beneficial enzymes, offer us better nutrition and allow our bodies to absorb vitamins (in particular C, and B12), minerals, nutritional value and omega 3s more effectively from foods.

- **They regulate the level of acidity** in the digestive tract and act as antioxidants. Fermented foods contain the same isothiocyanates found in cruciferous vegetables, and therefore are able to fight and prevent cancer.

Beneficial Fermented Foods and Recipes

Sauerkraut: Fermented cabbage.

To make sauerkraut:

1 medium cabbage, cored and shredded

1 tablespoon caraway seeds

2 tablespoon sea salt

In a bowl, mix cabbage with caraway seeds and salt. Pound with a wooden mallet for about 10 minutes to release juices. Place in a quart sized, wide mouth Mason jar and press down firmly until juices come to top of the cabbage. Cover jar tightly and keep at room temperature for about three days before transferring to cold storage. This sauerkraut improves with age.

Ginger Ale: Ginger is a root with pungent and flavorful flesh that eases digestive discomfort and is an effective remedy for nausea and vomiting. Ginger not only has anti-inflammatory properties, but also may provide protection against some cancers. Ginger is so highly concentrated with gingerols and other beneficial nutrients that only a small amount is needed in the recipes. Ginger ale is a refreshing drink that can be taken between meals for its benefits.

For making Ginger Ale:

1-inch piece of ginger root, peeled

1 medium tangerine, quartered

1 pint of red grapes, with seeds

2 cups of watermelon, with rind, cubed

4 ounces of sparkling mineral water

Push ginger root, tangerine, grapes, and watermelon through a juicer. Add mineral water to juice and stir well. If you use a strong blender in place of the juicer, use some of the sparkling mineral water to get the ingredients going and add the remaining water once the ingredients are blended together. Strain if preferred.

Pickled Garlic: Garlic has been used to treat arthritis and cancer. Today, garlic has been proven to contribute to cardiovascular health and to boost the immune system.

For making pickled garlic:

12 heads garlic

2 tablespoons dried oregano

4 tablespoons salt

1/2 cup water

Remove the outer skin of the heads of garlic, place in a 300-degree oven and bake until heads open and cloves can be easily removed. In a half cup of water, add oregano and salt, mix well and pour over garlic. The top of the liquid should be at least one inch below the top of the jar. Cover and keep at room temperature for three days before transferring to cold storage.

Kombucha: Although frequently referred to as a mushroom, kombucha is not a mushroom; it's a symbiosis of bacteria and yeast. When sugar and black or green tea are added to kombucha, a fermentation process results in the "tea" — a liquid containing vinegar, B vitamins and a number of other chemical compounds. Kombucha is most commonly prepared by taking a starter sample from an existing culture and growing a new colony in a fresh jar. The kombucha culture is the live substance which is put into the sweet tea to ferment and convert it into kombucha tea. The culture is probably best known as a kombucha mushroom, though this is an incorrect definition. The kombucha culture has been known as mushroom, lichen and many other things but the best and most accurate definition we have today is a SCOBY "symbiotic culture of bacteria and yeast."

For making Kombucha:

3 quarts filtered water

1 cup sugar

4 tea bags of organic black tea

1/2 cup kombucha culture (can be purchased online)

1 kombucha "SCOBY"

Bring water to boil. Add sugar and simmer until all dissolved. Remove from heat, add the tea bags, and allow the tea to steep until water has completely cooled. Remove the tea bags. Pour cooled liquid into a Pyrex bowl and add 1/2 cup kombucha culture. Place SCOBY on top of the liquid. Cover the bowl loosely with cloth or towel and transfer to dark place, away from contaminations. In 7 to 10 days kombucha will be ready. Remove the SCOBY and transfer the liquid to a glass container and store to refrigerate. It must be brewed in a clean glass container, as it contains self preserving anti-bacterial properties.

Kombucha has properties that aid in both weight gain and weight loss. For aid in weight loss drink kombucha before meals, and for weight gain, drink after meals.

Caution: Some people may have allergic reaction to kombucha; start with a small taste to observe the allergic reaction or any adverse effects.

Kefir: Kefir is a cultured, enzyme-rich food filled with friendly micro-organisms that help balance your "inner ecosystem." More nutritious and therapeutic than yogurt, it supplies complete protein, essential minerals, and valuable B vitamins. The beneficial yeast and friendly bacteria in the kefir culture consume most of the lactose (or milk sugar). Eat kefir on an empty stomach first thing in the morning before (or for) breakfast and you'll be delighted to find it can be easily digested — as numerous people who have been lactose intolerant for years have discovered.

Some facts about kefir

- **Kefir grain** is the actual culture with which you culture milk. It is not a grain like wheat but a slimy culture that resembles cauliflower florets.

- **Kefir** is the term for the milk-like product that has been fermented with kefir grains.

- **Kefir whey** is the thin liquid you get from straining kefir through linen. The other component is curd or cream cheese.

- **Kefir cream** is cream that has been cultured using kefir or kefir grains.

- **Kefir butter** is butter that has been cultured from cream using kefir.

- **Kefir** is quite different to yogurt and does not require the same precision in culturing it.

Coconut Water Kefir: It completely stops your cravings for sugar, aids digestion of all food, and has a tonifying affect on the intestines, even flattening the abdomen. It contains high levels of valuable minerals, increases energy and gives you an overall feeling of good health.

To make the coconut water kefir: Buy four coconuts and punch holes in the end where the eyes are. Pour the coconut water into clean glass jars. To one pint of liquid (about 4 coconuts) add a packet of kefir starter culture. Let this sit about 24-48 hours. You will know your kefir is ready when the color changes to a milky white. Usually there is a bit of bubbling or foam on the top. This means the sugar has all been removed. It will taste tangy and tart.

You can use about 1/4 cup of kefir from the first batch to "transfer" friendly bacteria to your next batch of kefir. You may do this up to seven times with one package of starter. When the weather becomes cold outside, warm the liquid to about 90 degrees before adding the starter. Then place the glass jar somewhere warm so the temperature remains steady at around 70 degrees. Allow enough room in the container for expansion as the coconut water ferments and becomes coconut

kefir. Cover and let set at room temperature for a day or two. The cooler it is in your home, the longer it will take to ferment. The water will become like a drinkable yogurt. When this happens, place it in the refrigerator. It will keep for several weeks. You may add vanilla, honey, or any flavoring and sweetening of your choice. Other flavoring you can use are ginger, fresh lemon or lime juice. You can purchase Kefir starter at the link below.
http://www.wildernessfamilynaturals.com/kefir_culture.htm

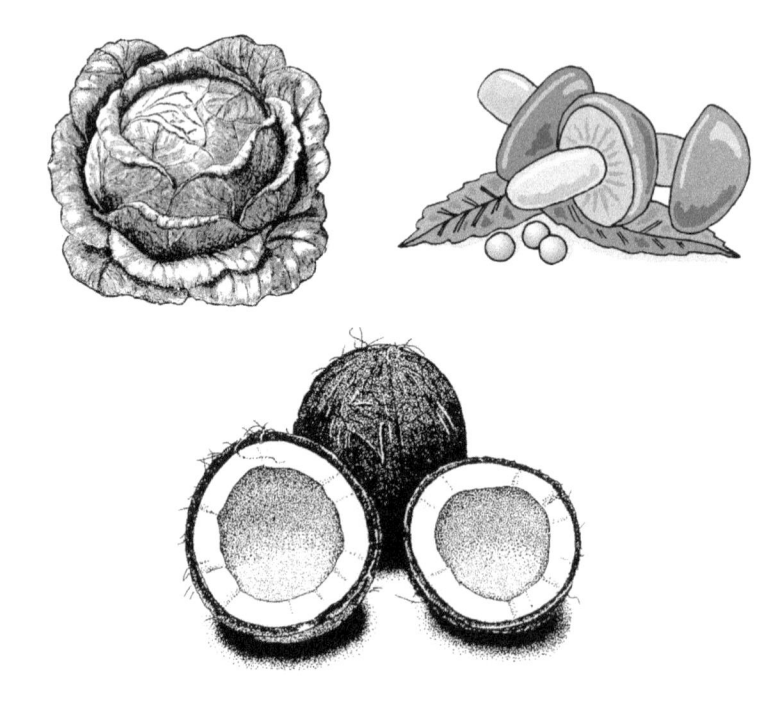

Beans, Lentils, and Legumes Guide

The Art of Cooking the World's Oldest Staple. Beans are a delicious high protein food. Cooking with beans sometimes brings hardships to many cooks, especially when you are cooking them from scratch. Soaking time varies with density of the beans. Knowing what spices to add is crucial, and the fear that beans may increase digestive upset in sensitive individuals scares many.

Beans are high in protein and fat, and lower in complex carbohydrates. They actually are enhanced by many spices, and can be added to many dishes to make delicious meals. They may be prepared in soups, as side dishes, or cooked with other foods. Beans provide a slow steady source of energy.

Legumes and beans are rich in enzymes, but also contain enzyme inhibitors. Unless deactivated by soaking and cooking properly, they can stress the digestive system. Soaking, culturing and fermenting all help deactivate enzyme inhibitors, thus making nutrients more readily available.

Beans fall into three categories, based on the cooking time

Beans	Time	Soaking	Cooking Time
Soft Beans Green lentils, red lentils, mung beans, split beans	None	45 to 50 minutes	1 hour
Medium Beans Small, light azuki, pinto, kidney, navy, lima, black, turtle and other medium sized beans	2 to 4 hours	1 1/2 to 1 3/4 hours	2 hours
Hard Beans Big, dark azuki, chick-peas, black, white, and yellow soybeans, and other hard beans	6 to 8 hours or overnight	3 1/4 to 3 1/2 hours	4 hours

Pressure-Cooking Beans

Beans	Time	Soaking	Cooking Time
Soft Beans Green lentils, red lentils, mung beans, split beans	None	30 minutes	45 minutes
Medium Beans Small, light azuki, pinto, kidney, navy, lima, black, turtle and other medium sized beans	1 hour	45 minutes	1 hour
Hard Beans Big, dark azuki, chick-peas, black, white, and yellow soybeans, and other hard beans	2 hours	1 to 1 1/4 hours	1 1/2 to 2 hours

Notes: Pressure cooking cooks beans faster, even when they are not soaked overnight. But soaking is recommended for better digestion. These times are approximate.

Some Useful Points Regarding Beans

- **Selecting and Storing Beans:** Keep beans in closed, airtight containers and store them in a cool, dark place. Preserved this way they retain their energy indefinitely. It is not a good idea to store different beans together in the same jar or container, as mixing may result in uneven cooking.

- **Washing Beans:** The drier the beans, the longer they need to be soaked and the more time is required on the stove or in the oven. Prior to cooking, pour beans in a plate and sort through for any stones or dirt. Then put in to a large pot, cover with cold water and quickly rinse two- three times; to remove dirt.

- **Soaking Beans:** Most beans, except lentils, split peas, and other light beans, require soaking. Some points to note in soaking beans:

- ▲ Soaking improves the digestibility of beans. Intestinal gas, which is commonly seen after eating beans is either due to lack of soaking, cooking that is too short or quick, insufficient chewing or overeating.

- ▲ To soak beans, add water to beans in a pot making sure to add enough to completely cover the beans plus a little more as the beans will swell (*see chart on the previous page*). This soaking water may be used for cooking as it will contribute to a richer taste to the final dish. Soaking in warm water makes the beans much softer and more digestible.

- **Seasoning Beans:** Beans should be seasoned near the end of the cooking, as this will allow the insides and the outsides to cook evenly. Salting beans at the beginning of cooking hardens the skin and makes for uneven cooking. Salt should also be added after the beans are cooked.

- **Cooking with Kombu:** A strip of kombu (sea vegetable) could be added when cooking beans. The combination improves the flavor of beans and adds minerals from the sea, making a more balanced dish. If time doesn't permit to cook dry beans, canned beans can be used. Eden brand beans are cooked with Kombu.

- **Cooking Beans:** The beans can be prepared in four different ways:

    a) **Shocking Method:** Put the soaked beans in a cast-iron pot, add 2 1/2 cups of water per cup of beans. Leave the pot uncovered to start and cook slowly over low heat until the water boils. Allow the water to bubble for a few minutes but do not let it boil strongly. Then cover the pot with a lid that fits down and covers pot well. As the beans cook over the low heat, they will expand in size and lid will jiggle as water comes back to a boil. At this time, just add enough cold water down to the side to stop boiling. Put the lid back on. Continue to add the cold water this way till the beans are 80 percent cooked (*see chart on previous page for approximate time*). At this point, add seasoning and 1/4 teaspoon of sea salt per cup of uncooked beans. After seasoning, cover the pot and cook until beans are done, adding more cold water when necessary. When beans are soft, turn up the heat to boil off any excess liquid. The result will be perfect beans, smooth, delicious, and easy to digest. The long, slow cooking, low heat and alterations of cold and hot water will bring out the bean's natural taste better than any other cooking methods.

b) Boiling Beans: This method calls for 3 1/2 to 4 cups of cold water per cup of dried beans. Bring the beans to a boil, lower the heat, cover the pot, and simmer until beans are 80 percent cooked. Uncover, season with about 1/4 teaspoon sea salt per cup of uncooked beans and other seasoning to taste. Cover the pot and cook until beans are soft. When done, remove cover, turn up the heat and boil off any excess water. Transfer the beans to a serving bowl and serve.

c) Pressure-cooking Beans: This method is recommended when one does not have much time. Simply wash the beans, soak them as long as possible, put them in a pressure cooker, and add two cups of water per cup of beans. Bring beans and water to pressure, reduce the heat to low, and cook until the beans are nearly done. Let the pressure come down, uncover and season with 1/4 teaspoon sea salt per cup of uncooked beans. Continue to simmer beans until any excess liquid has evaporated.

d) Baked Beans: Baked beans in a ceramic pot or crock are delicious. To prepare, clean and soak the beans, put in to a pot and cover with 4 to 5 cups of cold water per cup of beans. Boil for 15 to 20 minutes to loosen the skins. Pour the beans and cooking water into a crock or baking dish, cover and put in to the oven. Bake the beans at 350 degrees until 80 percent cooked, then add 1/4 teaspoon sea salt per cup of uncooked beans and add other seasoning to taste. Add more water if necessary and continue to cook until beans are soft and creamy.

CHAPTER THREE

The Practical Guide To Healthy Living

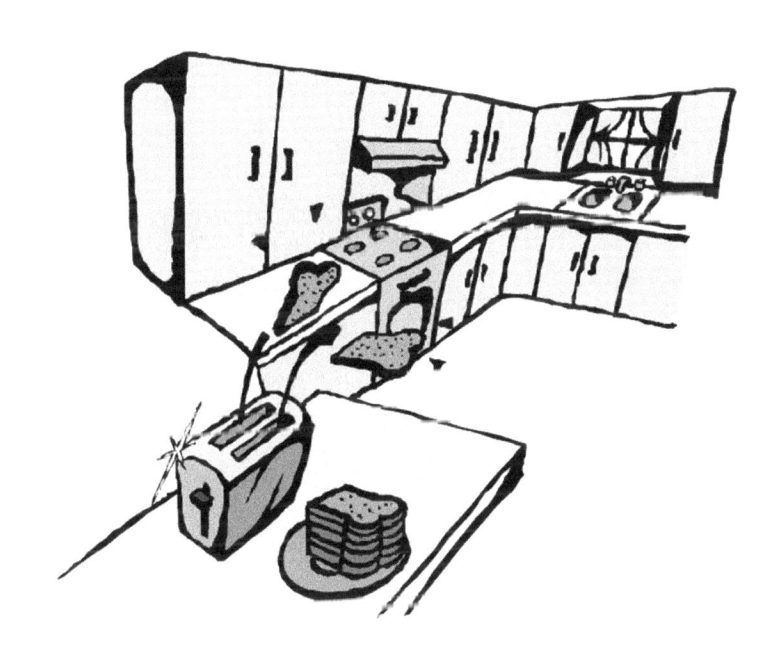

Preventing Cross-Contamination in the Kitchen

Cross-contamination occurs when an allergenic food or ingredient finds its way into the diet of a sensitized person. This could happen "accidentally" and many times does happen when the person cooking the food is not aware of many situations where cross contamination can be avoided. This is especially important in implementing a gluten-free casein-free (GFCF) diet.

Many children with ASD benefit from avoiding gluten and casein in their diets, although there is no medical literature yet to prove that diet is the key for all children on spectrum. However, it has been observed and reported by parents that certain symptoms for many children on the spectrum do improve after the implementation of the diet.

When following the GFCF diet, it is crucial that cross contamination be avoided. Gluten sensitivity is individualized. Some people are less bothered by traces of gluten than others, as evidenced by lack of reactions. However, for some children, including those with celiac disease, a trace of gluten can be extremely problematic. Reactions can sometimes be associated with pain and discomfort for children, who are very sensitive due to GI disturbances, such as inflammatory bowel disorder or chronic intestinal disorder.

Tips and Hints
to Avoid Cross-Contamination

- Don't prepare gluten-free foods on the same surface used to prepare foods with gluten unless the surface has been thoroughly cleaned. *(In restaurants, ask the chef to wipe down the grill before preparing your order.)*

- Make sure utensils have been thoroughly cleaned after preparing gluten-containing foods. Even better, have separate sets of utensils for gluten-free food preparation.

- Don't use the same toaster for both gluten-free bread and regular bread. If your home isn't entirely gluten-free and you can only have one toaster, purchase a toaster oven instead of a conventional toaster and purchase extra trays from the manufacturer. Another way is to place parchment paper on the bottom of the trays.

- Don't use the same sifter for gluten-free and gluten-containing flours. Clearly label the gluten-free sifter to avoid mistakes.

- Don't deep-fry gluten-free foods in the same oil used to fry breaded items. This is a particular risk in restaurants. You'll need to ask whether breaded and unbreaded items are fried in the same oil.

- **Caution:** Try to avoid using gluten-containing flours in kitchens where gluten-free food is prepared. Wheat flour can stay airborne for many hours and contaminate surfaces, utensils, and uncovered gluten-free food. **In general, foods prepared in any place that is not gluten-free are at risk for contamination.**

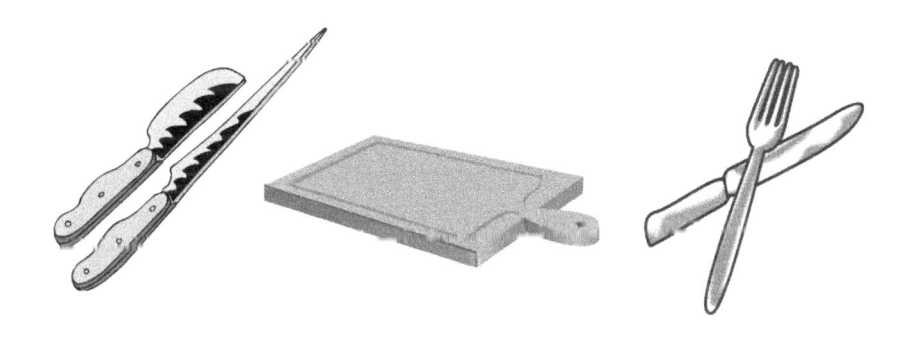

Healthy Eating Habits – Tips & Hints

- Food should be chewed thoroughly. Set aside time each day for meals. It's best to eat several small meals with small portions than to eat two or three large meals a day.

- Ideally, infants and young children should drink about one-half ounce of water for each pound of body weight per day. This helps ensure that important nutrients in food are being digested well, and it also maintains healthy pH in the body. This is a guide, not a goal, but it is important to encourage fluids throughout the day.

- Distractions should be avoided while eating, such as TV, radio, or reading. In children with special needs — especially those with oral motor issues — reinforcers such as videos or music can be used as an enhancement to introduce new foods or foods with varied texture. Make eating an enjoyable time. Colorful, child sized tableware can also be helpful.

- At each meal, offer a variety of raw and cooked vegetables. Be adventurous with menu choices. Be creative with your cooking, if your child doesn't like vegetables they can be disguised by shredding or pureeing them, and adding to food.

- Limit the intake of sugar. Prepare wholesome snacks from non-reactive food alternatives. Avoid commercially prepared "junk foods" and "fast foods" that contain a high sugar/trans fat content and empty calories.

- Children model their parents, even in nutrition. Set a good example by eating a healthy diet, which will encourage your child to do the same.

- **To improve healthy eating habits consider:**

    - Avoiding poor eating habits: Eating in the car, at the kitchen sink, at an open refrigerator door, eating while watching TV, eating while talking on phone, eating after 8 p.m.

    - Embracing good eating habits: Serving meals at the kitchen or dining room table, regular meal times, and eating without TV or other distractions.

- **Choosing restaurants:** Eating in fast food restaurants is not advisable. But if you want to eat out, remember to choose simple foods. Ask the manager for help in choosing the foods for your child, especially if he or she is on a restricted diet. Never hesitate to ask the restaurant chef about any food question, and also ask if a simple healthy meal can be prepared, even when it is not in their menu. Exploring a restaurant before dining there is a viable option.

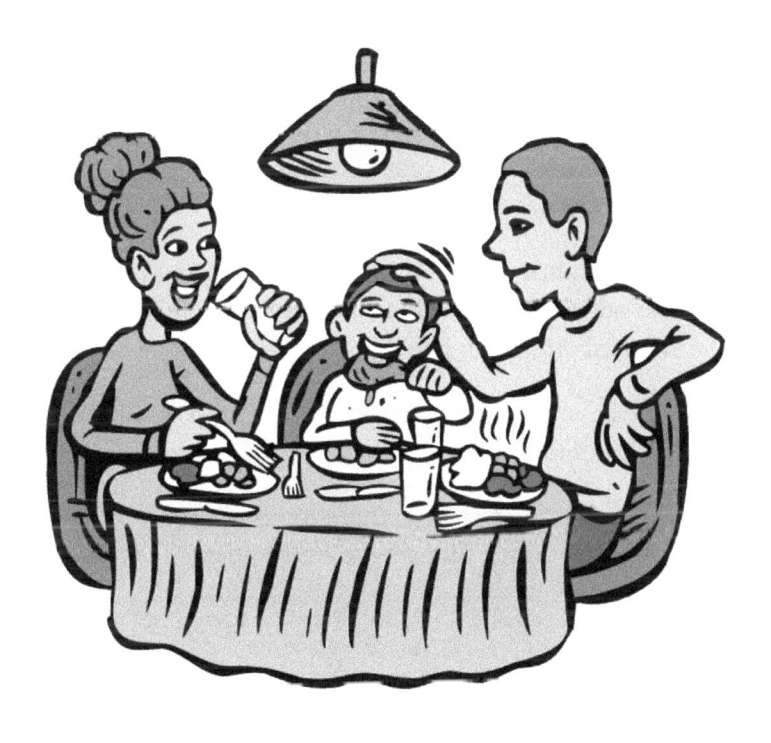

Hidden Food Allergens

Know your facts, and learn to read labels (which don't tell the entire story):

- Ingredients are listed on food packages by weight in descending order. This means the first ingredient listed on the label will have the highest concentration in the food.

- Some ingredients may not be listed by their specific names (*e.g.*, flavoring, color, spices, enzymes, MSG, etc.) and maybe an ingredient within an ingredient.

- Fat percentages (i.e., fat-free) are based on weight, not calories.

- Fat contents have to be noted carefully. There should be no hydrogenated or partially hydrogenated oils/trans fat in food.

- Look for 100 percent whole grain organic products that are not enriched and not processed.

- Look for sugar content. Fruit juices and fruit juice sweetened items should not contain added sugar or high fructose corn syrup. Sugar added to food has detrimental effects on health.

- Food colorings and additives should not be in food. Choose natural flavors over additives in food.

- If the list of ingredients is long, there are probably a lot of chemical additives in the product, and should be avoided.

Unhealthy Hidden Ingredients

This table below lists food items which are commonly consumed. This will help you identify ingredients that often are hidden in other food substances to which your child may react.

Food	Check Labels Carefully for These Hidden ingredients
Corn	Corn oil, corn meal, cereals, bread, corn flour, cornstarch, popcorn, hominy, grits, corn chips, tortillas, bleached white flours; cheeses; baking powder, coffee cream, candy, chewing gum, pancake syrup, jams, jellies, preserves, cake mixes, baking mixes, sauces, fish sticks, baked goods; peanut butter, processed meats, hot dogs, ice cream, salad dressings, margarines, Chinese foods (gravy with cornstarch), soups, cream pies, crackerjacks; carbonated drinks, soda water, fruit drinks, instant tea, vinegar, soybean milk, alcoholic beverages, sweetened deep frying mixtures, and glucose products; dates, canned foods, chili mix, gelatin desserts, gelatin capsules, graham crackers.
Cow's Milk	Butter, buttermilk, casein, all cheeses except hard cheeses such as cheddar, swiss, parmesan, provolone. Some cocoa-chocolates, cottage cheese, cream, cream cheese, evaporated milk, half and half, ice creams, imitation milk products, lactic milk, margarine, milk-chocolate, non-fat dry milk, processed cheese, skim milk, sour cream, sour half & half, whey and yogurt.
Eggs	**Whole eggs and food containing egg:** Baked goods, Bavarian cream, breaded foods, cake flours, batter used for frying foods, creamy fillings, puddings, custard, breakfast cereal, bouillon, cake flour mixes, prepared frostings, cookies, divinity, egg beaters, fondant, French toast, fritters, hollandaise sauce, ice cream, malted cocoa drinks (Ovaltine, Ovamalt), egg noodles, macaroni, muffins, meat loaf, meat balls, macaroons, marshmallows, mayonnaise, meringues, omelets, pancakes, pretzels, baking mixes, salad dressings, sausages, sherbets, soufflés, soups, tartar, waffles.
Soy	**Foods Containing Soy:** Bean sprouts, cellulose, glycerin, hydrolyzed vegetable protein, lecithin, miso, nitroglycerine, soybeans, soy dairy products, soy nuts, soy sprouts, soy sauce, tofu, some infant formulas, baby foods, baked goods, candy, cereals, coffee substitute, Crisco, custards, dry lemonade mix, hamburger mixes, ice cream, steak sauce, liquid protein foods, lunch meat, margarine, mayonnaise, cooking oil sprays, seasoning, salad dressings, sausages, soups, vitamins, weight loss products, Worcestershire sauce.

Food	Check Labels Carefully for These Hidden ingredients
Wheat	Biscuits, bologna, bouillon cubes, cakes, cereals, cookies, cooked meat dishes, chocolate candy, corn bread, crackers, doughnuts, dumplings, coco malt, flour-rolled meats, flour, gin, gluten breads, bagels, gravies, pancakes, ice creams, liverwurst, macaroni, matzo, spaghetti, pasta, durum, semolina, rolls, couscous, prepared soups, breading, waffles, muffins, crepes, French fries, baking flour, tortillas, meats
Yeast	Yeast is added to many, many products. Read labels on all baked goods, soups, vitamins, canned goods, etc. Baker's yeast is found in breads, bagels, buns, rolls, pastries. Brewer's yeast is found in all alcoholic beverages.

Guide to Natural Sweeteners

The desire for the sweet is inborn and instinctual. Our first food, mother's milk, is naturally sweet and, from an evolutionary standpoint, sweets are highly advantageous to one's survival. In the early days of man when survival was critical, the sweet plants were usually safe to eat. Inspite of its advantage, we should not overdo sugar. The best advice is to limit the intake of sugar and never to eat something that contains high amounts of sugar.

Consumers' concern in recent years to avoid fat has benefited sugar, which is often a key ingredient in products promoted as "fat-free." Today, sugar also appears to have a more positive image than was the case a decade or two ago. Sugary sweets create havoc on the healthy body. Commercial sweet products not only contain refined sweeteners like corn syrup or sugars, but are also loaded with highly processed white flour and hydrogenated oils.

Individual reactions to sweeteners, even natural sweeteners, vary. Many individuals experience a rapid rise in blood sugar when they consume one sweetener but not another. Some physicians have found that fructose in corn syrup consistently provokes a more severe reaction in certain individuals than sucrose in table sugar. Because reactions vary, caution must be used with sweet foods and sweeteners.

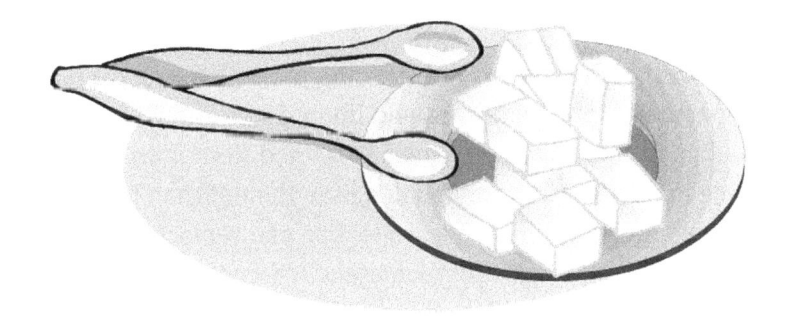

Refined Sugar vs. Natural Sweeteners

Refined Sugars are loaded with empty calories. They satisfy hunger on a short term basis by providing lots of energy, but they also generate lots of heat. These energy and heat producing factors, when not burned, get stored in the body as fat, which leads to other diseases in the body. Refined sugar carries only negligible amounts of bodybuilding and repairing materials.

Natural Sweeteners contain high amounts of minerals and other nutrients. They are actually defined as sweet foods from which nutrients have not been removed. There are many natural sweeteners that provide nutritional benefits. Listed below are nutritious natural sweeteners, but the critical point to remember is that reactions even to natural sweeteners are individualized.

- **Raw Honey:** Honey is loaded with nutrients found in plant pollens and is also rich in enzymes that digest carbohydrates. For this reason it is allowed in the Specific Carbohydrate Diet (SCD) — *see Chapter 5*. Honey does not upset the blood sugar levels as severely as refined sugars. It also offers incredible antiseptic, antioxidant, antibacterial, antiviral, antifungal and cleansing properties for our body and health. *(Always buy honey that says "raw" on the label.)*

- **Maple Syrup:** Maple syrup is a mineral-rich sweetener made from the sap of maple trees. It gives wonderful flavor to cream-based desserts and many baked goods, such as muffins and pancakes. Maple syrup is unlikely to cause an allergic reaction the same way nuts and fruits may do. It is safe for everyone.

- **Agave:** Agave syrup is formed after the juice of the agave plant is extracted from its core. It is then heated and filtered to form syrup. Unlike the crystalline form of fructose, which is refined from corn, agave syrup is fructose in its natural form, and is a little thinner than honey. It can be substituted for honey in recipes, and also can replace sugar in other recipes, although less is needed. Approximately 3/4 cup of agave is the equivalent of 1 cup of table sugar. The syrup ranges in color from light to dark and contains iron, calcium, potassium, and magnesium. It has a low glycemic level, so is safer to use than table sugar.

- **Date Sugar:** More a food than a sweetener, this is an unprocessed sugar made from dehydrated dates that are ground into small bits. Date sugar is high in fiber, and contains a list of vitamins and minerals, including iron. It does not dissolve easily, and is therefore unsuitable for many desserts. Its high tryptophan content makes it an ideal sweetener for hyperactive children, as this amino acid has a calming effect. Date sugar tastes good in porridge.

- **Molasses:** Molasses is a thick by-product of the processing of the sugar beet or sugar cane into sugar. It has a strong taste and moderate sweetness. It contains many minerals, especially iron, calcium, zinc, copper and chromium.

- **Sorghum Syrup:** A sweetener made from sweet sorghum made by boiling the sorghum syrup. Sorghum syrup contains B vitamins and minerals such as iron, calcium and phosphorus. It may be used instead of maple syrup.

- **Brown Rice Syrup:** It is made by combining barley malt and brown rice, and cooking the mixture until all the starch is converted to sugar. The mash is then strained and cooked down to syrup, which is only 20 percent as sweet as sugar. Brown rice syrup is considered to be one of the healthiest sweeteners in the natural food industry, since it is produced from a whole food source and comprised of simple sugars. Brown rice syrup is excellent for a bit of sweetness on toast, whole grains, sweet potatoes or squash, or in tea. It blends well to sweeten salad dressings, soups, and sauces. **Since it does contain barley malt, it is not a part of the gluten-free diet.**

- **Fructose and High Fructose Corn Syrup:** It comprises any of a group of corn syrups that has undergone enzymatic processing to increase its fructose content, and is then mixed with pure corn syrup (100 percent glucose), becoming a high-fructose corn syrup. It is used in various types of food, from soft drinks and yogurt to cookies, salad dressing and tomato soup. Studies have not conclusively demonstrated what impact high-fructose corn syrup may have on children's health. The researchers are concluding that there is evidence that children who consume sweetened beverages have a higher incidence of being overweight. **It should be totally avoided.**

- **Concentrated Fruit Juices:** Concentrated fruit juice is a relatively new sweetener, and one that is rapidly gaining popularity among manufacturers. It is highly refined, and at 68 percent soluble sugar, is relatively concentrated. The ratio of fructose to glucose or sucrose will vary according to the fruit from which it is derived. Through reduction, filtration and evaporation, the color, acidity, and most of the flavor are removed, leaving an end product with little similarity to the original juice. **Its preference to white sugar is debatable.** Concentrated fruit juice can still cause erratic blood sugar levels if consumed in large amounts. The food industry uses fruit juice concentrates in jams, canned fruits, beverages and some baked goods.

Avoiding sugar and keeping it away from children can be a challenging task for parents. The first challenge is that sugar is readily available and has made its way into all the things you buy for children, such as juices, candies, muffins, pancakes etc.

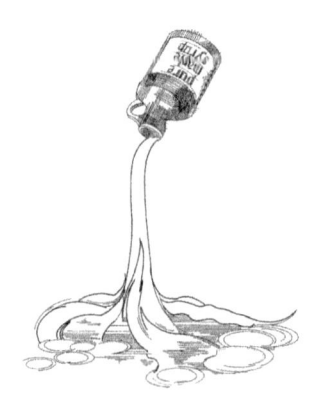

Impact of a High-Sugar Diet

In addition to throwing off the body's homeostasis, excess sugar may result in a number of other significant consequences. The following is a listing of a few of sugar's metabolic effects:

- Sugar can suppress the immune system.

- Sugar depletes trace minerals in the body.

- Sugar can affect behavior in children.

- Sugar can increase fasting levels of glucose and swings in blood sugar.

- Sugar can cause problems with the gastrointestinal tract.

- Sugar contributes to obesity.

- Sugar stimulates the growth of Candida. (yeast)

- Sugar causes dental caries.

Tips for Limiting Children's Sugar Intake

- Don't keep sweets around the house. They can be used sparingly as a reinforcer if that is one of the preferred choices for your child. Use it wisely.

- Never shop when you are hungry. You are likely to buy foods that are high in sugar, as you yourself will be craving something to get instant energy.

- Prepare your children's school lunches. Most schools now have have strict nutritional policies that limit or ban foods. Still, in some cafeterias, the sugary beverages are available.

- Refined sugar should be eliminated from your child's diet as much as possible. When serving sweets, make it a nutritional treat. Homebaked treats such as cookies and muffins can contain healthier sweeteners, pureed fruit instead of refined sugar. Proteins and fats can be added to the food along with natural sugar such as blended fruit to make a healthy food.

Notes:

Planning Lunch Box Meals That Kids Enjoy

Snacks can be prepared at home using alternative flours and the "list of ingredients allowed" in the children's least reactive food list. Here are some tips which can be useful while packing the lunch box for kids.

Tips for Lunch boxes

Food safety is important, especially when food will not be refrigerated for several hours. Bacteria grow rapidly on food at room temperature. A healthy lunch can become a live colony of harmful bacteria in a period of three to four hours at room temperature. If food cannot be kept warm or cold, follow the suggestions below:

- **Invest in a lunch box** that has blue ice frozen inserts to keep food cool.

- **Freeze beverages and place in lunch box.** They will thaw by lunch time and keep other foods cool.

- **Bring hot lunch in a thermos.** Soups, stews and casseroles are nutritious full meals. A glass-lined or stainless-lined thermos will keep foods hot or cold safely.

- **Keep at least two drinks in child's lunch box.** Include 100% juice, if allowed, and a water bottle. Drinking plenty of water is helpful in many ways. Make child's habit of drinking water throughout the day.

- **Choose a water bottle** that does not leach plastic carcinogens into water, and to be sure check the recycling symbol on your bottle. If it is a #2 HDPE (high density polyethylene), or a #4 LDPE (low density polyethylene), or a #5 PP (polypropylene), your bottle is fine. The type of plastic in which water is usually sold in most supermarkets is usually a #1, and is only recommended for one time use. Do not refill it. It is better to have a reusable water bottle, and fill it with your own filtered water from home.

- **Wrap children's sandwiches in waxed paper.** Do not use plastic or foil in direct contact with the food. Wrap the sandwich with wax paper and then you can cover it with foil or plastic.

- **Include at least one nutritious food.** Along with favorite things that children like, such as chips, cookies, etc., always have one nutrient dense nutritious food in the lunch box. It can be in the form of a protein (chicken drumstick) or nutrient dense nuts/seeds.

- **The lunch box should have** at least one fresh fruit serving; avoid using pre-packed fruits that are not loaded with sugar.

- **Make the child's lunch creative.** Cookies, sandwiches, pancakes, etc, can be cut into animal or other shapes to make lunch more attractive. Children with ASD do not like to try new things, so making the lunch creative can help them try something new.

- **Food should never be heated in the microwave,** especially in plastic containers. When having a picnic or party it is best to us biodegradable PLA picnic ware and compost it afterwards. It's available locally.

For more information on BPA and safe plastics, visit the National Geographic site, www.thegreenguide.com.

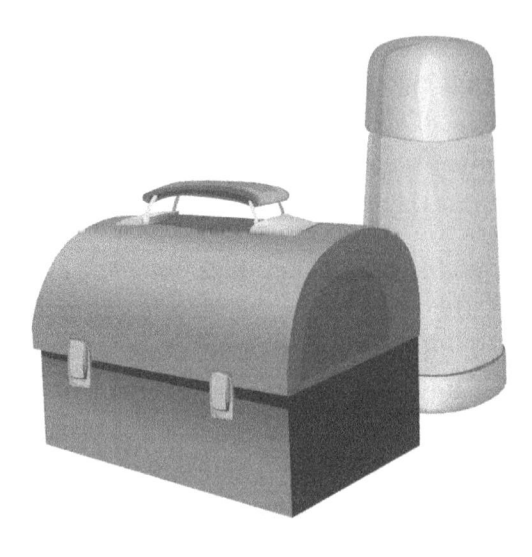

NOTES:

Notes:

CHAPTER FOUR

Kitchen Savvy and Cooking Aids

Tips and Hints

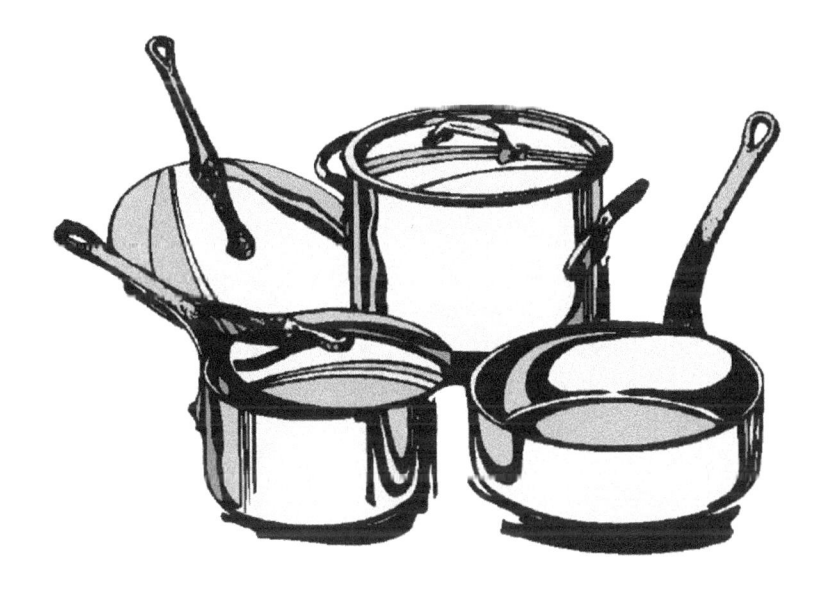

Suggested List of Cookware for Healthy Cooking

Modern day kitchen utensils, such as non-stick cookware, are designed to make cooking faster, but they can also be blamed for modifying the nutritional content of the food which can be detrimental to health. Healthy cookware is characterized by the way its surface reacts with food. The key is to find a material that is inert, meaning it does not affect the quality, taste or safety of the food. This chapter offers tips and hints to help you prepare healthy meals for your child and whole family.

- **Stainless Steel Cookware:** This can easily be a first choice of cookware to use. Stainless steel is actually an alloy of metals including steel, carbon and chromium. The reason stainless steel is called "stainless" is because of its ability to resist corrosion. It has the advantage of no known interaction with food.

- **Cast Iron Cookware:** Cooking in cast iron is known to increase the dietary source of iron. Cast iron skillets are great for frying and stir frying vegetables. These pots can easily be taken care of, too. There is no need to wash these utensils with soap. Simply rinse with hot water and wipe with a paper towel. Food cooked in a seasoned iron skillet never gets stuck or burned, so it can be a better choice over non-stick pans. These pans need to be seasoned, using high heat-stable oils like olive or coconut oil, or else they will rust.

- **Glass Cookware:** This kind of cookware is made from a transparent glass-ceramic material that withstands temperature extremes and offers real convenience and versatility. The same pot may be used for range top, oven, broiler (without cover), refrigerator, freezer, and microwave. This non-reactive, non-porous glass-ceramic will not absorb food odors or flavors, or react with foods. It is ideal for water-based cooking and for dishes that require stirring. It is dishwasher safe, and can be cleaned easily by hand. Pyrex and others make quality glass cookware, but it is important to note that overheating or quickly cooling this type of cookware can cause it to shatter. Do not use extremely high heat when cooking on the stovetop.

A good idea when using this cookware for long cooking times on the stove is to use a heat deflector placed on top of the burner for added protection and uniform heating.

- **Enamel Cookware:** This is a fused glass surface material that can last a lifetime when handled with care. It is possibly the best choice to cook with. Buy the best you can afford, as the inexpensive ones are easily scratched or chipped, and can leach the inner surface contents into the food. Enamel cookware with a non-stick lining is not a good choice.

- **Earthenware and Clay Pot Cookware:** These pots hold moisture and allow even cooking of a variety of foods. Foods cooked in earthenware are moist, tender and flavorful. Clay pots have nutritional value and need to be soaked in water before use. Most have a lid. As the pot is heated, steam builds up inside and the food is steamed until tender. Less water may be used since foods also release water when cooked.

- **Soapstone Cookware:** Soapstone is a natural quarried stone that, due to its mineral composition of talc and magnesite, has the extraordinary ability to hold heat longer than conventional cookware and kitchenware. It is great for low-fat cooking, is virtually non-stick after curing, and imparts no odor or taste, to food. It does not react with acidic foods, and is stovetop, grill and oven safe. It is easy to clean and lasts for generations.

- **Pressure Cooker:** Foods are cooked much faster by pressure cooking than by other methods, and use much less water than boiling, so dishes can be ready sooner. Less energy is required than when boiling, steaming or oven cooking. Since less water is necessary, the foods cook faster. The food is cooked above the boiling point of water, killing bacteria and viruses. The pressure cooker can also be used as an effective sterilizer for jam pots and glass baby bottles, for example, or for water while camping. With pressure cooking, heat is very evenly, deeply, and quickly distributed. This is a good cookware option; however it is not ideal when the food has to be cooked slowly at low temperatures.

Suggested List of Cookware to Avoid

- **Teflon:** Even when heated at normal temperatures, Teflon outgases and can cause danger to humans. For this reason, and because coating can also flake off into your food and expose you to toxic metals beneath the coating, Teflon pans and skillets should be discarded.

- **Non-Stick Cookware:** There has been a growing amount of research claiming that other non-stick utensils contain certain chemicals and heavy metals that can dissolve in food while cooking. Try to limit the use of these utensils or, if possible, completely eliminate them from the kitchen.

- **Aluminum:** More than half of the cookware on the market today is made from aluminum because it is a good conductor of heat. It is used frequently in non-stick pots and pans. Recent studies, however, have shown that food cooked on aluminum surfaces form aluminum salts. Since aluminum has been connected with brain disorders such as dementia, Alzheimer's, Autism, behavior abnormality, poor memory and impaired motor and visual coordination, aluminum cookware should be avoided.

- **Microwave and Microwave Cookware:** It is rare to find any American home without a microwave oven, but unfortunately most families use them for much more than just making popcorn, reheating meals and preparing prepackaged foods. Microwave cooking changes the molecular structure of food. Microwaves are now part of the modern day kitchen, but, if possible, avoiding them completely would be ideal.

Cooking Pans

- A little salt or flour placed in a frying pan will prevent splattering.

- When braising meats, add a few sticks of celery, lining the bottom of the pan, to keep food from sticking.

- Vinegar brought to a boil in a new frying pan will prevent foods from sticking.

- When you are scalding milk, prevent sticking by rinsing your pan in cold water before putting milk in it.

- Pots and pans with flat bottoms keep the burner heat from escaping.

- Use tightly fitting lids on pans. Foods cooked in a covered pan will begin to boil or steam quicker so you can use lower temperature settings. On the stovetop, start with high heat and lower the setting when food starts to bubble or boil.

Kitchen Accessories Guide

NOTE: **Kitchen accessories can be a source for cross-contamination. As indicated below, it is good to have two sets when cooking for someone on a special diet.**

- **Kitchen Scissors:** Kitchen Scissors, used for snipping herbs and a variety of other tasks, have to be cleaned and sterilized.

- **Wooden Spoons:** Use separate spoons when cooking for a child with food sensitivity. They need to be cleaned after each use as they can be a source of pathogens. They can be sterilized in a microwave.

- **Cutting Board:** Wooden cutting boards are non-slippery and therefore great for cutting, but they should be cleaned after each use as they are likely to harbor pathogenic bacteria. It is better and also more convenient to use glass cutting boards that can be put in the dishwasher to clean. To avoid cross contamination, one should have two boards, one for meats and one for vegetables and fruits.

- **Knives and Peelers:** Sterilize knives and peelers often. Keep separate knives for meat, fruits and vegetables and clean well after each use.

- **Baking Accessories:** Using mixing bowls and baking dishes made of glass, ceramic, or stainless steel is safe and ideal for baking. A glass liquid measuring cup is preferred over plastic cups. Stainless dry measuring cups and spoons are preferred over plastic as well. Since cookie sheets and muffin pans are generally made of non-stick materials or aluminum, it is recommended to line the baking pans with parchment paper and to use individual cupcake liners for baking in muffin tins.

- **Additional Accessories:** Can opener, pizza wheel, and bamboo steamers. Try to keep two sets, one for the child with a special diet, and one for the rest of the family. (Be sure to clean the can opener wheels after every use.) You can also opt for additional cooking accessories that can make cooking easier for you. If not possible, the dishwasher set on sanitation cycle will be hot enough to get rid of bacteria. Using an extra rinse cycle can also guard against stubborn food residue left on dishes, pots & untensils.

Small Kitchen Appliance Suggestions

Special Note: Small Kitchen Appliances can also be a source of cross contamination. It is crucial that they either be separated or handled with care when your child is on special diet.

- **Blenders:** A very useful tool. This low cost appliance makes soup cooking a breeze. It can also be used for making smoothies, blending fruits and vegetables, and grinding soaked lentils to make the batter for pancakes.

- **Juicers:** A juicer can be handy tool. Juicing is a proven technique that provides the incredible healing power of common fruits and vegetables. Juicing is easy, safe, and inexpensive, and an easy way to treat or prevent many health-related problems. It is also an effective way of providing children with vital nutrients from fruits and vegetables if they do not like to eat them raw.

- **Mini Mill:** This is useful for grinding spices and seeds (flax, sesame, etc). Freshly ground spices have more prominent taste and offer very profound flavors.

- **Handheld Mixer:** This useful appliance can mix a variety of ingredients effectively with little effort.

- **Dehydrators:** This time-honored food preserving method can either be an alternative to canning and freezing or a complement to these methods. This is useful when you have an abundance of a particular fruit or vegetable that can be dehydrated for later use. With modern food dehydrators, drying food is simple, safe and easy to learn. Dried food is great in traditional recipes and can save you a lot of time in the kitchen during meal preparation

- **Food Processor:** This "helping hand" can make cooking fun and less time consuming. It can be used for a variety of purposes from chopping, slicing, and grating to mixing and blending.

- **Lemon Juicer:** A great small hand appliance used to extract lemon juice and keep seeds out of the food. A useful tool used in cooking many healthy recipes.

- **Ice Cream Maker:** This useful but optional, tool can be used to make homemade ice cream for your kids. If your child loves ice cream and is on a restricted diet, make ice cream with rice or almond milk and a few nuts for a healthy alternative to sugary treats.

Tips for Using Food Storage Containers

- **Glass and Stainless Steel Food Containers:** Glass or stainless steel containers are less likely to alter the taste of refrigerated food than plastic containers.

- **Glass Beverages Containers:** For storing lacto-fermented beverages, use glass beverage containers with an airtight seal such as mason jars. **Fresh juices should be consumed as you make them**. If you need to store them, use glass containers because fresh juices have live bacteria that can react with plastic.

- **Wide-Mouth Quart-Size Glass Containers:** They are very handy in storing sauces or other homemade fermented foods. They can also be used to store soups, stock or other liquid.

- **Ceramics and Pottery Containers:** These are preferable to plastics. These containers tend to be artistic and well suited to display while containing food. They can be found without lids and with lids that seal. Ceramic containers can be used to store food leftovers, are easy to clean, and some can be heated in an oven.

- **Wood Containers:** Choose these wisely. Many paints, oils and finishes are toxic and not safe to be next to food. Some wooden containers are suitable for storing foods that are still wrapped or otherwise protected. A few companies sell bamboo products that are safe, but frequently they do not have a lid. Wood containers should not be frozen or placed in the oven.

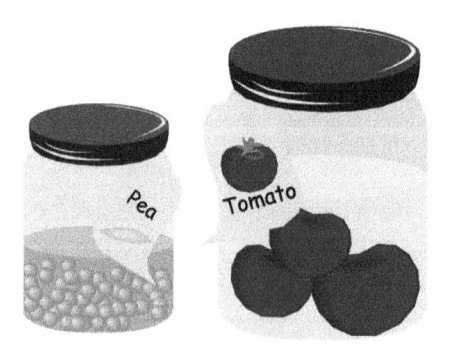

General Kitchen Tips & Hints

- **Wash all fruits and vegetables** to remove dirt and other residue. Soak them in hydrogen peroxide liquid (1 teaspoon per gallon) for 10 minutes and rinse well.

- **Keep kitchen uncluttered** and counters clean. Store only frequently used items on the kitchen counter, leaving as much working space as possible.

- **Keep all food preparation areas spotless.** Wipe counters after each cooking task to provide space for the next meal. This makes cooking more fun, rather than more work.

- **Have easy access to tools and utensils.** Always thoroughly wash the cutting boards, knives, and countertops that come in contact with food.

- **Dishwasher powder/liquid** can be extremely poisonous, so should be handled with great care. Use half the recommended amount, as these powders/liquids can get into the food we eat, and can be extremely dangerous for young developing children. Try to use natural or eco-friendly detergents for the dishwasher.

- **Refrigerate and cover food** as soon as possible. Foods do not always need to be cooled before being refrigerated. Bacteria grow very rapidly when food is left out at room temperature, and especially when it is exposed to air for a long period of time. It's the in-between stage that is bad. Refrigerate within two hours.

- **Clean the refrigerator often.** Throw out leftover and old purchases, especially foods that are past their expiration date. Wipe off the shelves and clean the meat and vegetable bins. Remove and scrub out the drip pan from under the appliance (which can harbor mold and mildew). Clean well under the refrigerator, too.

Cooking Efficiency

- If possible, always plan for the next two meals ahead.

- When cooking foods, think about increasing the amount so that extras can be frozen for the time when quick meals are needed.

- Learn to read all ingredient labels on cans, boxes, jars and packages. Many commercially prepared foods can have hidden ingredients and additives that can have harmful effects.

- Choose fresh and frozen foods over canned food. The inside lining of some cans may have some harmful metals that can erode and contaminate the food.

- Ideally, fresh foods and vegetables should be eaten within two to four days. Avoid microwave and high heat in cooking, since important nutrients can be lost, thus making food less nutritious.

- Prepare meats, fish and poultry as fresh as possible. Avoid fast foods and processed food, as they have many preservatives that are not good for health.

- Avoid overcooking vegetables. Cook just until crisp-tender. Add raw vegetables to the diet as much as possible; they make meals more interesting. This may not be possible if your child has low oral muscle tone.

- To peel large amounts of garlic, place whole bulbs in oven and bake at 300 degrees until the individual cloves open. Remove from oven and pick out individual cloves.

- Avoid using commercial table salt. Instead, use Sea Salt. It contains many useful minerals such as calcium, potassium, magnesium and several trace minerals that are needed by the body.

- Always skim the stock, sauces, soups, legumes and stews to remove impurities that will rise to the top. Seasonings and other spices should be added after skimming.

- Juices drained from meat should be added back to the sauce or stew, as they are a rich source of important amino acids that should not be wasted.

- The ideal diet should have plenty of fruits and vegetables. Aim for at least 50 percent raw or enzyme-enhanced foods. Whole foods like gluten-free whole grains, nuts and seeds, can also be added to the diet. Processed foods should be avoided because they are enzyme poor and may add potential carcinogens.

- For health benefits, lunch or dinner should start with a dish containing a lot of enzymes. This would include eating a salad or soup. This aids in digestion by restoring the enzymes buffer.

- If the meal you serve consists entirely of cooked foods, then a lacto-fermented condiment should be added to the diet. Probiotics in food ensures a healthy immune system.

- Start the day with gluten-free whole grain dishes, such as pancakes or muffins, eggs or nut milk. Ready-made breakfast cereals produced by the process of extrusion (flakes, special shapes, puffed grains) should be avoided.

- Unsaturated fatty acids found in commercial cooking oils should be avoided. They are needed by the body in only small amounts, and are in adequate supply in vegetables, nuts and even in meats. Excessive processed fatty acids can have devastating effects on the body, leading to degeneration and early aging. Instead, incorporate into the diet oils with good sources of fat, such as olive oil, coconut oil, safflower or sunflower oil.

Ideas for Baking

- Dip measuring spoons or cups into hot water before measuring butter or oils. The fat will slip off without sticking.

- Slippery foods are easier to hold if you dip your fingertips in a little salt first.

- To hold wax paper in place when rolling dough, dampen the counter before placing the paper on it.

- If a recipe calls for honey (which many of our recipes do), look for the color. Dark color means the taste will be strong. If you're looking for something silky and sweet for a muffin or fresh-baked breads, look for the lightest color available.

- When you have to add any citrus juice to a recipe that you are baking, wrap the fruit in cheesecloth and squeeze it directly in the bowl or pot. The seeds will be trapped and you will have one less dish to wash.

- A preheated oven ensures good results and can sometimes be credited for the success of recipe. The right oven temperature is the key to browned meat or rising baked food. Use a thermometer to calibrate the oven.

- In an oven, cook as many dishes at once as possible. Foods with a cooking temperature within 25 degrees of each other can be cooked simultaneously.

- If you have an oven light, check food through the oven door's window. Each time you open the oven door, the temperature can drop 25 to 50 degrees.

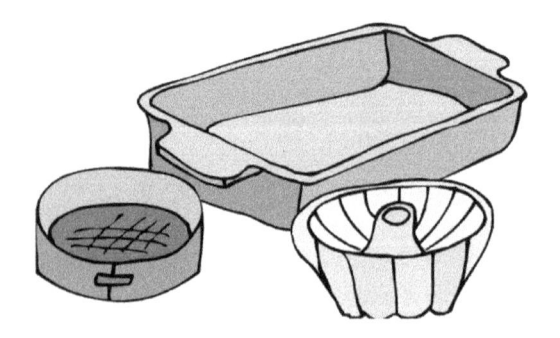

Kitchen Safety Tips & Hints

Cooking requires assembling ingredients, measuring in the right proportions, mixing, steaming, and baking, often in a chaotic atmosphere, especially if you're feeling rushed or when cooking around children. Here are some useful guidelines for avoiding injuries in the kitchen:

- Tie back loose hair and don't wear hanging jewelry.

- Roll up sleeves when working in the kitchen.

- Sharp knives need special care. The sharper the knife, the better the results. Always work with blade directly away from the hand, and do not become distracted from the task. Don't leave sharp cutting tools in the bottom of the sink, or at the edge of the counter. Also, place sharp knives and pointed utensils sharp side down in the dishwasher utensil rack.

- Don't leave spoons in hot pans.

- Turn panhandles toward inside of stove to avoid it accidentally falling.

- Remove lids carefully to avoid being burned by any steam.

- Don't use any wet potholders. They can transmit heat and result in severe burns.

- Make sure food processors are turned off before changing the blades, or before putting them away.

Notes:

Chapter Five

Diet and Dietary Planning

Introduction to Diets

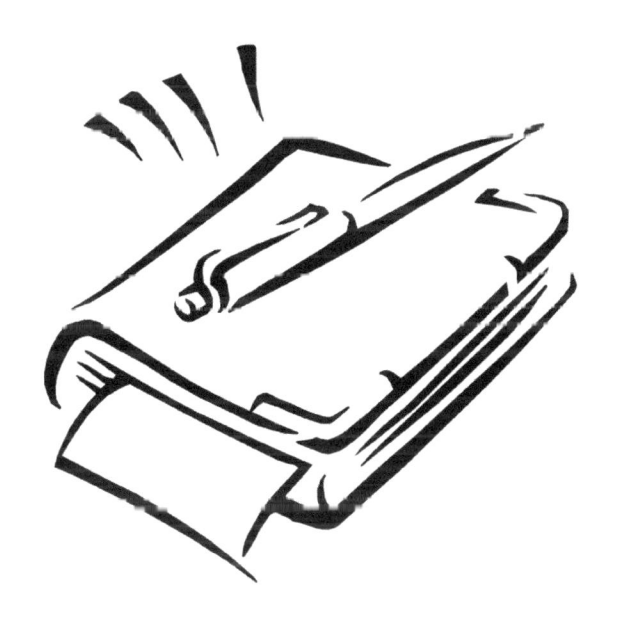

CHILDREN WITH ASD and developmental disorders often have co-occurring, and perhaps treatable, problems. Neuro-Metabolic disorders, endocrine dysfunction (thyroid disorders), immunologic and gastrointestinal problems (celiac disease, reflux, colitis, etc.) may also be present.

Nutrition deficiencies can result from these co-occurring problems or may even be the cause of them. This section of the book focuses on diet as a means of treating nutritional deficiencies which have been identified in some children. The proper diet can improve a child's gastrointestinal problems, which in turn may improve overall health, reduce stress, and contribute to the family environment as a whole.

Food Sensitivity and Food Intolerance: Many individuals have food allergies and intolerance issues. This is especially true of children with ASD and other developmental disorders.

- **A food allergy** occurs when the body's immune system mistakenly thinks that a harmless substance (meaning whatever food you happen to be eating) is harmful. In response, the body creates antibodies to that food, so that whenever one eats that food, the body releases massive amounts of chemicals that can trigger allergic reactions, typically in the respiratory system or gastrointestinal tract.

- **Food Intolerance** happens or appears when your digestive system has trouble processing foods. This may in part be caused by insufficient digestive enzymes or by imbalances in the gut. Symptoms of food intolerance include gastrointestinal distress and behavioral problems.

Someone who is allergic to a substance, such as food, will typically react to it in a very short time, whereas someone with intolerance can react hours and even days later. This is important to keep in mind, because symptoms of allergies and intolerances can be similar. Because symptoms are so common, it sometimes becomes difficult to distinguish between them.

Systems Affected by Food Allergy/Food Intolerance

- Gastro-intestinal (stomach and intestines)
- Respiratory (lungs and breathing)
- Dermatological (skin diseases)
- Neurological (pain, memory and mood)
- Musculoskeletal (muscle and bone disorders)
- Reproductive (genital and fertility issues)
- Immune responses (ability to fight infection)

Gluten and Casein-Free Diet (GFCF Diet)

Gluten is a protein found in wheat, rye, barley, kamut, spelt, triticale, and any derivatives of these grains. This includes malt grain starches, hydrolyzed vegetable proteins, grain vinegar, soy sauce, and natural flavorings.

Gluten is a problem because it is one of the most complex proteins consumed by man. It is a very large molecule compared to other food molecules, and for that reason is difficult for the digestive system to break down. Problems begin when it reaches the small intestine. In sensitive individuals, gluten interrupts the lining of the gut, which acts as a natural barrier to pathogens. This "Leaky Gut Syndrome" allows foreign particles (whatever is in the gut, including bacteria) to cross into the bloodstream, setting the body's immune system on high alert, resulting in the symptoms.

Gluten Intolerance and Celiac Disease: Gluten intolerance is a broad term that includes all kinds of sensitivity to Gluten. It is common that only a small fraction of gluten-intolerant people test positive on the Celiac Disease test. Most tests are negative or inconclusive. The correct term for these people is Non-Celiac Gluten Sensitive (NCGS). This may account for as much as 15% of the population.

Celiac Disease (CD) is the first type of gluten sensitivity for which diagnostic testing was devised — in the 1940s. It is a lifelong, autoimmune intestinal disorder found in individuals who are genetically susceptible. Damage to the mucosal surface of the small intestine is caused by an immunologically toxic reaction to gluten, and interferes with the absorption of nutrients. Celiac Disease (CD) is unique in that a specific food component, gluten, has been identified as the trigger.

This disease is also known as a disease of malabsorption. When a person with celiac disease eats foods, or uses products containing gluten, his immune system responds by damaging tiny, fingerlike protrusions, called villi, lining the small intestine.

These villi allow nutrients to be absorbed into the bloodstream. Without healthy villi, a person becomes malnourished, regardless of the quantity of food eaten.

Symptoms of Gluten Intolerance and Allergy

- Chronic diarrhea or constipation
- Abdominal distension
- Poor appetite
- Poor weight gain or growth
- Muscle wasting
- Vomiting
- Irritability
- Weight loss
- Anemia
- Weakness
- Fatigue
- Fuzzy thinking
- High pain tolerance
- Self-injurious behaviors

Casein is a protein found in all things dairy, regardless of the source.

The difference between dairy, lactose and casein

Dairy refers to the food made from milk, cream, and milk products. Casein is one of the proteins found in milk, and lactose is the sugar in milk. The point to remember is dairy-free is not always casein-free, and lactose–free is not casein-free, either.

Some children with ASD have chronic diarrhea, and, as a consequence of this, they might be washing away the enzyme lactase, which digests lactose. They may be actually lactose-intolerant and not dairy-intolerant, but may be both. When your child has allergies to milk, learn to read labels because many non-dairy foods contain casein in some form or ingredient. One such example is calcium caseinate, a form of casein. Lactose- free milk is readily available in supermarkets.

Cow's milk is 80 percent casein and only 20 percent whey protein. This may account for the fact that cow's milk is repeatedly ranked among the top eight offenders for food allergies. Mother's milk is 80 percent whey and only 20 percent casein, which may prove that we are naturally geared more towards whey than casein in milk digestion.

Symptoms of Casein (Milk) Allergy: An allergy is by the body's reaction to an allergen. The symptoms of a milk protein allergy fall into three types:

Skin Reactions	Stomach and Intestinal Reactions	Nose, Throat and Lung Reactions
Itchy red rash Hives Eczema Swelling of lips, mouth, tongue, face or throat Allergic "shiners" (black eyes)	Abdominal pain and bloating Diarrhea (usually very runny) Vomiting Gas/wind Cramps	Runny Nose, Sneezing Watery and/or Itchy eyes Coughing Wheezing Shortness of breath

Both Gluten and Casein, may cause physical and neurological reactions in children with ASD, resulting in such behaviors as hyperactivity, irritability, lethargy, headaches, fatigue, self-injurious behavior, fuzzy thinking, weakness, obsessive-compulsive problems, and eye-hand coordination difficulties.

Decision about implementing the diet: The GFCF diet should be the foundation upon which further nutritional interventions should stand for children with special needs. The GFCF diet not only helps to resolve the constipation and diarrhea symptoms, but also improves cognitive function and reduces severity of behavioral symptoms for many children.

Theories Regarding Gluten and Casein and Children with ASD

The Leaky Gut Theory

Many autistic individuals have permeable intestinal tracts, possibly due to viral infections, yeast infections, and reduction in phenol sulfur transferase (PST, which lives in the intestinal tract and protects it from being too permeable). If the digestive process is impaired, gluten and casein digestion becomes critical and causes problems such as:

- Increased intestinal permeability

- Allows overgrowth of bacteria, parasites, viruses, yeasts and fungi that causes intestinal inflammation

- Irritation causes "tight junctions" between intestinal cells to loosen and allow large particles to enter blood stream (leaky gut)

Opioid Effect Theory

Gluten and casein in the intestinal tract break down from the protein state to a smaller unit called peptides. Some researches surmise that many cases of autism may result from an immune system dysfunction that affects the body's ability to break down certain proteins and to combat yeasts and bacteria. These proteins, which are not broken into smaller peptides, may pass through imperfections in the intestinal tract and act like morphine (opioid derivative) in the body. Casomorphin and gliadinomorphin are two such peptides that resemble opium-like drugs. They can pass through the blood-brain barrier and have a negative impact on the brain. It has been suggested that peptides from gluten and casein may have a role in autism, and that the physiology and behaviors of autism might be explained by excessive opioid activity linked to these peptides. This is reasoned because some studies show that the peptides in question are found in unusually high amount in the urine of some autistic individuals.

Negative reactions when first starting GFCF diet: There are a few negative reactions when first starting the diet, like upset stomach, anxiety, clinginess, dizziness, aches and pains and ill temper. These may be a withdrawal effect, since the body is reacting to the absence of gluten and casein. However, this may be a good sign and the precursor to a positive response in the future. A trial period of at least three months is recommended

Both positive and negative results are usually more noticeable in younger children than in older ones. If the child has severe negative reactions, withdraw offending foods in stages, over a period of two weeks or more, to lessen the severity.

Gluten and Casein-Free Diet: Guidelines for Parents

- Elimination of casein, followed by gluten-containing foods, is easier to implement.

- Removing milk and wheat takes away many nutrients. Children's nutrient levels have to be tested and supplemented accordingly. Any deficiency can add to problems.

- Substitute the same foods the child likes (e.g., pancakes), with alternative GFCF options (GFCF pancakes). *See our gluten-free flour options discussion in Chapter 9 and breakfast recipes in Chapter 10 for much healthier options that are easy to make and highly nutritious.*

- Be patient — your child might refuse to eat for a few days due to withdrawal, craving or merely control tactics. Believe in the diet, and he or she will eventually comply.

- GFCF diet substitutes such as cookies, crackers, candy, and cakes are loaded with sugar, so look for low sugar foods. Homemade desserts and snacks are a good option, where sugar content is limited and foods can be made with more nutritional ingredients.

- Be careful with corn and soy as alternate choices when going GFCF, as both are highly allergenic foods.

- When going GFCF, plan for frequent meals for children. When milk and wheat are removed, digestion improves, but children tend to feel hungry more frequently. When hungry, their craving for high sugar foods can increase because these provide instant energy. Meal planning will help provide children with nutrient-rich foods.

- Learn to read food labels to identify any hidden ingredients. A strict GFCF diet often brings improvements. Ask questions at restaurants, manufacturers or vendors, where your child loves to eat, to learn of any hidden triggers not listed on their offerings.

- Other caregivers, like grandparents, teachers, therapists or babysitters, need to be included in the plan. All should be informed about the foods that are allowed and not allowed. It is safest to pack the appropriate foods and snacks so that you can minimize any dietary infractions.

Low Oxalate Diet (LOD)

Oxalates are present in plants and fruits and in virtually all seeds and nuts. Ordinarily, the gut won't absorb much of the oxalates from the diet; however under the conditions of "Leaky Gut," a lot of dietary oxalates are absorbed.

Oxalate Crystals: When we consume foods that are high in oxalates, the oxalates in the intestine combine with calcium, magnesium and zinc to form crystals. This binding of minerals in the GI tracts leads to their impaired absorption. Oxalates crystals are then deposited throughout the body, in the brain, liver, kidneys, bowels and even bone marrow.

Effect of Oxalate Crystals on the Body: Oxalate is a highly reactive molecule. When it is present in high amounts, it can lead to oxidative damage in the body.

Oxalates and Children with ASD: Oxalates levels in the urine of ASD children are observed to be much higher than in normal children. When there is a leaky gut, or when there is prolonged diarrhea or constipation, excess oxalate from foods can be absorbed and become a risk to other cells in the body. Children with autism manifest conditions that may increase their sensitivity to oxalates.

High Oxalates Foods List

- **Greens:** Spinach, swiss chard, beet greens, collards, kale, parsley
- **Nuts and Seeds:** Almonds, cashews and peanuts
- **Legumes**: Soybeans, tofu, white beans
- **Grains:** wheat, spelt, kamut
- **Fruits:** blackberries, blueberries, raspberries, strawberries, currants, kiwi fruit,concord-purple, grapes, figs, tangerines, and plums
- **Vegetables:** celery, green beans, rutabagas, leeks, and summer squash
- **Others:** cocoa, chocolate, and black tea

Considerations about Implementing a Low Oxalate Diet (LOD)

Parents can consider implementing the Low Oxalate Diet (LOD) when they have tried other diets like GFCF, SCD (Specific Carbohydrate Diet), and PFSF (Phenol and Salicylates Free diet) with minimal to no results and still there are behavioral and digestive problems persistent with children. **Parents can consider implementing this diet with their children, if the children have some of the symptoms listed below:**

- Urinary problems, night bed wetting or pain during urination

- Sensation or feeling of pain in the genital areas

- Frequent bowel movements, gastrointestinal pain or other discomfort felt within minutes or hours after eating high-oxalate foods

- Continued diarrhea or constipation symptoms even after implementing other diets

- Craving for high-oxalates foods

- Child having delayed growth in height and weight, even when child is seemingly consuming a healthy diet. It has been noted that children on a LOD experience a rapid growth spurt.

- Children with obsessive and compulsive problems. Less rigid behaviors are seen in children after implementing LOD.

Low Oxalate Diet: Guidelines for Parents

- This is a difficult diet that allows few food choices. But it is worth it to try for a period of at least three months for children who have not benefitted much from other diets.

- There are some supplements that are recommended to support LOD, such as taurine, vitamin A, calcium and magnesium citrate and zinc. Supplement with vitamin B6, since it is a cofactor for one of the enzymes that degrade oxalate in the body, and has been shown to reduce oxalate production. **(Consult with your health care practitioner before taking any of the above mentioned supplements)**.

- Increase water intake to limit oxalate stress in the body.

- Yeast and fungi cause high oxalate stress in the body; hence use of probiotics may also be helpful in degrading oxalates in the intestine. Lactobacillus acidophilus and bifido bacterium lactic have enzymes that degrade oxalates.

- Epsom salt baths have been reported by parents to have reduced symptoms caused by high oxalate stress.

- Sodium bicarbonate or Alka-Seltzer Gold can help with behaviors.

- **Lemon juice:** Helps with digestion when given before eating and may help balance pH issues.

Phenol-Free Diet
(Phenols, Salicylates, Amine and Feingold)

Phenols are chemicals found in practically all foods we eat. This category contains quite a few subgroups, both food and non-food. Amines and salicylate are examples. The phenols, salicylates and amines cause problems in some children, especially those with deficits in certain biochemical pathways, such as the sulfation pathway.

Phenols and polyphenols are not completely unwanted, since they have antioxidant qualities and protective functions. Many children with ASD have a deficiency in the sulfation pathway, which makes it desirable to limit phenols from the diet.

The Role of the Sulfation Pathway within the Body:

- It nourishes the GI tract by contributing to formation of mucins, the lack of which may lead to inflammation, permeability and leaky gut syndrome.

- Sulfation produces hormones that trigger secretions of digestive enzymes from the pancreas, and bile from the gall bladder.

The problem arises when phenols and salicylates consume a lot of sulfate in the body in order to be broken down. In other words, the phenols and salicylates compete for the body's sulfate stores. This adds to the GI tract problem of the children with ASD.

Feingold Diet: The Feingold diet eliminates a number of artificial colors and artificial flavors, aspartame, three petroleum-based preservatives, and (at least initially) certain salicylates.

Additives: Food additives are used to preserve flavor or improve the taste and appearance of food. Some natural additives have been used for centuries. For example, foods are preserved by pickling (with vinegar), salting as with bacon, preserving sweets or using sulfur dioxide in some wines. The real problem started when, with the advent of processed foods in the second half of the 20th century, many more synthetic additives were introduced. These were added to products to increase shelf life. Today, a typical child in the United States is exposed to these powerful chemicals everyday. It is no wonder children are now facing diseases and conditions which were never heard of, or which were extremely rare.

Considerations about Implementing Phenol-Free and Salicylate-Free Diet

Considerations about implementing the Phenol-Free diet are tricky at best, as they are based more on observing behaviors. There are no specific tests to determine if phenols are the real problem with your child.

But there are many components that can be taken into account to help parents make the determination, such as:

a) Reaction to phenol foods *(see following list of symptoms)*

b) Reaction to Tylenol or acetaminophen and artificial ingredients (such as hyperactivity, compulsive behavior, sleep disturbance, aggressive behaviors)

c) High levels of sulfate in the blood and urine

d) Family history of neurological disorders, including ASD

e) Self-injurious behavior present in child, especially if a GFCF diet has not shown improvements

Symptoms Of
Phenols and Additives Stress

Behavioral Problems	Learning Problems	Health Problems
Marked Hyperactivity Constant motion Running instead of walking Inability to sit still Inappropriate wiggling of legs/hands **Impulsive Actions** Disruptive behavior Unresponsiveness to discipline Unkindness to pets Poor self-control Destructive behaviors Throws or breaks things Little or no recognition of danger to self Inappropriate noises Interrupts often Excessive talking Loud talking Abusive behavior Unpredictable behavior **Compulsive Actions** Aggression Perseveration/repetitive Touching things or people Chewing on clothing Chewing objects Scratching and biting Picking/pinching skin **Emotional Concerns** Low frustration tolerance Depression, frequent crying Demands immediate attention Irritability Overreaction to touch, pain Sensitivity to sound and lights Panics easily Nervousness Low self-esteem Mood swings Suicidal thoughts	**Short Attention Span** Impatience Distraction Failure to complete projects Inability to listen to whole story Inability to follow directions **Neuro-Muscular Involvement** Accident-prone Poor muscle coordination Difficulty writing, drawing Dyslexia/reading problems Speech difficulties/delays Difficulty with playground activities, sports Eye muscle disorder (nystagmus, strabismus) Tics (unusual or uncontrollable movements) Seizures **Cognitive and Perceptual Disturbances** Auditory memory deficits (difficulty remembering what is heard) Visual memory deficits (difficulty remembering what is seen) Difficulty in comprehension and short term memory Disturbance in spatial orientation (up-down, right-left) Difficulties in reasoning (simple math problems, meaning in words)	**Frequent Physical Complaints** Ear infections Asthma Bedwetting (enuresis) Daytime wetting Stomach aches Headaches, migraines Hives, rashes (urticaria) Eczema Leg aches Constipation, diarrhea Congestion Seizures (especially if combined with migraine or hyperactivity) **Sleep Problems** Resistance to going to bed Difficulty falling asleep Restless / erratic sleep Nightmares, bad dreams

Phenol and Additives-Free Diet: Guidelines for Parents

Because phenols are present in virtually all foods we eat, it is almost impossible to eliminate them completely. The good news is that, when we reduce the phenol content by consuming a low-phenol diet, we can still get benefits in children.

There are certain guidelines for parents to keep in mind:

- Phenols, salicylates and additives are a problem that typically needs to be addressed after the Gluten Free / Casein Free (GCFC) diet has been started. Generally, it is recommended to limit foods high in phenols or salicylates, and additives about two to six months after you start a GFCF diet.

- **Amines** are another class of food that is associated with phenols. Refer to *Chapter 7* for "Food Amine and Salicylates Content List" to see if the child is allergic or intolerant to this class. For example, a banana is a low phenol food, but is high in amines. (Banana is one of the favorite foods for many children, especially for children with ASD.) If your child exhibits hyperactive symptoms after eating a banana, eliminate it completely, then re-introduce it after implementing the low phenol diet for a period of four to six months.

- **Mega doses of vitamin B6 and/or Pyridoxal-5-Phosphate**, found in a few vitamin supplements, can aggravate the PST problem of some children (make it even more difficult for the child to process phenols), so if you are supplementing with mega doses of vitamins B6 and/or P5P, you may consider reducing the dosage.

- Along with implementing the Phenol Free diet, consider supplementing with phenol assist enzymes which will help break down any other phenol consumed in foods. Some parents have found supplementing **with molybdenum** has helped with phenol sensitivity. One study found urinary sulfite to be elevated due to a lack of molybdenum.

- The enzymes in raw foods will improve phenol tolerance in children.

- Supplements that add sulfates are helpful. Many parents report that **Epsom salt baths** are beneficial in helping their child's body handle phenols.

- **Keep a food journal.** Track what your child eats and watch behaviors. Negative reactions to high phenol foods happen within 30 minutes of food consumption, and this is where a journal can help you track reactions.

Specific Carbohydrate Diet (SCD Diet)

The Specific Carbohydrate Diet (SCD) is a strict grain-free, lactose-free, and sucrose-free meal plan. It was developed by Sydney Valentine Haas, MD. Elaine Gottschall helped to popularize the diet after using it to help her daughter recover from ulcerative colitis. Gottschall continued research on the diet and later wrote her own book, *Breaking the Vicious Cycle: Intestinal Health Through Diet*.

Approach to Specific Carbohydrates Diet (SCD Diet): There are specific carbohydrates that can be troublesome for the digestive system. Many people suffer from gastric distress, which ranges from mild to more serious disorders, such as Crohn's Disease, Ulcerative Colitis, Diverticulitis, Irritable Bowel Syndrome (IBS), Chronic Diarrhea and Celiac Disease. The purpose of the SCD Diet is to eliminate specific carbohydrates which contribute to the gastrointestinal problems, and to help restore a healthy digestive system.

The Specific Carbohydrate Diet is a Scientific Diet: SCD Diet is a Scientific Diet that is based on chemistry, biology, and clinical studies. The selection of foods on the Specific Carbohydrate Diet is based on:

- The chemical structure of the foods.

- Carbohydrates classified by their molecular structure.

- The allowed carbohydrates have a molecular structure that is small enough to be transported across the small intestinal surface into the bloodstream.

- These carbohydrates do not need to be broken down by various processes of the digestive organs, such as by the pancreas or the intestinal cells' surface enzymes.

Thus the foods allowed are easier to digest.

- **Principles of the Specific Carbohydrate Diet (SCD Diet):** Specifically selected carbohydrates that require minimal digestion are allowed. They are well absorbed, leaving virtually nothing for intestinal microbes to feed on. As the microbes decrease from lack of nourishment, their harmful by-products diminish. The activity of mucus-producing cells diminishes, and carbohydrate digestion is improved.

- The Specific Carbohydrate Diet corrects malabsorption, thereby allowing nutrients to enter the bloodstream and be available to the cells, consequently strengthening the immune system.

- Some individuals cannot digest carbohydrates, most likely due to damage to the small intestine mucosa. This maldigestion leads to malabsorption of disaccharides (unabsorbed complex sugars), which cause bacteria and yeast overgrowth as they feed on these unabsorbed complex sugars. These bacteria destroy enzymes, further inhibiting carbohydrate metabolism and creating additional damage to the small intestine, completing a "vicious cycle". The Specific Carbohydrate Diet helps to eliminate this problem.

SCD "Legal" vs. "Illegal" Foods: There is a wide range of permissible foods allowed on the SCD diet. Permitted foods are SCD "legal" and non permissible foods are "illegal." It is important to understand that just because a food is allowed doesn't mean it will be tolerated. If you go slowly, adding new things gradually and in small amounts, you will be able to observe if a negative reaction occurs. Keeping a food journal and recording the results is helpful. Rotation of tolerated foods is not required but it may be useful if your child is very sensitive and has many reactions to food.

SCD Diet: Possible Negative "Die-Off" Reactions: A negative reaction could happen immediately or two days later. It is suggested to introduce each food one at a time and for up to four days, so the offending foods can be easily identified and eliminated. It is common to see some initial, temporary negative reactions, such as sleep disturbances and behavioral changes such as irritability, tantrums, short tempered, increased "stimmy" behaviors, hyperactivity, inability to focus, headaches or dizziness. Also, nausea or vomiting, bowel movements changes (constipation or diarrhea), runny nose, cough and flu-like symptoms, achy joints, back pain, and skin rashes have been seen. To avoid or decrease these symptoms, gradually lower the amount of starches and sugars at least one week before starting this diet. These negative reactions are temporary, and benefits usually follow in many cases.

Specific Carbohydrate Diet (SCD Diet) and Children with ASD: The Specific Carbohydrate Diet has gained popularity in the autism community, as there have been many anecdotal reports from parents with children with ASD who have dramatically improved after being on the Specific Carbohydrate Diet.

Many children with ASD have bacterial and fungal overgrowth problems, bacterial imbalance, gut inflammation, and chronic diarrhea and/or constipation problems. The Specific Carbohydrate Diet helps heal the intestinal tract and has proven to be a successful dietary intervention in treating children with ASD. Some researchers have linked gut pathogens (the microorganisms in the gut) to digestive problems and impairment of brain function. Our digestive systems are linked to our immune, endocrine, circulatory and central nervous systems. When the digestive system has been improved, remarkable changes in an individual's physical, mental and emotional health often follow.

Specific Carbohydrate Diet: Guidelines for Parents

- SCD allows for some dairy products such as homemade cheeses and yogurt. (*See the recipe in "Homemade Specialties" in Chapter 9*). If a child has casein sensitivity, dairy products should be carefully re-introduced or continued.

- Slowly introduce probiotics, enzymes and yogurt. Use activated charcoal capsules if you think your child is having a possible initial negative or "die-off" reaction. (*Die-off is usually caused by the toxins released by the gut pathogens as they die off and leave the body*).

- SCD Diet limits starches. Nut flours are used extensively in place of grains in the recipes. Nuts are high in copper. A zinc supplement, in proper ratio to offset the copper, should be discussed with your physician.

- Many fruits are allowed on SCD, but watch for fruits that are very high in sugar because these can cause hyperactivity. Many fruits are also high in phenol and oxalate content that can cause problems in many children.

- If the child seems to have chronic digestive issues, accompanied by pain and discomfort, it is worth trying this diet for a short period of time, along with GFCF diet.

- Try Epsom salt baths. Fill the bathtub with lukewarm water waist deep, then add 1 cup of salts and soak for 20 minutes. Adjust the amount of salts based on your child's tolerance. For example, use 1/2 cup if sensitive, or 2 cups if tolerated.

- Remember that well-formed stools are a good indicator of a healthy gut. Look for changes in stool color. Pale stool color indicates lack of bile salts; fetid odors can indicate changes in gut pathogens.

- For some ASD individuals, the SCD Diet has worked well when other diets have not effected marked improvements.

NOTES:

Notes:

CHAPTER SIX

Other Diet Options

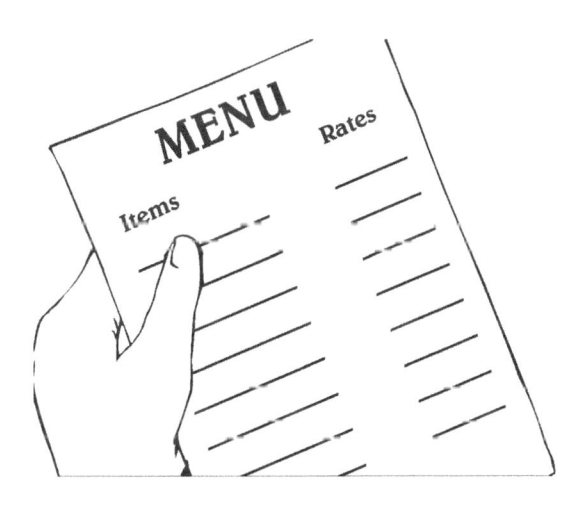

The following are additional diet options that are known to have health benefits. They are not designed to be implemented alone, but when used in conjunction with any of the four major diets discussed in earlier chapters, they can help your child.

The Raw Food Diet

The Raw Food Diet is based on unprocessed and uncooked plant foods, including fresh fruits and vegetables, sprouts, seeds, nuts, grains, beans, dried fruit, and seaweed. This diet enlists the principle of enzymes, which are live and easily digested.

Sprouting Grains, Nuts and Seeds: Soaking and sprouting are used often in raw food preparation. It has been seen that heating food above 116 degrees F° destroys enzymes that can assist in the digestion and absorption of nutrients. Cooking is also believed to diminish the nutritional value and "life force" of food.

Benefits of eating sprouted food in the diet: Sprouting increases vitamin B contents in food, especially B2, B5 and B6. Sprouting neutralizes phytic acid, a substance present in the bran of grains that inhibits the absorption of calcium, magnesium, copper and zinc. Sprouted grains should be a regular feature of the diet. They can be used in salads, sandwiches, vegetable dishes, breakfast cereals, and in breads and baked goods.

Raw Food Diet and Children with ASD: The Raw Food Diet should be incorporated with other diets. For children with ASD, a raw foods diet alone can be difficult, since digestion of raw foods is difficult for a compromised digestive system. Sprouting and soaking increase the nutrient and digestive properties of food. A raw food should be incorporated in at least one meal, no matter which special diet is being considered for ASD children.

Health Benefits of Raw Food Diet

- Balance pH of body
- Heals the gut
- Removes yeast
- When used in conjunction with other diets, allergenic reactions to food reduced with time
- Provides enzymes, which improves digestion
- Detoxification process promoted
- Better energy level
- Higher nutrient value of food

Food Rotation Diet

The Food Rotation diet proves beneficial when a person has food allergies. It has been observed that if a person has multiple food allergies, one of the best ways to help himself is to rotate foods, or eat a rotation diet.

A Rotation Diet is a system of

- Controlling food allergies by eating similar foods on the same day and then waiting four days before eating them again. Such a diet can help those with food allergies in several ways.

- Rotating diets may help prevent the development of allergies to new foods. Any food, if eaten repetitively, can cause food allergies in allergy-prone individuals or people with "leaky guts."

- A rotation diet helps you identify sensitivities to foods that your child may have, and which you may not have suspected were problems.

Food Rotation proves beneficial in children who have allergic or sensitivity reactions to food. For example, if a wheat allergy is suspected, the chid may be fed rice as an alternative. After some time, however, a rice allergy can occur. A rotation diet helps in this situation. Food is rotated regularly so that individuals can have varieties of foods without developing new allergies. This increases the food choices for children, whose choices are limited due to allergies in the first place.

Health Benefits of Food Rotation Diet

- Allows one to eat foods to which they have borderline allergic tendencies.

- Allows having a variety of foods, which is good for both mental and physical health.

- Proves beneficial with allergenic or sensitizing foods that cannot be avoided because the child's diet is limited.

- Allows the eating of a food to which an individual has allergic reactions, if eaten on rotation basis, once per week, or every four days.

Food Elimination Diet

This is the short-term testing diet that will involve eliminating problematic foods for two weeks. Then, one food at a time is re-introduced in small servings. In a food journal, reaction to food which could be troublesome should be recorded. If a problem is identified the offending food is eliminated. A new food is introduced every three days.

This diet should be considered if the following symptoms are seen in children: diarrhea, constipation, hyperactivity, lethargy, aches and pains, depression, irritability, aggression, restlessness, speech-delay, tantrums and obsessive-compulsive problems.

A food journal is the key in this diet. Parents need to learn to identify the signs of their children's food sensitivities. There is a pattern in their reactions to the problem foods, including inappropriate laughter, hyperactivity and skin rashes. Other behavioral and physical signs may be specific to your child. Parents need to have dedicated time to complete the journal process. It may take a month or more.

Health Benefits of the Food Elimination Diet

- This is sometimes the first cleaning-up process before following any specific diet.
- Helps to identify food sensitivities in children, even before testing.
- Problem foods could have further devastating effects on an already compromised digestive system. This provides relief.
- Simply through an elimination process, children may be able to handle other foods more easily.

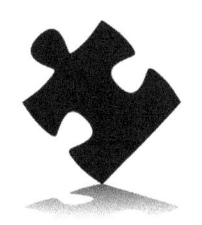

Chapter Seven

Special Diets: Food List and Resources

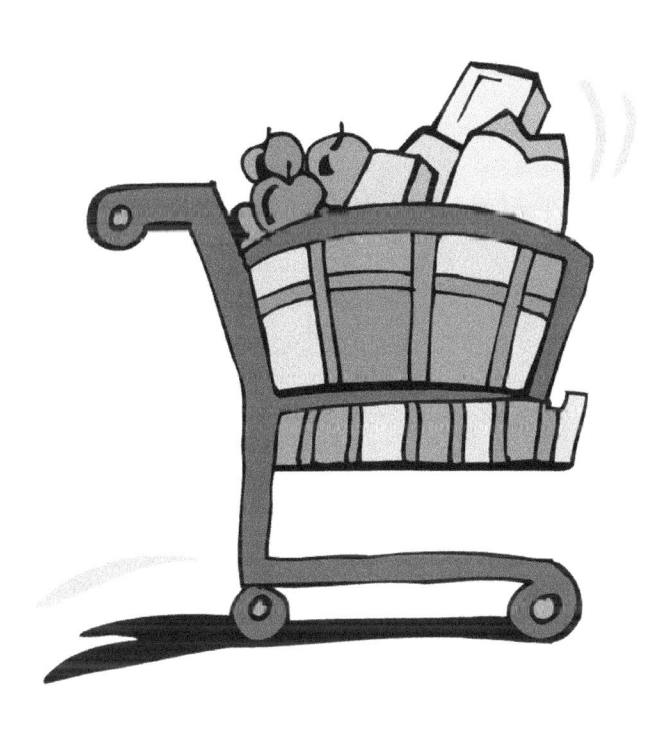

This chapter is a reference for parents who want to implement a particular diet for their children. Efforts have been made to create a comprehensive list. Website resources have been included for parents who want some additional information.

Gluten-Free & Casein-Free (GFCF Diet) Food List

	Foods to Avoid	Choices to Make (Healthy Alternatives)
Gluten	Wheat Oats Rye Spelt Kamut Barley Bulgar Candy (sugar) Crackers (wheat) Snacks (wheat) Cream soups Malt sweeteners Salty dressings and dips	Amaranth Millet Quinoa Rice (brown and white) Buckwheat (kasha) Gluten-free breads Gluten-free pastas Corn (alternate, not totally healthy choice) Gluten-free baking flours (garbanzo, rice, buckwheat, millet, amaranth, lentils, nut flours) Gluten-free ice cream/cones
Casein	Cow's milk and products Cheese having cow's milk Yogurt Ice creams Cottage cheese Cream cheese Cream, sour cream Whipped cream Butter and margarines Lactose-treated milk Buttermilk Condensed powder Evaporated milk Acidophilus dairy milk and yogurt	Rice milk Almond milk Hazelnut milk Hemp seed milk Potato milk Coconut milk Rice milk ice cream Homemade nut milk Hemp seed protein shakes Casein-free ice creams

Gluten Free and Casein Free Resources/Shopping List

Web-based Wholesale and Retail Distributors for Dietary Interventions

Ener-G Foods – This is one of the foremost producers of foods for diet-restricted individuals. They provide a wide range of ready-made foods and mixes that are wholesome, nutritious, delicious, and risk free. They have healthy food alternatives for people on special diets. www.ener-g.com.

Kinnikinnick Foods – This Canadian Company has many baked gluten-free and casein-free items. It is one the oldest companies, with a wide range of product options for people with dietary restrictions. www.kinnikinnick.com.

Bob's Red Mill – Natural Foods produces more than 400 products, including a full line of certified gluten free and organic products. With a wide variety of whole grain products, from flours and hot cereals to baking mixes and grains, Bob's Red Mill has "whole grain foods for every meal of the day." www.bobsredmill.com/home.php.

The Really Great Food Company – Offers baking mixes for people with special dietary needs, including gluten-free, wheat-free, soy-free, dairy-free and casein-free baking mixes. www.reallygreatfoods.com.

Glutino & Gluten Free Pantry – This manufacturer and distributor specializes in gluten-free products. They offer frozen foods, baking mixes, many snacks alternatives, cookies and breads. This company is dedicated to being gluten free, but be careful to read if products contain casein and corn. www.glutino.com.

Ian's All Natural Foods – Offers allergen-free (Wheat Free/GF Recipe) specialty food products designed for kids with special dietary needs. These nutritious and tasty products are made without wheat, gluten, casein, milk, eggs or nuts. They have gluten free chicken nuggets, chicken patties, chicken fingers, Mac & Cheese, Mac & Meat Sticks, French Bread sticks and Chocolate Chip Cookies – all things children really enjoy. www.iansnaturalfoods.com/index.html.

Food for Life – They have a wide selection of wheat-free, gluten-free and yeast-free bread loaves. www.foodforlife.com/index.html.

Enjoy Life Foods – They carry a variety of allergy-friendly and gluten-free foods, including a selection of cookies, granolas, snack bars, bagels, trail mixes, chocolate chips, and chocolate bars. www.enjoylifefoods.com/index.php.

Foods by George – These foods can be found in the frozen foods section of health food and grocery stores. They have a good selection of foods that are wheat and gluten free, soy free, corn free, lactose, dairy and casein-free. www.foodsbygeorge.com.

Tinkyada – Offers good tasting stone-ground, gourmet class, whole grain rice pastas. Pasta made by this company comes in all forms, including spaghetti, spirals, penne, shells, grand shells and elbows. They contain no wheat, gluten, corn, egg, soy, dairy, casein, meat, nuts or peanuts in them. http://tinkyada.com.

Dairy Substitutes & Sources

There are quite a few healthy alternatives to cow's milk. Most of these products are fortified with calcium and vitamin D, but supplementation may still be in order since children with ASD usually need higher dosages, and also may have absorption issues. The products listed below are GF/CF unless noted, but ingredients are subject to change, so please read the labels and check the ingredients. Always read labels carefully. Call the manufacturer if you have any doubts or need further information.

Vance DariFree: Vance's™ DariFree™ milk substitute is great for drinking, pouring on cereal, cooking, and baking. DariFree™ is made from specially processed potatoes, and qualifies as a non-allergenic milk alternative. It contains as much calcium as milk and is a source of other nutrients. Since DariFree™ is FREE of gluten, casein, protein, soy, tofu, rice, cholesterol, lactose, preservatives, MSG, and mono-diglycerides, it can be enjoyed by most people who have special dietary needs. Phone: (1-800-497-4834). Available from www.VancesFoods.com.

Better Than Milk: This tofu beverage is both gluten and casein free. It tastes quite good, and can be used in breads and other recipes that need "dry milk." Its options include Soy Original and Chocolate and, Rice Original. The products may be ordered on the Amazon website at www.amazon.com.

Eden Blend: This drink is easily found in grocery and health food stores. It contains water, brown rice, soybeans, kombu (seaweed), carageenan, sea salt and carbonate. The Eden's Rice milk is sweetened with rice syrup that uses barley enzyme for processing. It offers Eden Organic Rice & Soy Beverage, Unsweetened Eden Organic Soy Milk. Phone (1-800-248-0320). (Store locator on website or purchase online at www.EdenFoods.com,

Pacific Ultra: This soy beverage has no gluten hidden in the rice syrup used as sweetener. It contains Lactobacillus acidophilus and L.bifidus. The products are available at local health food and whole foods stores.

Pacific Natural Foods: It has alternative milk choices such as organic hazelnut, rice, almond, soy varieties. Available from www.PacificFoods.com.

Hempseed Milk: The most nutritious of all alternative milk.

Silk® Soymilk: Available in grocery stores and Starbucks nationwide, this comes in a variety of soymilk flavors. More information at www.silksoymilk.com.

Tree of Life: It offers Harmony Farms Non-Dairy Beverage, Soy Original Enriched, Soy Vanilla Enriched, Soy Original Non-Enriched, Soy Original Vanilla Non-Enriched, Rice Original Enriched, Rice Vanilla Enriched, Rice Original Non-Enriched and Rice Vanilla Non-Enriched. Phone 1-800-260-2424. See store locator at www.TreeofLife.com.

Blue Diamond Growers: They offer creamy, smooth texture and hint-of almond taste to make a delicious non-dairy beverage, Almond Breeze. It comes in Original, Vanilla and Chocolate flavors. A store locator will be found at www.BlueDiamondGrowers.com.

Grainaissance, Inc. Shakes: Grainaissance has been dedicated to making great-tasting, nutritious products from brown rice. Their products include Vanilla Gorilla Amazake Rice Shake, Amazake The Amazing Shake, Almond Shake, Oh So Original Rice Drink, Amazing Mango Rice Drink, Banana Appeal Rice Drink, Go Hazelnuts Rice Drink and Chocolate Almond Rice Drink Store locator on website at www.GrainAissance.com.

Thai Kitchen: Makes Thai Premium Pure Coconut Milk. Store locator at www.ThaiKitchen.com.

WestSoy Plus: This drink is flavorful, and although the color is on the yellow instead of white, it looks appetizing. It is thick and delicious. The beverage is also available in fat free, no fat and lite-fat versions. If soy is tolerated it is a very healthy drink. You can buy this product online at www.Westsoy.biz.

So Delicious: Unsweetened coconut milk available in the dairy case in a half gallon carton.

Low Oxalate Diet Food List

There are some healthful foods that are high in oxalates, such as some fruits, vegetables, seeds and nuts. This diet can be challenging to implement at first, but still is worth trying due to the benefits reported by parents. This diet should be implemented for a limited time.

Foods to Avoid: The foods listed in the table below are too high in oxalates.

Oxalate Contents Food List
Foods (Over 10 mg = 1/8 tsp)

Fruits (Over 10 mg)	Legumes, Nuts and Seeds	Grains	Sweets	Condiments	Vegetables	Beverages
Blackberries	Beans, green, waxed, dried	Bread, whole wheat	Fig Newton	Cinnamon, ground	Beetroots	Fruit Juice (4oz)
Blueberries	Peanuts	Cheerios (1 cup)	Fruitcake (1 slice)	Pepper (over 1 tsp/day)	Celery	Cranberry Grape
Concord Grapes	Pecans	Graham crackers	Marmalade	Ginger (over 1 tbl /day)	Collards	Orange Tomato
Red Currants	Peanut butter	Graham flour		Soy sauce	Dandelion greens	Chocolate Milk
Figs (dried, raw)	Sesame seeds	Corn Grits		Parsley, raw	Eggplant	Coffee Brewed
Gooseberries	Soybean curd (tofu)	Kamut		Turmeric	Escarole	Berry Juices
Kiwi	Soya proteins	Oatmeal			Green beans	Ovaltine
Lemon peel	Sunflower seeds	Popcorn (4 cups)			Kale	Tea
Lime peel	Walnuts	Soybean crackers			Leeks	Hot cocoa
Orange peel	Cashews	Spelt			Okra	Instant coffee
Raspberries, red and black	Almonds	Stone ground flour			Parsley	
Rhubarb		Wheat bran			Parsnips	
Star fruit		Wheat germ			Peppers, green	
		Whole wheat flour			Pokeweed	
		Yellow Dock			Popcorn	
					Potatoes	
					Potatoes, sweet	
					Rhubarb	
					Rutabagas	
					Sorrel	
					Spinach	
					Turnip greens	

Phenol-Free Diet Food List

Phenols are chemicals found in basically all foods we eat. It is virtually impossible to avoid phenols completely. To achieve the benefits of this diet, the foods to be avoided are those which have high to very high phenol contents. Refer the food list below. *– Also high in amines*

Fruit	Vegetables	Nuts and Snacks	Sweets	Herbs, Spices and Condiments	Drinks	Fats and Oils
Apple, Granny Smith and Jonathan Avocado* Grapefruit Kiwi fruit* Lychee Mandarin* Mulberries Nectarine Passion fruit* Peach Pomegranate Watermelon Apricot Blackberries Blackcurrants Blueberries Boysenberries Cherries Cranberries Currants, dried Date* Grapes* Guava Loganberries Orange Pineapple Plum Prune Raisins, dried Raspberries Redcurrants Rock melon Strawberries Sultana, dried Tangelo Tangerine Youngberries	Alfalfa sprouts Artichokes Broad beans Chili Cucumbers Eggplant* Radish Tomato* Water chestnuts Watercress Zucchini Green Bell Peppers Chicory Endive Gherkin Hot pepper Olives* Radish Tomato products*	Almond Muesli bars Savory flavored chips and snacks	Fruit flavors Honey Honey flavors Jam (except pear) Liquorices Mint-flavored sweets Peppermints	Allspice Bay leaf Caraway Cardamom Cinnamon Cloves Coriander Cumin Ginger Mixed herbs Mustard Nutmeg Oregano Pepper Pimiento Rosemary Tarragon Turmeric Vinegars (e.g., cider, red, and white wine) Aniseed Cayenne Commercial Gravies & sauces Curry Dill Fish Meat Tomato paste*	All tea types Fruit juice, other than pear juice Cordials Fruit-flavored drinks	Coconut oil Olive oil (they are moderate to high)l

Specific Carbohydrate Diet Food List
Foods "Legal" and "Illegal"

Food	Legal/Illegal	Note
Agar-agar	Illegal	Agar Agar is a vegetarian gelatin substitute produced from a variety of seaweed vegetation.
Agave syrup	Illegal	Agave syrup — sometimes called agave nectar — is a natural sweetener that is marketed as a healthy alternative to processed sugars, as well as an alternative to honey, corn syrup and similar liquid sweeteners.
Algae	Illegal	We do not use algae (Spirulina) because IBD involves the immune system and algae can aggravate an already disturbed immune system.
Allspice	Legal	As long as you're just using Allspice as a cooking spice, it's legal.
Almond butter	Legal	Almond butter with no sugar added is allowed.
Almond milk	Legal	May be tried after being on the diet for 6 months.
Almond oil	Legal	Almond oil is extracted from the kernels of dried almonds.
Almonds	Legal	Nuts sold in mixtures are not allowed, as most are roasted with a starch coating. Nuts should only be used as nut flour, in recipes, until diarrhea has subsided.
Aloe Vera	Illegal	It contains mucilaginous polysaccharides, and also increases the release of tumor necrosis factor which is associated with IBD inflammation and increased immune stimulation.
Amaranth flour	Illegal	Amaranth is a grain substitute, contains starches, and so is not allowed.
Anchovies	Legal	Anchovies are small silvery fishes, native to the Mediterranean, and have been used as a food fish for centuries.
Apple Cider	Legal	It is brown and not clear as apple juice is. It should be just straight pressed apple. It is usually pasteurized in order to kill bacteria. Cider should be diluted with water before drinking.

Food	Legal/Illegal	Note
Apple juice	Illegal	Apple juice usually has sugar added during processing, but cider is allowed (see above listing).
Apples	Legal	Most of the apple's fiber is contained in its skin, as is the majority of its quercitin. Apples are a good source of dietary fiber and vitamin C.
Apricots	Legal	An apricot is a small sweet fruit with a golden orange color. A ripe apricot can be recognized by its fairly firm skin, and it will be plump and juicy when it is at its best.
Arrowroot	Illegal	It is a mucilaginous herb. Mucilaginous herbs are loaded with starch. This starch is food for the pathogens that the SCD Diet is designed to starve out.
Artichokes (French)	Legal	They are the green artichokes that you steam, then dip the leaves in lemon butter and scrape off with your teeth. They have edible hearts and an inedible choke.
Artichokes (Jerusalem)	Illegal	They are actually a tuber, and are not legal.
Ascorbic acid	Legal	Should be nothing but vitamin C.
Asiago cheese	Legal	May be used occasionally. Asiago is a traditional farmhouse and creamery unpasteurized hard cheese. Originally made of ewe's milk, now is made with cow's milk only. There are types of Asiago: first one (mistakenly taken for Pressato) is a lightly pressed cheese made from whole milk matured for 20-30 days. The other (Asiago d'Allevo) is the mature cheese made with skimmed milk. Long and slow maturation process creates fruity, slightly sharp cheese with a compact, granular interior full of small holes. Matured over two years, becomes intensely flavored. Can be grated and used as a condiment.
Asparagus	Legal	Fresh or frozen is allowed. Canned vegetables are not allowed.
Aspartame	Legal	When symptom free, one aspartame-sweetened soft drink per week is allowed.
Aspartic acid	Legal	Aspartic acid is a non-essential amino acid and is found in abundance in plant proteins, especially in sprouting seeds, but can be manufactured in the body.
Astragalus	Illegal	They contain polysaccharides and so are illegal.

Food	Legal/Illegal	Note
Avocados	Legal	Avocados are high in the "good fat" (monounsaturated) making them a heart-healthy food that lowers cholesterol and reduces the risk of heart disease. These monounsaturated fats also help keep the receptors in your brain sensitive to serotonin, which helps with mood. Additionally, avocados are high in vitamins (particularly vitamin E) and other nutrients that help to maintain good health.
Avocado oil	Legal	Good for mayonnaise and salad dressings but might not withstand heat very well
Bacon	Legal	Smoked bacon that has been fried very crispy is allowed once per week. Look for sugar-free bacons which are also low in sodium.
Baker's yeast	Illegal	A commercial preparation consisting of dried cells of one or more strains of the fungus Saccharomyces cerevisiae, used as a leavening in baking.
Baking powder	Illegal	Baking powder contains sodium bicarbonate, but it includes the acidifying agent already (cream of tartar), and also a drying agent (usually starch).
Baking soda	Legal	Baking soda is pure sodium bicarbonate.
Balsamic vinegar	Illegal	It's not that balsamic vinegar is illegal, it's that what you can get in the store isn't really balsamic vinegar and most have sugar added to them.
Bananas	Legal	They must be ripe with black spots on the skin.
Bark tea	Illegal	Bark tea (Pau d'Arco) contains steroidal saponins and is both an immune booster and a laxative.
Barley	Illegal	Barley is a wonderfully versatile cereal grain with a rich nut like flavor and an appealing chewy, pasta-like consistency.
Bay leaf	Legal	Bay leaf is often included as a pickling spice. Best used in soups, sauces, stews, daubes and courts-bouillons; an appropriate seasoning for fish, meat and poultry.
Basil	Legal	Basil also complements vegetables such as eggplant, zucchini, squash and spinach. When added within the last half an hour of cooking, basil enhances the flavor of vegetable and legume (split peas, lentil) soups. Most salads, especially those with tomato, benefit greatly from the addition of fresh basil.

Food	Legal/Illegal	Note
Bean flour	Illegal	Bean flour made from beans or lentils, soaked prior to grinding, have more nutritional value and health benefits.
Bean sprouts	Illegal	Bean sprouts are the tender edible shoots of germinated beans. Most people think of mung bean sprouts when bean sprouts are mentioned, but a wide assortment of seeds, nuts, grains, and beans can be sprouted.
Bee pollen	Illegal	Pollen is irritating to a damaged gut. Clear, pure, pasteurized honey is okay. Cloudy honey (still containing the pollen) should be avoided.
Beef	Legal	Fresh and frozen are allowed as long as nothing has been added during processing; check the labels carefully.
Beer	Illegal	Beer is the world's oldest and most widely consumed alcoholic beverage and the third most popular drink overall, after water and tea. It is produced by the brewing and fermentation of starches, mainly derived from cereal grains — the most common of which is malted barley, although wheat, maize (corn), and rice are widely used.
Beets	Legal	Beets are frequently consumed either pickled or in borscht. These colorful root vegetables contain powerful nutrient compounds that help protect against many health conditions.
Berries	Legal	Berries of all kinds are legal.
Black beans	Legal	May be tried when symptom free. Dried legumes must be prepared according to the instructions in the book, (*Refer to our section on lentils, legumes and seeds in Chapter 2.*)
Black eye beans	Illegal	Black-eyed beans have a smooth texture and pea-like flavor and are good when mixed with other vegetables. They are low in fat, and when combined with grains, beans supply high quality protein which provides a healthy alternative to meat or other animal protein.
Black radish	Legal	It is very fibrous, so go slowly and be careful.
Blue cheese	Legal	May be used occasionally. *Note:* Use with caution with Casein Allergy/Intolerance.
Bok choy	Legal	Bok choy is much like cabbage and is legal but you should not use a member of the cabbage family until you are well on your way to getting better. In other words, do not use if you still have diarrhea and gas.

Food	Legal/Illegal	Note
Bologna	Illegal	Bologna is often accused of being composed of "mystery meat," but it is actually made from either beef, pork, or a combination of both meats. Some higher-end bologna products may contain more exotic meats such as veal, goat or even moose. Meat used in the production of bologna is generally ground to a fine paste before processing, then extruded into a natural or artificial casing.
Bouillon cubes	Illegal	Bouillon cubes and instant soup bases are not permitted.
Brandy	Illegal	Brandy is a spirit produced by distilling wine, the wine having first been produced by fermenting grapes. Brandy generally contains 36 to 60 percent alcohol by volume.
Brazil nuts	Legal	Nuts sold in mixtures are not allowed, as most are roasted with a starch coating.
Brick cheese	Legal	May be used freely on SCD diet. Brick cheese is a semi-hard, cow's milk cheese originating in Wisconsin. The cheese has a number of small and irregular holes and an open texture. The flavor is a mixture of sweet, spicy and nutty. As it ripens, it becomes almost as strong as limburger. The name brick cheese is said to have come from the fact that bricks were once used to weight the curd and press out the whey.
Brie cheese	Legal	On SCD diet can be used occasionally. Brie is a creamy cow's milk cheese from France which is well known around the world. Sometimes called the "Queen of Cheeses," Brie is a delicious dessert cheese, usually served at room temperature or even slightly warmed. It has a distinctive rich, creamy flavor which is deliciously mild and complements fruit, high quality bread, and anything else the cheese can be smeared onto.
Broccoli	Legal	Broccoli is a member of the cabbage family, and is closely related to cauliflower. Its Italian name means "cabbage sprout." Broccoli provides a range of tastes and textures, from soft and flowery (the floret) to fibrous and crunchy (the stem and stalk).
Brussels sprouts	Legal	Brussels sprouts look like perfect miniature versions of cabbage since they are closely related; both belong to the Brassica family of vegetables. Brussels sprouts are rich in many valuable nutrients.

Food	Legal/Illegal	Note
Buckwheat	Illegal	People think that buckwheat is a cereal grain; it is actually a fruit seed that is related to rhubarb and sorrel, making it a suitable substitute for grains for people who are sensitive to wheat or other grains that contain protein glutens.
Bulgur	Illegal	Bulgur is a quick-cooking form of whole wheat that has been cleaned, parboiled, dried, ground into particles and sifted into distinct sizes. Often confused with cracked wheat, bulgur differs in that it has been pre-cooked. Bulgur holds a place in recipes similar to rice or cous cous but with a higher nutritional value. Best known as an ingredient in tabouli salad, bulgur is also a tasty, low-fat ingredient in pilaf, soup, bakery goods, stuffing or casseroles. It is an ideal food in a vegetarian diet because of its nutritional value and versatility. It is excellent as a meat extender or meat substitute in vegetarian dishes.
Burdock root	Illegal	Burdock is a root that is found in Europe in Asia. It contains inulin (FOS) Fructo-Oligo-Saccharide and mucilage.
Butter	Legal	*Caution:* Children who are casein-intolerant or allergic can not handle butter well.
Butter beans	Illegal	Butter beans, sometimes called lima beans, are a seed, and are considered a vegetable. They are of the genus and species Phaseolus lunatus, and have two main varieties. The first variety is a large slightly curved flat green bean that those in the Southern US would refer to as lima beans or the lima type. A second type of P. lunatus has smaller seeds and is often called the sieva type. When Southern U.S. cuisine mentions butter beans, they are referring to the smaller sieva seed.
Buttermilk	Illegal	Cultured buttermilk is probably the easiest and most fool proof fermented milk product to make nothing more than the tart liquid left after the butter is churned. Buttermilk is low in fat. It's sometimes tolerated by people with lactose intolerance since some of the lactose is fermented by bacteria. The acidity of buttermilk also explains its long refrigerator shelf life.
Cabbage	Legal	You should not use a member of the cabbage family until you are well on your way to getting better. In other words, do not use if you still have diarrhea and gas.

Food	Legal/ Illegal	Note
Camembert cheese	Legal	May be used occasionally. Camembert cheese is made with cow's milk curdled and inoculated with bacteria. The curds are packed into cheese molds, yielding a crumbly cheese which softens as it ripens, eventually forming a cheese with a velvety white rind and a slowly oozing center. As a general rule, Camembert cheese should be served at room temperature or warm, as this brings out the buttery, slightly salty flavor of the cheese. The gooey nature of the cheese makes it very easy to spread, as well.
Cannellini beans	Illegal	Cannellini beans are large and have that traditional kidney shape. With a slightly nutty taste and mild earthiness, they have a relatively thin skin and tender, creamy flesh. They hold their shape well and are one of the best white beans for salads and ragouts.
Canned fish	Legal	Canned in oil or water is acceptable, but check the labels carefully. Do not buy products containing "broth." Usually the low sodium varieties do not contain "broth."
Canned fruits	Legal	Fruits canned in their own juice are allowed.
Canned vegetables	Illegal	There are no canned vegetables permitted; they must either be fresh or frozen.
Canola oil	Legal	**Legal, but not recommended.**
Cantaloupe	Legal	Cantaloupe with its refreshingly rich flavor and aroma and minimal number of calories is the most popular variety of melon. Cantaloupes are also referred to as a netted melon because they have a ribless rind with a distinctive netted skin.
Capers	Legal	Capers are sometimes confused with the brined and dried fish called anchovies since both are harvested from the same regions and are processed similarly. Capers are actually immature buds plucked from a small bush. They have been a part of Mediterranean cuisine for thousands of years. In fact, capers were often used as informal currency among merchants traveling ancient trade routes. Capers became favorite additions to fish sauces and marinades, along with brined and dried anchovies.

Food	Legal/Illegal	Note
Carob	Illegal	Carob chips are an edible product, similar to chocolate chips, made from carob. They are used in baking and in trail mixes, often serving as a substitute for chocolate chips. The color is the same as that of dark chocolate, although the taste is markedly different, with slightly nutty and bitter overtones. Their appearance is nearly identical to a regular chocolate chip. They are made using carob powder, which has the same look, color and texture as baking cocoa.
Carrageenan	Illegal	Carrageenan is seaweed and high in polysaccharides, therefore illegal.
Carrots	Legal	Easy to pack and perfect as crudités for that favorite dip, the crunchy texture and sweet taste of carrots is popular among both adults and children. The carrot has a thick, fleshy, deeply colored root, which grows underground, and feathery green leaves that emerge above ground.
Cashews	Legal	Nuts sold in mixtures are not allowed, as most are roasted with a starch coating.
Cauliflower	Legal	Cauliflower is sometimes hard to digest and should be tried cautiously after some progress has been made on the diet.
Celeriac/celery root	Legal	Introduce slowly in diet, it is very fibrous, even when it is steamed or mashed.
Celery	Legal	Celery's crunchy texture and distinctive flavor makes it a popular addition to salads and many cooked dishes.
Cellulose (in supplements)	Legal	Cellulose in your supplements is okay and virtually impossible to avoid.
Cellulose gum	Illegal	The gum structure is because of the carbohydrates structure in it that forms a latticework to give its sticky-like, glue-like consistency. It has proven to be hard to digest and problem arises when it moves down to the lower small intestine and colon and certain type of microorganism thrives on just that very disaccharide.
Cereals	Illegal	Cereal comes from grains, in natural form (as in whole grain,) and they are a rich source of vitamins, minerals, carbohydrates, fats, oils and protein. However, when refined by the removal of the bran and germ, the remaining endocarp is mostly carbohydrate and lacks the majority of the other nutrients.

Food	Legal/Illegal	Note
Chard	Legal	Chard (red, green, rainbow and Swiss). Chard is similar to spinach/celery so it is legal. It is also a bit like cabbage, so use with caution if gas is still a problem.
Cheddar cheese	Legal	May be used freely on SCD diet. Cheddar cheese is a semi-hard cow's milk cheese which can vary in taste from mild to extra sharp. Many consumers associate the color orange with cheddar cheese, due to a long tradition of adding dyes to the cheese to change the color. In fact, cheddar cheese is naturally a creamy to pale white, although orange cheese has become much more common. Cheddar cheese also has a wide range of flavors, depending on how it is made and how long it is aged.
Cherimoya	Legal	Cherimoya is a compound fruit that is conical or somewhat heart-shaped. The skin, thin or thick, may be smooth with fingerprint-like markings or covered with conical or rounded protuberances. The sweet, juicy, white flesh is melting, and very fragrant. The fruit is of a primitive form with spirally arranged carpals, resembling a raspberry. Also known as custard apple or sharifa.
Cherries	Legal	Loaded with vitamins, minerals and other essential nutrients, cherries are more than a sweet snack — they're a powerful, bite-size health booster.
Chestnut flour	Illegal	The chestnut is referred to as Un-Nut because its characteristics are really not like a nut at all. A "real" nut has 45 to 55 percent fat content. Chestnut flour is closer to 1 percent fat. A "real" nut is low in carbohydrates. Chestnut flour is about 78 percent carbohydrate. It is a wonderful alternative to those who are sensitive to or allergic to wheat, and because it is gluten free, it's perfect for those with Celiac Disease.
Chestnuts	Legal	May be tried when symptom free. However, if you buy dried chestnuts, soak them and cook them until soft.
Chevre	Illegal	Chevre is a generic term which denotes a cheese made from the milk of goats.
Chickory root	Illegal	Chickory root is not legal and cannot be used instead of coffee beans because it contains large amount of fructooligosaccharides.

CHAPTER 7: SPECIAL DIET: FOOD LIST AND RESOURCES

Food	Legal/Illegal	Note
Chick peas	Illegal	Chick peas are perhaps better known by the name garbanzo beans. They are roundish, beige to light green. Chick peas can be ground and used as flour, called gram flour. Chick peas are considered a starchy carbohydrate, and are a great staple for people with diabetes. They do not elevate glucose when consumed, thus they rate well on the glycemic index.
Chlorella	Illegal	It is blue-green algae similar to spirulina.
Chocolate	Illegal	Chocolate has become one of the most popular flavors in the world. It is a common ingredient in many snacks and desserts, including cookies, cake, ice cream, pudding, pie and candy. It's sugar content is also a concern.
Cilantro	Legal	An herb with wide delicate lacy green leaves and a pungent flavor. The seed of the cilantro plant is known as coriander. Although cilantro and coriander come from the same plant, their flavors are very different and cannot be substituted for each other.
Cinnamon	Legal	Cinnamon is spice commonly used in cakes and other baked goods, milk and rice puddings, chocolate dishes and fruit desserts, particularly apples and pears.
Citric Acid	Legal	Citric acid is used as a flavoring in many formulations of vitamin C. Citric acid as an additive is okay.
Club soda	Legal	Club soda may be identical to plain carbonated water or it may contain a small amount of table salt, sodium citrate, sodium bicarbonate, potassium bicarbonate, potassium citrate, potassium sulfate, or disodium phosphate, depending on the bottler.
Cocoa powder	Illegal	Cocoa powder is made when chocolate liquor is pressed to remove three quarters of its cocoa butter. The remaining cocoa solids are processed to make fine unsweetened cocoa powder.
Coconut	Legal	Fresh or unsweetened, shredded coconut and coconut flour are all legal.
Coconut milk	Legal	May be tried after being on the diet for 6 months.
Coconut oil	Legal	Withstands heat well, good for frying/cooking,

Food	Legal/Illegal	Note
Coffee	Legal	Coffee should be made very weak. Instant coffee is not allowed.
Coffee (instant)	Illegal	Coffee is a brewed beverage prepared from roasted seeds, commonly called coffee beans, of the coffee plant. Due to its caffeine content, coffee has a stimulating effect in humans.
Collard greens	Legal	Of the cabbage family; introduce late in the diet.
Colby cheese	Legal	Colby cheese is a semi-hard cow's milk cheese. May be used freely.
Cordials	Illegal	Liqueurs (also known as Cordials) are sweet, flavor-infused spirits that are categorized according to the flavoring agent (i.e., fruits, nuts, herbal and spice blends, creams and such).
Corn	Illegal	Corn is hard to digest for children with food sensitivity. It is used for food and animal feed, or is processed to make food and food ingredients (such as high fructose corn syrup (HFCS), corn starch and lysine supplements).
Corn oil	Legal	Corn oil, which is extracted from corn germ, has high polyunsaturated fatty acid content and oxidative stability. Its largest single use is in bottled oil for consumer use, followed by margarine and industrial snack-frying operations.
Corn syrup/HFCS High Fructose Corn Syrup	Illegal	Corn syrup is a sweetener made by processing corn starch with enzymes or acid to create a dextrose solution. High fructose corn syrup (HFCS) is further processed to increase its sweetness. Since HFCS is more stable and cheaper to produce than ordinary sugar, it has largely replaced sugar in processed foods and soft drinks.
Cornstarch	Illegal	Corn starch is just what it sounds like: starch derived from corn. It is ground from the white endosperm at the heart of a kernel of corn. It is used as a thickening agent in cooking.
Cranberry juice	Legal	Knudsen's Cranberry Juice does not have sugar added, so this is an option to consider. Juice should be diluted with water before drinking, in the ratio of 2:1 (juice: water).
Cream	Illegal	It is illegal because it contains lactose. Cream can be added to milk and then fermented to make SCD 24-hour yogurt as the lactose will be used up in the fermentation. Cream has less lactose than milk and the more fat it contains the less lactose it has.

Food	Legal/Illegal	Note
Cottage cheese	Illegal	Cottage cheese is a loosely packed cow's milk cheese distinguished by its slightly bland taste and the whey which is left in with the cheese curds. The cheese is designed to be eaten fresh, and is highly perishable.
Cream of Tartar	Illegal	Cream of tartar is the common name for potassium hydrogen tartrate and is essentially an acidic salt. Cream of tartar is found in some baking powder, and is often used to help stabilize egg whites, or to produce creamy frostings and candy.
Cream cheese	Illegal	Cream cheese is made from a combination of cream and milk, and is not matured or hardened, as are other cheeses. It becomes slightly firmer by the introduction of lactic acid.
Croscarmellose sodium	Illegal	Croscarmellose sodium is a very commonly used FDA-approved pharmaceutical additive. Its purpose in most tablets, including dietary supplements, is to assist the tablet in disintegrating in the intestinal tract at the required location.
Cucumbers	Legal	A healthy snack children like a lot.
Custard apple	Legal	Also known as sharifa or cherimoya.
Date sugar	Illegal	May be tried after being on the diet for quite some time and being symptom free, but it is not recommended.
Dates	Legal	Medjool and California dates are allowed. They must be loose and not have anything added.
Decaf products	Illegal	Decaffeinated products are not legal since the manufacturing process may introduce questionable ingredients or reactions.
Dextrose (contained in commercial products)	Illegal	The problem with the dextrose and fructose being sold in granulated form, as well as the dextrose contained in commercial products, is that it is not pure dextrose, which should be the same as the single sugar, glucose, found in fruits and honey.
Dried milk solids	Illegal	Powdered milk is a manufactured dairy product made by evaporating milk to dryness. One purpose of drying milk is to preserve it; milk powder has a far longer shelf life than liquid milk and does not need to be refrigerated, due to its low moisture content.

Food	Legal/Illegal	Note
Durum Flour	Illegal	It's a type of wheat grain flour.
Echinacea	Legal	Especially if it is in alcohol, but even it is in pill form with a bit of lactose. It can be very helpful in cold or flu.
Edam cheese	Legal	It is a Dutch cheese. May be used occasionally.
Eggplant	Legal	Eggplants belong to the nightshade family of vegetables, which also includes tomatoes, sweet peppers, and potatoes. They grow in a manner much like tomatoes, hanging from the vines of a plant that grows several feet in height. While the different varieties do range slightly in taste and texture, one can generally describe the eggplant as having a pleasantly bitter taste and spongy texture.
Eggs	Legal	Use organic free range organic eggs. Eggs from hens raised on pasture are far more nutritious than eggs from confined hens in factory farms.
Ethanol	Legal	Ethanol is alcohol (the kind in gin, etc.).
Evaporated cane juice	Illegal	Fancy name for sugar.
Ezekiel 4:9® bread	Illegal	Sprouted grain breads are illegal.
Fava beans	Illegal	Fava beans are one of the oldest plants under cultivation. They have a distinct flavor and creamy texture that makes them a great addition to a wide variety of dishes.
Fenugreek	Illegal	Dried seeds should be lightly roasted before using (don't overdo it though, or they will become bitter). After roasting, they are easily ground. A small amount will complement many other spices, but too much can be overpowering.
Feta Cheese	Illegal	Feta may be used after about 6 months of improvement, but used only in small amounts. Feta is a Greek cheese traditionally made from the milk of goats, although feta from the milk of cows and sheep is also available.
Filberts (hazelnuts)	Legal	Nuts sold in mixtures are not allowed, as most are roasted with a starch coating. Nuts should only be used as nut flour, in recipes, until diarrhea has subsided.
Figs	Legal	Figs unpolluted by chemicals or additives are legal. Use caution with dried form as it has tiny hard seeds which can be hard on the intestines.

Food	Legal/Illegal	Note
Fish	Legal	Fresh and frozen are allowed as long as nothing has been added during processing; check the labels carefully.
Flax seed oil	Legal	The oil itself, in very small amounts, may be helpful. It is not to be heated.
Flax seed	Illegal	Has lignin which is found when the whole seed (and its stiff coat) are ground up. It may be harmful for people just starting out on SCD. Also, some bacteria feast nicely on lignin, which is tough, like bark.
Flour	Illegal	Flours come from organic grains of wheat, oats and rye, from seeds like amaranth, sorghum and quinoa, and nuts like cashew, pistachio and almond. They flours from grains are all illegal; however, flours from nuts and seeds are acceptable.
FOS	Illegal	Also known as fructooligosaccharides. As the use of Inulin/FOS as an additive in the food industry has increased, the reports of allergic responses have also increased. They remain indigestible, and typical side effects depend on individual level of tolerance. The list of known side effects includes flatulence, bloating, cramps, abdominal pain, and diarrhea.
Fowl	Legal	All types including turkey, chicken, duck, goose, pheasant, pigeon, etc.
Frozen orange juice (concentrate) and fresh	Illegal	If orange juice is just frozen and has no additives, then it is legal; however, frozen orange juice is normally concentrated before freezing and the process used to concentrate it makes it illegal.
Fructose (granulated)	Illegal	Granulated fructose (or even liquid) that is sold as "fructose" has a mixture of other trisaccharides, etc. in it. It is extracted from corn. Purity is an issue.
Fruits (canned)	Legal	Fruits canned in their own juice are allowed.
Garbanzo beans	Illegal	This is another name for chick peas.
Garfava flour	Illegal	Made from two types of beans, Garbanzo beans and Fava beans; neither are SCD legal.

Food	Legal/Illegal	Note
Garlic	Legal	Use fresh garlic; garlic powders have starch added as anti-caking agents. You may also make your own garlic powder from fresh garlic by dehydrating it and grinding it.
Guar gum	Illegal	Guar gum can best be described as a natural food thickener, similar to locust bean gum, cornstarch or tapioca flour. Guar gum is said to have significantly more thickening power than cornstarch.
Gelatin (unflavored)	Legal	It is a denatured protein that has lost its tertiary structure, although it is not the best protein.
Ghee	Legal	This is clarified butter.
Ginger	Legal	Ginger is a spice whose leaves, seeds, or other plant parts are used for flavoring food or as a condiment.
Gjetost cheese	Illegal	Gjetost is made from the whey or buttermilk which is heated very slowly until the water has evaporated and the milk sugar forms a kind of brown caramelized paste. At this stage, milk or cream may be added to change the fat content of the product.
Glucose candy	Illegal	Contains granulated glucose.
Glycerin/Glycerol	Legal	Since glycerin is not a sugar to begin with, the "ol" at the end does not make it a sugar alcohol (see below). Glycerin is considered to belong to the fat family. So is glycerol.
Goatein	Illegal	It is a Protein powders that contains Bifidobacteria Bifidum. Protein powders are a bad idea in any case as they're generally oxidized cholesterol; i.e., damaged by heat.
Gorgonzola cheese	Legal	May be used occasionally. A pasteurized cow's milk cheese that is ivory-colored with blue-green veins running through it.
Gouda cheese	Legal	May be used occasionally. Made from cow's milk. Can be made from part-skim or whole milk, and can be aged from a few weeks to over a year.
Granulated glucose	Illegal	It is known to contain other sugars in addition to glucose.
Grape juice	Legal	White or dark grape juice is allowed. We use Welch's bottled grape juice, as it has been checked out and does not have sugar added. Avoid frozen grape juice, it usually has sugar added. Juice should be diluted with water before drinking.

Food	Legal/Illegal	Note
Grapefruit	Legal	Tart and tangy with an underlying sweetness, grapefruit has a juiciness that rivals that of the ever popular orange and sparkles with many of the same health promoting benefits.
Grapefruit juice	Legal	Fresh is allowed, with no added sugars.
Grapes	Legal	The combination of crunchy texture and dry, sweet, tart flavor has made grapes an ever popular between-meal snack as well as a refreshing addition to both fruit and vegetable salads. It is a very sweet fruit, so it should be used with caution.
Grape seed oil	Legal	Grape seed oil is extracted from the seeds of grapes, typically wine grapes.
Green tea	Legal	Limited to 2 cups per day.
Gruyere cheese	Legal	Gruyere is in the family of Swiss cheeses, a group of semi-firm pale cheeses stippled with small holes or air pockets.
Gums	Illegal	All gums are illegal.
Haricot beans	Legal	These are legal and are the same as navy beans.
Havarti cheese	Legal	May be used freely. Havarti is a creamy semi-firm Danish cheese, named after the farm where it was developed at the turn of the twentieth century. It is a mild cheese, similar somewhat to Tilsit or Gouda in flavor, and is peppered with small holes and irregularities.
Hazelnuts (filberts)	Legal	Nuts sold in mixtures are not allowed, as most are roasted with a starch coating. Nuts should only be used as nut flour, in recipes, until diarrhea has subsided.
Hemp seed, hemp protein powder	Illegal	Hemp plants are cultivated for industrial use and harvested for their fibers, seeds, oils, and meal. Industrial hemp seeds are available in different forms. They can be sterilized, toasted, roasted, or cracked. Hemp can be pressed into oil or hulled into meal.
Honey	Legal	Honey is one of the oldest sweeteners known to man, and it has been extensively consumed and written about historically. Early observers noted that the flavors of honey were influenced by the area in which the honey collected and the season, and early apiarists placed their beehives in strategic locations to improve the quality of their honey.

Food	Legal/Illegal	Note
Horseradish sauce	Legal	If homemade; if manufactured, use only if you know they have no added illegal ingredients. Sometimes served with salmon fillets, steak or even grilled vegetables, creamed horseradish sauce is a great alternative to other condiments.
Hot dogs	Illegal	Commercially produced hotdogs will normally be illegal but a recipe for SCD-legal hot dogs will be found at www.scdiet.net/scdfood.htm
Ice cream	Illegal	Commercially prepared ice cream is not allowed. However, there are many wonderful recipes for homemade ice cream. Refer to our recipe in the desserts chapter.
Inulin	Illegal	Inulin is a FOS (*see descriptive listing above*) and is illegal.
Iron supplements	Illegal	Do not get vitamins with iron; they encourage all kinds of infections especially in the gut, and iron has had much research done on it for other diseases. No oral iron. Just eat the liver pate and if you like liver, eat it once a week.
Isoglucose	Illegal	It is a new sweetener likely to be used in many products in future. It comes from crops which are high in a fructose-type-starch such as inulin, fructooligosaccharides.
Jalapenos	Legal	A favorite among cooks for their spicy flavor, jalapenos are very easily seeded for use in recipes. When smoked and dried, jalapenos are known as chipotles.
Jicama	Illegal	Jicama is actually a legume. It is a crispy, sweet, edible root that resembles a turnip in physical appearance.
Juice from concentrate	Illegal	Juice from concentrate is normally illegal because when it is reconstituted they often add other things (like sugar). Often additives are not listed on the label.
Kale	Legal	Kale is an archaic type of cabbage that grows loosely furled leaves, rather than forming a head. The leaves of kale have a distinctive ruffly appearance that distinguishes the plant from a close relative, collard greens. Kale tends to be a little bit bitter in flavor, although this bitterness is tempered by washing, cooking, and using younger leaves. Kale is also extraordinarily nutritionally rich, even among the leafy green vegetables.
Kefir	Illegal	Kefir is a yeast fermentation which produces alcohol. So the yogurt made from Kefir grains will have a good deal of alcohol. It is a healthy food, but use with caution, and not until child is well.

Food	Legal/Illegal	Note
Ketchup	Illegal	Commercially prepared ketchup contains sugar and is not allowed. Refer to our condiments recipes section for a homemade ketchup recipe.
Kidney beans	Legal	All types may be tried when symptom free. Dried legumes must be prepared according to the instructions in this book and confirmed in the book, Breaking the Vicious Cycle.
Kimchi	Legal	It is pickled, fermented vegetables, usually cucumbers, cabbage, etc. Legal so long as it is not thickened with starch-like thickeners and sweetened with additional sweetener.
Kiwi fruit	Legal	A kiwi, sometimes marketed as a kiwi fruit or Chinese gooseberry, is brownish-green in color.
Kohlrabi	Illegal	It is a cross between the cabbage family and the turnip family. It is one of those foods that should not be tried until well into the diet and doing well. Then it should be introduced slowly.
Kudzu (or kuzu)	Illegal	It is a mucilaginous herb. Mucilaginous herbs are loaded with starch. This starch is food for the pathogens that the SCD is designed to starve out.
Kumquats	Legal	A kumquat is a fruit which resembles a miniature orange. It is sometimes mistaken for a citrus fruit. It is often candied or used to make preserves and jelly.
Lactaid milk	Illegal	Lactaid milk is the same as lactose hydrolyzed milk. The rate of flow of galactose to the liver when one drinks lactose hydrolyzed milk is high. With lactose hydrolyzed milk, you are ingesting the two sugars, glucose and galactose, at the same time.
Lactose hydrolyzed milk	Illegal	Same as Lactaid Milk (see above).
Lamb	Legal	Fresh and frozen are allowed as long as nothing has been added during processing; check the labels carefully.
Leek	Legal	Leeks are root vegetables that look quite similar to onions, to which they are related. Their flavor is onion-like but much milder. Leeks are a great source of fiber in your diet, and may actually help lower cholesterol. They're also packed with important vitamins and minerals.
Lecithin	Legal	Derived from soy (illegal). There is plenty of good lecithin in egg yolks.

Food	Legal/ Illegal	Note
Lemons	Legal	Lemons are oval in shape and feature a yellow, texturized outer peel. Like other citrus fruits, their inner flesh is encased in eight to ten segments.
Lentils	Legal	These are dried legumes. Refer to "Beans, Lentils and Legumes Guide" in Chapter two for preparation instructions.
Lettuce	Legal	All varieties of lettuce are legal.
Licorice	Illegal	A spice whose leaves, seeds, or other plant parts are used for flavoring food or as a condiment. Licorice is both a demulcent and a laxative.
Lignin	Illegal	Lignin is a complex organic polymer found in the tissues of plants. Digestion of lignin is difficult, and undigested lignin particles can become food for certain microorganisms.
Lima beans	Legal	Dried or fresh are permitted. Dried legumes must be prepared according to the instructions. Refer to "Beans, Lentils and Legumes Guide" in *Chapter 2* for preparation instructions.
Limburger cheese	Legal	May be used occasionally. Limburger cheese is a shockingly odorous cheese which originated in Belgium. Limburger's distinct odor is partly due to the fact that it is a washed rind cheese.
Limes	Legal	The word "lime" is used to refer to a large group of green citrus fruits with a tart, intense flavor.
Liqueurs	Illegal	Liqueurs (also known as Cordials) are sweet, flavor infused spirits that are categorized according to the flavoring agent (i.e., fruits, nuts, herbal and spice blends, creams and such).
Macadamia nuts	Legal	Macadamia nuts are rich, flavorful nuts. The nuts may be eaten out of hand, roasted, or ground into nut butter. Many people pair macadamia nuts with white chocolate in confections, and they can also be found in nut mixes and other desserts.
Macadamia oil	Legal	This is heat-stable oil.
Magnesium citrate	Legal	Legal as a supplement ingredient.
Magnesium stearate	Legal	Legal as a supplement ingredient.

Food	Legal/Illegal	Note
Maltitol, Maltisorb, & Maltisweet	Illegal	Like sorbitol, mannitol, and xylitol, these are all sugar alcohols and are not SCD legal. They fall under the category of indigestible carbs and sugars, which allows companies to label things "sugar free," even though they are providing nutrition to the bacteria that live in your digestive tract.
Maltodextrin	Illegal	Maltodextrin is the worst of the small molecules of sugars. It is a very short chain of glucose molecules (derived from starch). The chances of digestion are practically nil. It therefore will feed bacteria because of its particular structure.
Manchego cheese	Legal	Manchego is made by heating milk with rennet and special cultures so that the milk curdles. The milk curds which are formed are subsequently pressed to remove whey, and then brined to encourage the cheese to form a hard rind.
Mangoes	Legal	Mangoes contain some of the same oils as do poison oak and poison ivy, and some people can have an allergic reaction to the oils on both the fruit skin and the leaves of the tree. In any case, the skin is not edible and is quite hard even when the fruit is ripe.
Maple syrup	Illegal	Maple syrup is a disaccharide and a viscous sweetener derived from maple tree sap. Many people use it in baking in place of sugar or other sweeteners; some use it in tea instead of honey, and it is frequently used as a topping for pancakes, waffles, and other breakfast foods.
Margarine types	Illegal	Margarine is produced using a combination of different vegetable oils. Some brands tend to use soybean oil, while others favor corn oil. As part of the preparation process, the oil undergoes hydrogenation. The drawback is that the process of hydrogenation converts some of the unsaturated fats in the oils to saturated fats.
Marshmallow	Illegal	It is a mucilaginous herb. Mucilaginous herbs are loaded with starch. This starch is food for the pathogens.
Mastic gum	Illegal	Mastic is a sticky substance exuded from the branches and trunk of the mastic tree.
Mead	Legal	If homemade and ingredients are honey and yeast, commercial is likely to have sugar added and is illegal.

Food	Legal/Illegal	Note
Meats	Legal	All fresh or frozen meats with no additives or processing are legal, including beef, lamb, pork, liver, kidney, oxtail and tongue.
Meats (canned)	Illegal	Canned meats are illegal.
Meats (processed)	Illegal	Most have additives such as starch, lactose and sugar; e.g., hot dogs, turkey loaf, sliced ham, bologna, and smoked meats.
Melatonin	Illegal	Melatonin is a natural hormone that is made by the pineal gland. Supplements for melatonin are readily available for people who would like to get back to a normal sleeping pattern the natural way.
Melon	Legal	All types are legal.
Milk	Illegal	Fluid milk of any kind is not permitted.
Millet	Illegal	Millet is a collective term for a variety of grasses that produce small, rounded seeds that are harvested for food.
Miso	Illegal	Miso is a paste made from a mixture of soybeans, a starch such as rice or barley, salt, a touch of water, and yeast.
Molasses	Illegal	Molasses is a thick, brown to deep black, honey-like substance made when cane or beet sugar is processed.
Monterey Jack cheese	Legal	May be used occasionally. Monterey Jack cheese is a cheese made from cow's milk, semi-firm with a creamy, mild flavor and a high moisture content.
Mozzarella cheese	Illegal	Mozzarella is made by heating milk with rennet to form curds. The curds are separated from the whey and then cut to encourage additional drainage before being allowed to sit.
MSG	Illegal	Regardless of whether it is SCD legal or not, try to avoid it. MSG can be a potent neurotoxin.
Muenster cheese	Legal	May be used occasionally. Muenster cheese is a smooth textured cheese with an orange rind and a white interior. This washed-rind cheese is made from cows' milk. The orange color is derived from vegetable coloring. It usually has a very mild flavor and smooth, soft texture.
Mung beans	Illegal	Mung beans are illegal on SCD diet. It is a nutritious food to incorporate in the diet if you are not on SCD. Refer to "Beans, Lentils and Legumes Guide" in Chapter 2 for preparation instructions.

Food	Legal/Illegal	Note
Mushrooms	Legal	Mushrooms are the fruit formed from underground fungi, many of which are edible.
Mustard (plain)	Legal	Mustard is legal as long as it doesn't contain illegal ingredients; read the labels carefully.
Natural flavors	Illegal	"Natural flavoring" can be used to refer to anything, including the chemicals coming from big "flavor" companies which sell chemicals to food processors.
Navy beans	Legal	Dried legumes must be prepared according to the instructions. Please refer to our beans, lentils and legumes guide in *Chapter 2*.
Nectarines	Legal	Nectarines are similar to peaches.
Nettles	Illegal	Adverse effects from consuming nettle tea can range from upset stomach to burning sensations in the skin, difficulty in urination, and bloating.
Neufchatel cheese	Illegal	Neufchatel cheese is snow-white, soft, and very spreadable, with a hint of crumble. As the cheese ripens, it becomes more pungent, develops a soft rind, and turns more crumbly.
Noni juice	Illegal	Noni juice is made from the fruit of the Morinda citrifolia, or noni tree. Noni juice is a supplement and not medicinal, therefore no dosage is associated with it. It is suggested that drinking noni juice on an empty stomach might be the best way to gain maximum benefits.
Nutmeg	Legal	Nutmeg is usually associated with sweet, spicy dishes — pies, puddings, custards, cookies and spice cakes. It combines well with many cheeses, and is included in soufflés and cheese sauces. In soups it works with tomatoes, split pea, chicken or black beans. It complements egg dishes and vegetables like cabbage, spinach, broccoli, beans, onions and eggplant.
Oats	Illegal	Oats are among the many annual grasses that produce grains consumed by humans.
Okra	Illegal	No okra (also called bhindi or drumsticks). Because they are a mucilaginous food, they are illegal.
Olive oil	Legal	Olive oil withstands heat well, is good for frying and is highly recommended.

Food	Legal/Illegal	Note
Olives	Legal	Olives are legal as long as they do not contain illegal ingredients; read the labels carefully.
Onions	Legal	Use fresh onions. Onion powders have starch added as anti-caking agents. You may also make your own onion powder from fresh onions by dehydrating them and grinding them yourself.
Orange juice	Legal	Fresh orange juice that does not have sugar added is allowed. While diarrhea is active, avoid having orange juice in the morning. We recommend Tropicana's Original Orange Juice, because it does not have sugar added.
Oranges	Legal	Juicy and sweet and renowned for its concentration of vitamin C, oranges make the perfect snack and add a special tang to many recipes; it is one of the most popular fruits in the world.
Oregano	Legal	An herb is a plant whose leaves, seeds, or flowers are used for flavoring food or in medicine. It's a main seasoning herb in Italish recipes. Other uses of herbs include cosmetics, dyes, and perfumes.
Pappadum	Illegal	An Indian snack made from lentils, they're like a chip. Also contains rice flour.
Papayas	Legal	When fully ripe, the papaya has a yellowish to orange skin that is somewhat hard and not edible. Unripe papayas may be used in some recipes, but generally are not consumed.
Paprika	Legal	Paprika is often used as a garnish, sprinkled on eggs, hors d'ouvres and salads for color. It spices and colors cheeses and cheese spreads, and is used in marinades and smoked foods. It can be incorporated in the flour dusting for chicken and other meats.
Parmesan cheese	Legal	May be used occasionally. Parmesan cheese is traditionally made by mixing whole morning milk with skimmed milk from the previous evening. The milk is heated and mixed with rennet to form curds, which are pressed in a cheese mold.

Food	Legal/Illegal	Note
Parsley	Legal	Fresh or dried parsley may be used in omelets, scrambled eggs, mashed potatoes, soups, pasta and vegetable dishes and in sauces to go with fish, poultry, veal and pork. It is included with garlic and butter for making garlic bread or simply garnishing a juicy, sizzling barbecued steak. Parsley is a key ingredient, along with mint in the healthy and nutritious Middle Eastern salad, tabouleh.
Passion fruit	Legal	Passion fruit by itself tends to taste tart. It is usually used with other types of fruit in recipes to lighten its tangy taste. Passion fruit, as well as its flower, is known for its aromatic scent. Because of its sweet smelling fragrance, it is sometimes added to food simply to enhance its aroma.
Parsnips	Legal/Illegal	Some children do well with them, others do not.
Pea flour	Illegal	No pea protein concentrate, no legume concentrate. This is very bad. It falls into the same category as bean flour. The type of starch in these legumes is uncertain. This is so because there are hundreds of different cultivars (species) due to breeding techniques.
Peaches	Legal	Peaches are tender, flavorful fruits that are popular on their own, and also in things like pies, preserves, and fruit salad.
Peanut butter	Legal	Natural peanut butter with no sugar added is allowed.
Peanut Oil	Legal	Peanut oil, which may be called groundnut oil. It is made from the legumes called peanuts, and it is known for its high smoke point.
Peanuts	Legal	Peanuts in the shell may be tried cautiously after 6 months on the diet if diarrhea is gone. Shelled peanuts are illegal. Nuts sold in mixtures are not allowed, as most are roasted with a starch coating.
Pears	Legal	Pears are juicy and sweet, with a soft, buttery yet some what grainy texture. Depending upon the variety, their paper-thin skins can either be yellow, green, brown, red or a combination of two or more of these colors.
Peas	Legal	A pea (sometimes inaccurately called a sweet pea) is small spherical seed. Although treated as a vegetable in cooking, it is botanically a fruit.

Food	Legal/Illegal	Note
Pecans	Legal	Nuts sold in mixtures are not allowed, as most are roasted with a starch coating. Nuts should only be used as nut flour, in recipes, until diarrhea has subsided.
Pectin	Illegal	It is a polysaccharide which gels in the presence of acid and sugar. It is used as a thickener in jams, and occurs naturally in some fruit, like apples. In apples, it is mostly in the peel. For someone beginning the diet, you normally would not get too much from eating an apple, because you would peel it. Pectin as an added ingredient is not legal, because it is a complex sugar.
Peppermint tea	Legal	Some brands add natural flavorings which would make them illegal, so check the ingredients carefully.
Peppers	Legal	Green, yellow, and red peppers are permitted. Also jalapeno peppers, habanera peppers, chili peppers, poblano peppers, relleno peppers, etc. are legal.
Persimmons	Legal	Persimmons are red to orange fruit grown on trees.
Pickles (dill)	Legal	Dill pickles are legal as long as they do not contain illegal ingredients; read the labels carefully.
Pine nuts	Legal	They are very hard to digest. Grinding them for pesto does not make them any easier on your gut. May be tried in small amounts after symptoms have subsided.
Pineapple	Legal	A pineapple is a tropical fruit with a sweet, slightly acidic flavor and very juicy flesh. Many people enjoy eating pineapple straight, or blending it with fruit in fruit salads. This fruit is rich in vitamin C, making it a great addition to the diet.
Pineapple juice	Legal	Fresh pineapple juice that does not have sugar added is allowed. We use Dole's unsweetened pineapple juice in the can, as it has been checked out and does not have sugar added. Juice should be diluted with water before drinking, in the ratio 1:1 (juice:water).
Pinto beans	Illegal	Even after soaking, the starch in pinto beans is hard for children to digest.
Pistachio nuts	Legal	They are legal, but avoid pink-dyed and salted ones.
Phosphatidylcholine	Legal	Another name for lecithin which is legal. Egg is a good source of phosphatidylcholine. If child is allergic to eggs, it can be taken in supplements form.

Food	Legal/Illegal	Note
Plantains	Illegal	Plantains are similar to their sweeter banana cousins, but they are much starchier in consistency and more bland in taste. Plantains grow in the same tropical regions as bananas, but they are not used for the same culinary purposes.
Plums	Legal	Plums are fleshy, smooth skinned stone fruits which have been cultivated for thousands of years. These flavorful, juicy fruits can be used in a wide range of dishes, from delicate fruit pastries to fruit salads.
Pomegranate concentrate	Illegal	Pomegranate is about the size of an orange, with a yellowish shell that turns a rich red color as it matures. Depending on the variety, pomegranate juice can be extremely sour or pleasantly tart with a degree of sweetness.
Pork	Legal	Fresh and frozen pork is allowed as long as nothing has been added during processing; check the labels carefully.
Pork Rinds	Legal	Use the plain pork rinds with no added flavorings and check the label carefully to make sure they don't contain illegal ingredients.
Port wine	Illegal	It is full of sugar.
Postum	Illegal	Postum was a coffee substitute manufactured by Kraft Foods. It was discontinued in 2007. Do not use any of the replica recipes for Postum that you may find on the Web.
Potatoes	Illegal	Both white and sweet potatoes are illegal.
Poultry	Legal	Fresh and frozen are allowed as long as nothing has been added during processing; check the labels carefully.
Primost cheese	Illegal	A Scandinavian cheese made from cow's milk with a soft spreadable texture providing a semi-sweet taste. The sweetness is derived by caramelizing the milk sugars of the whey as it is made. Also known as Mysost cheese, this cheese is very similar to Gjetost cheese, except that Gjetost is made from a combination of goat and cow's milk or strictly goat's milk.
Protein powder	Illegal	Protein powders are made from four basic sources: whey (from milk), egg, soy and rice. They are illegal on diet, due to starches.

Food	Legal/Illegal	Note
Provolone cheese	Legal	An all-purpose semi-hard Italian cheese with a firm texture and a mild, smoky flavor. The thin, hard rind is golden-yellow and shiny. Italian-style provolone can be made with buffalo or cow's milk, or a mixture of the two. Sometimes it's lightly smoked.
Prunes	Legal	Prunes are a dried type of plum, very sweet and moist. They are usually black to brown in color and replete with wrinkles.
Psyllium husks	Illegal	They are loaded with cellulose and lignin that support bacterial growth. The cellulose in vegetables and fruit is handled well, but concentrated form such as husks is a problem.
Pumpkin	Legal	Fresh pumpkin is legal, canned pumpkin is not allowed. Butternut squash may be used as a substitute for pumpkin in baking.
Pumpkin (canned)	Illegal	Canned pumpkin is illegal. Butternut squash may be substituted for pumpkin in baking.
Quinoa	Illegal	Since Quinoa is 60 percent starch, it is illegal.
Quorn™	Illegal	Quorn™ is the brand name of a premium line of all-natural, meat-free frozen foods made from fungi.
Raisins	Legal	Try them cautiously.
Rhubarb	Legal	Rhubarb is a vegetable with a unique taste that makes it a favorite in many pies and dessert. Rhubarb is rich in vitamin C and dietary fiber.
Rice	Illegal	Both brown and white rice are illegal.
Rice bran oil	Illegal	Rice bran oil is natural oil that is created using the hull of the rice grain. Considered to be rich in antioxidants and several vitamins, rice bran oil is used for cooking as well as in the creation of creams and other skin care product.
Rice flour	Illegal	Both brown and white rice flour are illegal.
Ricotta cheese	Illegal	Ricotta is a type of whey cheese, a very flexible and delicious dairy product, starring in lasagna, cannoli, and many other delicious dishes which require the use of a soft, mild cheese product.

Food	Legal/Illegal	Note
Romano cheese	Legal	May be used occasionally. Romano cheese is a traditional Italian, rich creamy yellow color cheese. It has a slightly granular texture and a sharp, tangy, salty flavor, and is usually grated over other dishes, although it can be eaten plain.
Roquefort cheese	Legal	May be used occasionally. Roquefort is a type of blue cheese that is renowned throughout the world as the King of Cheeses.
Rosemary	Legal	Both the flowers and leaves of rosemary are used for garnishing and cooking. Crush or mince the spiky leaves before sprinkling over or rubbing into foods.
Rutabaga	Legal	Caution: Go slow and be careful. The rutabaga is a root vegetable which is often confused with a turnip because it resembles an oversized turnip. Rutabaga greens are typically eaten like spinach, although they are sometimes mashed together with boiled rutabaga roots.
Rye	Illegal	Rye is a hardy grain crop. The distinctive flavor of rye makes it a frequent additive to breads.
Saccharine	Legal	The main ingredient in the popular pink-packets of "Sweet N Low," saccharine is one of the more well-known sugar substitutes.
Safflower oil	Legal	Safflower oil is oil pressed from the seeds of the safflower plant, a member of the sunflower family. There are two distinct types of safflower oil, each with very different uses. Monounsaturated safflower oil, high in oleic acid, is used as heat-stable cooking oil. Polyunsaturated oil, high in linoleic acid, is used as cold oil.
Sago starch	Illegal	A starch that is extracted from the sago palm, used in baking, and as a thickener for soups and puddings. The starch is also used in making some types of noodles. Sago starch is available in Asian markets.
Sage	Legal	Sage is an herb with oblong gray-green leaves which are used in cooking and herbal medicine. The herb has a pungent, mildly astringent, and slightly bitter to peppery flavor which accents many foods including roasts, soups, savory sauces, and stuffing.

Food	Legal/Illegal	Note
Sake	Illegal	The word sake in Japanese can refer to any alcoholic beverage, but, in general, it is used in English to mean a specific type of rice alcohol, also known as nihonshu. Sake is sometimes called rice wine, but in truth it is not a wine, nor is it exactly a beer, nor a spirit. Sake is a rather unique type of fermented alcohol.
Salt	Legal	Ordinary iodized table salt sometimes contains dextrose, but is legal because it is important to get iodine. Look for iodized sea salt as a preferred choice.
Sashimi	Legal	Sashimi is raw fish sliced very thin and served with a variety of garnishes and sauces. Sashimi is always made with saltwater fish, because many freshwater fish species contain parasites which could cause intestinal distress if eaten. (Japanese sushi-style raw fish is served all by itself without rice.)
Sauerkraut	Legal	*Caution:* Go slow, introduce in later stage of the SCD diet. Sauerkraut is a fermented cabbage dish. It has a tangy, zesty flavor and is often used as a garnish, especially with meats like sausage, also is added to salads, sandwiches, and other foods.
Scotch whisky	Legal	Only have it occasionally. Scotch whisky is one of the heather-flavored ales made from barley malt that the Picts and their prehistoric ancestors brewed.
Seaweed	Illegal	Seaweed is high in polysaccharides and therefore illegal.
Seed butters	Legal/Illegal	*Caution:* The amounts would vary on individual child tolerance. A little can be a lot for some children but many others tolerate them well. The usage would depend individually.
Seed flour	Illegal	Seeds are permissible after 3 months with no symptoms. Flours are illegal as they would surpass the usage amount limits that could not be well tolerated by children with sensitive GI issues.
Seeds	Legal	Permissible after 3 months of no symptoms.
Sesame seeds	Illegal/Legal	Sesame seeds, like other edible seeds, are illegal at the beginning of the diet but may be added later with caution after a few months of initial success. You can grind your own or purchase pure sesame butter (tahini) to make your own tahini preparations.

CHAPTER 7: SPECIAL DIET: FOOD LIST AND RESOURCES

Food	Legal/Illegal	Note
Sesame oil	Legal	Sesame oil (also known as gingerly oil or til oil) is an edible vegetable oil derived from sesame seeds. Besides being used as cooking oil in South India, it is often used as a flavor enhancer in Chinese, Taiwanese and Korean dishes.
Sharifa	Legal	Also known as custard apple or cherimoya.
Shellfish	Legal	Fresh and frozen are allowed as long as nothing has been added during processing; check the labels carefully.
Sherry	Illegal	Sherry is a fortified wine. Once Sherry is fermented it is fortified with brandy. At this point, some Sherry has more yeast added and some does not. Sherry is similar in some ways to other fortified wines.
Silica	Legal	Legal as a supplement ingredient.
Silicon Dioxide	Legal	Legal as a supplement ingredient.
Slippery elm	Illegal	It is a mucilaginous herb. Mucilaginous herbs are loaded with starch. This starch is food for the pathogens so is not allowed to be consumed on SCD diet.
Smoked meats	Illegal	Smoked meats are loaded with sugar during the smoking process.
Sodium benzoate	Legal	Legal as a supplement ingredient.
Sodium starch glycinate	Illegal	Starches are illegal on diet.
Sorbitol	Illegal	Sorbitol, mannitol, and xylitol are all sugar alcohols and are not SCD legal. They fall under the category of indigestible carbs and sugars, which allows companies to label things "sugar free," even though they are providing nutrition to the bacteria that live in your digestive tract.
Sour cream	Illegal	Sour cream is a dairy product made primarily of cream. Adding bacteria derived from lactic acid makes sour cream sour. This is similar to yogurt, but yogurt tends to use other bacteria to ferment milk.
Soy	Illegal	There is increasing evidence of the detrimental effects of Soy. Soya beans have many undesirable substances, and much chemical processing is required to separate and produce other products. Even after fermentation, it's doubtful that these substances will be removed entirely. In any manufacturing process, we are reliant on what the manufacturer tells us.

Food	Legal/Illegal	Note
Soy lecithin	Legal	Derived from soy (illegal). There is plenty of good lecithin in egg yolks.
Soy sauce	Illegal	Soy sauce is a fermented soy product and also contains wheat so it is illegal.
Soybean milk	Illegal	Soy milk is a beverage made from soybeans. It was first developed in Asia, along with numerous other soy based foods such as tempeh, tofu, and soy sauce, and has since spread to the rest of the world. Many vegans and vegetarians drink soy milk in preference to cow's milk, as do people with lactose intolerance.
Soybean oil	Illegal	Soybean oil is cooking oil that is extracted from soybeans. Like other cooking oils, soybean oil can be used in such culinary tasks as frying, seasoning, and baking.
Soybeans	Illegal	Soybeans are legumes which grow throughout much of the world and constitute one of the world's major food crops. They are turned into a wide array of foods, including tofu, miso, soymilk and tempeh.
Spearmint tea	Legal	Spearmint tea isn't a tea at all, because it lacks the leaves of Camellia sinensis, the tea plant. It is more properly a tisane, a distillation of leaves, flowers, twigs, roots, or bark from sources other than the tea plant. One of the key distinctions between a tea and a tisane is that tisanes lack caffeine. However, teas and tisanes are prepared in the same way, and many people use the term "tea" to describe tisanes.
Spelt	Illegal	Spelt is a grain in the wheat family. Spelt can also be eaten by some individuals with gluten intolerance. It has a delicious and characteristic nutty taste that is unlike the milder flavor of wheat.
Spices	Legal	Spices of all kinds may be used, but avoid spice mixtures; buy spices separately.
Spinach	Legal	Spinach is a dark green leafy vegetable. Its leaves are tender, with a faintly bitter flavor. The plant is naturally rich in vitamins A and C, folate, calcium, and iron, which leads many people to regard spinach as a super food and a valuable addition to the human diet.

Food	Legal/Illegal	Note
Spirulina	Illegal	Spirulina is blue - green alga which is used as a nutritional supplement in many regions of the world. It is illegal, since in conditions like IBD which involves the immune system, Spirulina can aggravate an already disturbed immune system.
Split peas	Legal	Dried legumes must be prepared carefully. Refer to the beans, lentils and legumes guide in Chapter two.
Sprouted grain bread	Illegal	The sprouted grain bread is just too risky. Starch is stored in the seed and, under the right conditions, temperature and moisture, the starch is broken down so that the circulatory system of the plant can get glucose from the starch (even plants cannot use starch until it is broken down into monosaccharides). If the sprout is allowed to grow quite high (differs in each grain seed) and nothing is left but the coat of the seed, theoretically, the sprout would be okay biochemically. However, you still have to be sure that the bread was made ONLY with sprouts and nothing added, which is usually not the case.
Squash	Legal	Both winter and summer squashes are legal.
Stevia	Illegal	Its molecular structure resembles a steroid and the effects are unknown.
Splenda	Illegal	Splenda is the trade name of sucralose. Refer to sucralose below for more information.
Stilton cheese	Legal	May be used occasionally. Stilton cheese is a type of blue cheese. It is a popular cheese, with a flavor milder than that of other blue cheeses, and is exported all over the world for a wide variety of table uses.
String beans	Legal	They are legal and are also referred to as Green Beans.
Sucralose	Illegal	Sucralose is a zero-calorie sugar substitute artificial sweetener.
Sulphates	Legal	When a fruit such as peaches (dried) and coconut is sulphated, it means it has been exposed to sulphur to keep the color from darkening. Some people are allergic to sulphated products but most of us are not bothered by them.
Sunflower oil	Legal	Sunflower oil is a type of vegetable oil which is pressed from oil-type sunflower seeds. This oil can be used in cooking and cosmetics, and is especially popular with people who prefer healthy fats.

Food	Legal/Illegal	Note
Sweet potatoes	Illegal	Sweet potatoes are tubers, distantly related to potatoes, and native to South America. They are often confusing to consumers since many sweet potatoes are labeled as yams in the U.S. In fact, true yams, first grown in Africa, are much larger, starchier and far less sweet. Sweet potatoes, on the other hand, can be very sweet, but sweetness depends upon the variety.
Swede	Legal	Another name for rutabaga.
Swiss cheese	Legal	May be used freely. Swiss cheese or fromage Suisse has holes in it due to the fermentation process which creates the cheese. Cheese is made by introducing bacteria to milk, which begins to curdle as the bacteria eat and produce lactic acid.
Tabasco sauce	Legal/Illegal	Tabasco sauce is a brand of hot sauce made from tabasco peppers, vinegar, and salt, and aged in white oak barrels for three years. It has a hot, spicy flavor and is popular in many parts of the world. Only the original red tabasco sauce labeled McIlhenny Company Tabasco Brand Pepper Sauce is legal, but as with all manufactured products check the ingredients. The other tabasco styles all have sugars and gums added.
Tagatose	Illegal	Tagatose is a functional sweetener. It is a naturally occurring monosaccharide, specifically a hexose. It is often found in dairy products, and is very similar in texture to sucrose (table sugar) and is 92 percent as sweet, but with only 38 percent of the calories.
Tamari	Illegal	It is made from soy.
Tamarind	Illegal	Tamarind is a fruiting tree native to Africa and widely planted throughout the world. The pulp of the fruit is the main portion of tamarind used in food production.
Tangerines	Legal	A tangerine is a citrus fruit, Citrus reticulata, which is smaller and less sweet than a classic orange. Tangerines are closely related to mandarins, and the two fruits are in fact considered the same species.
Tapioca	Illegal	Tapioca is a starch which is used as a food thickener extracted from the cassava root. It is a starch, therefore illegal.

Food	Legal/Illegal	Note
Tapioca flour	Illegal	The flavor of tapioca is fairly neutral, making it an excellent choice of thickener for both sweet and savory foods. Tapioca has little nutritional value. And being starch, it is illegal.
Tarragon	Legal	Tarragon is a Eurasian herb in the Aster family. Tarragon's use is also well-known in tarragon vinegar and in béarnaise sauce, a sauce made with egg yolks, butter, vinegar, wine, and shallots and used for eggs, fish, meat, and vegetables.
Taro	Illegal	Very similar to potatoes, it has too much starch in it.
Tea	Legal	Ordinary black tea, instant tea, Ojibwa tea (Essiac), many herbal teas, teas made from bark, etc., are full of polysaccharides and are illegal. Peppermint and spearmint herb teas are legal, and you can make a tea from ginger which is also legal.
Thyme	Legal	Thyme is a culinary herb, used widely in European cuisine. It has a faintly lemony flavor which goes well with vegetables, poultry, fish, meats, stuffings, and sauces. It's available in both fresh and dried form at many markets.
Tofutti cheese	Illegal	They are soy based and also most of the products have casein. Soy being illegal makes this cheese illegal as well.
Tofu	Illegal	It is made from soy.
Tomato juice (canned)	Legal	Tomato juice is legal so long as it has only salt added.
Tomato paste (canned)	Illegal	Tomato paste is legal so long as it has only salt added.
Tomato purée (canned)	Illegal	Tomato puree is legal so long as it has only salt added.
Tomato sauce (canned)	Illegal	Tomato sauce is legal so long as it has only salt added.
Tomatoes	Legal	Fresh tomatoes are acceptable, but canned tomatoes are illegal.
Triticale	Illegal	Triticale is a hybrid of wheat (Triticum) and rye (Secale).
Turbinado	Illegal	It is liquid cane sugar, therefore it is illegal.
Turnips	Illegal	A turnip is an edible tuber with the spicy flavor of a fresh young turnip and turnip greens. Turnips are illegal as no tubers are allowed on SCD.

Food	Legal/ Illegal	Note
Vanillin	Legal	Vanillin is the chemical found in vanilla that gives it its distinct flavor and smell. It can be synthesized artificially, but it can also be extracted and purified from the vanilla bean. So vanilla bean extract already has vanillin in it.
V8 Juice	Illegal	It is also made from concentrate tomatoes and has added sugar.
Vegetables (canned)	Illegal	Canned vegetables are not permitted; they must either be fresh or frozen to be acceptable on diet.
Vegetable stearate	Legal	Stearate is a fat (stearic acid) so vegetable stearate is fat from some vegetable.
Vinegar	Legal	Red and white wine vinegars as well as white and cider vinegars are allowed, but check the label for any added illegal ingredients. Balsamic vinegar is not allowed since it has added sugar.
Vodka	Legal	Only have it occasionally. Traditionally, vodka may be made from virtually anything; vodkas can be found made from grapes, soy, beets, potatoes, and corn, In addition to the more common wheat and rye varieties.
Walnuts	Legal	Nuts sold in mixtures are not allowed, as most are roasted with a starch coating. Nuts should only be used as nut flour, in recipes, until diarrhea issues has subsided for your child (if they have any known issues).
Walnut oil	Legal	Walnut oil is oil derived from Walnuts. It is not cooking oil; high heat destroys its delicate flavor. Where it does shine is as an ingredient in a salad dressing or a fresh pasta sauce or to give a final splash over a finished dish.
Wasabi	Legal	Wasabi is a relative of the watercress family and an elusive little root. Like horseradish, it is a root, or rhizome, and it is grated or sliced for use in cooking. It is legal on diet, as long as it is in its natural state and hasn't had fillers added by a manufacturer. Read the labels carefully.

Food	Legal/Illegal	Note
Water chestnuts	Legal	They should be avoided in the beginning stages of the diet. The water chestnut is a type of aquatic plant cultivated for its edible root. In cooking they are used to add texture and flavor. They have a faintly sweet flavor which retains through cooking, along with the crunchy texture. Unlike many vegetables which soften as they are heated, water chestnuts stay firm, adding a crunchy feel to the dishes.
Watercress	Legal	Watercress, a green in the mustard family, is related to collards and kale. It is known for its peppery taste, so often used to spice up sandwiches and added to salads, where it is usually combined with some vegetable or greens having a milder flavor or with citrus fruit. It can also be wilted and served as a green, used to season dumplings or savory mousse, or served as an ingredient in soups ranging from Chinese watercress soup to cold cream of watercress soup to potato, leek, or watercress soup.
Watermelon	Legal	Watermelon is almost 92 percent water. It is most often enjoyed as served in slices but it can also be added to smoothies, fruit salads, or even grilled in round slices called watermelon steak.
Wheat	Illegal	Wheat is a type of grass grown all over the world for its highly nutritious and useful grain. It is one of the top three most produced crops in the world, along with corn and rice. It is high in starch so it is illegal in diet.
Wheat germ	Illegal	Wheat germ is a part of the wheat kernel. It contains 23 nutrients, and has more nutrients per ounce than any other vegetable or grain. Wheat germ is very high in protein. It contains around 28 percent protein and has more protein than can be found in most meat products.
Winc	Legal	Very dry wine is legal. Wine is an alcoholic beverage often made of fermented grape juice. The natural chemical balance of grapes is such that they can ferment without the addition of sugars, acids, enzymes or other nutrients.
Xanthan Gum	Illegal	Xanthan gum is a polysaccharide used as a food additive and rheology modifier. It is produced by fermentation of glucose or sucrose by the Xanthomonas campestris bacterium. It is also used as a substitute for wheat gluten in gluten-free breads, pastas and other flour-based food products.

Food	Legal/Illegal	Note
Xylitol	Illegal	Sorbitol, mannitol, and xylitol are all sugar alcohols and are not SCD legal. They fall under the category of indigestible carbs and sugars, which allows companies to label things "sugar free," even though they are providing nutrition to the bacteria that live in your digestive tract.
Yams	Illegal	Yams are sprawling tropical vines with edible tubers. Being tubers, they have starch content so are considered illegal.
Yogurt (commercial)	Illegal	Eating commercial yogurt is not permitted. Commercial yogurt may be used as a starter for making homemade yogurt.
Yogurt (homemade)	Legal	Homemade SCD compliant yogurt is permissible. (Refer to our recipe in *Chapter 9*.)
Yucca Root	Illegal	Yucca (also known as manioc or cassava), is a white, starchy tropical vegetable. It is a dietary staple usually eaten boiled, steamed, and in flour form as thickeners or additional ingredients for noodles, cakes, and pastries.
Zucchini	Legal	Zucchini is a type of summer squash, also known as Courgette.

Notes:

CHAPTER EIGHT

Aspects of Oral Motor Development

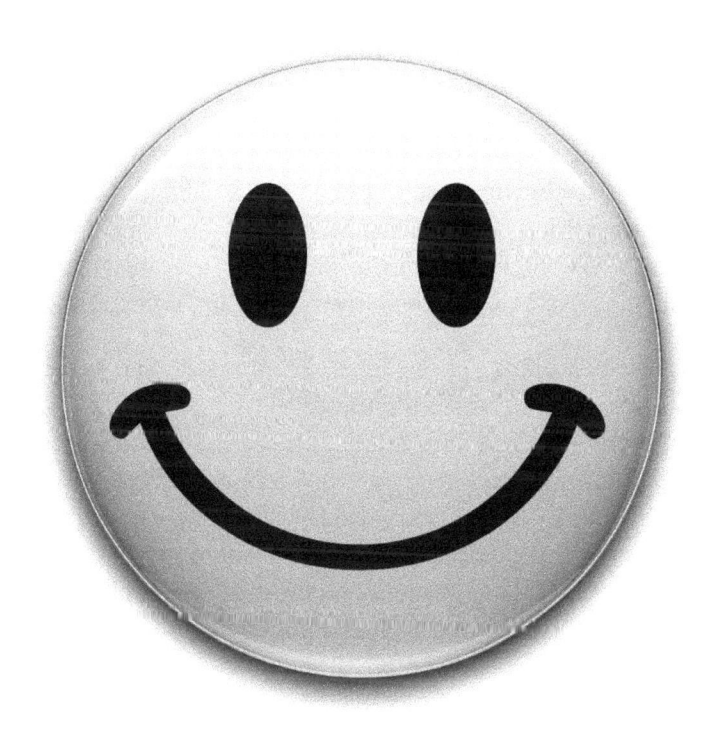

FEEDING PROBLEMS ARE COMMON IN CHILDREN with ASD so that overall nutrition can be compromised by the child's preference for certain foods and unwillingness to try new foods. Many parents complain that their child has a limited diet, and prefers crunchy foods such as pretzels or crackers that are offered as a snack food. Often these become the main food source. It is common to reject meats, foods with lumps, and most fruits and vegetables. This type of child will usually have difficulty imitating words and phrases, and will produce a limited variety of speech sounds. They are likely to reject tactile input, such as brushing their teeth. These problems must be addressed first, through oral motor therapy, so that accepting new foods can be a part of the treatment program. Introducing more nutritious foods can follow.

The brains of many children with ASD are unable to process sensory input, causing them to receive too much or too little. The child who receives too much input will become overloaded. Too little sensory information may cause a child to crave more. This is seen in all sensory systems, including the oral cavity.

In typical development, oral-motor skills, feeding skills, and speech/language skills all develop together and build on each other. The child uses the same muscles for eating as he does for speaking. Therefore, a meal or snack as part of an oral-motor program can assist in increasing oral stability, mobility, and awareness, not to mention the benefits of how the introduction of new and different textured foods can improve overall health and nutrition.

Many children enjoy chewing crunchy solids because they provide stimulation, and facilitate improved chewing skills and jaw stability. Foods such as pretzels, carrots sticks, apples, chips, toast, crunchy cereals and rice cakes are common favorite snack foods. With this in mind, a parent or therapist can use a healthier choice of food, such as carrot sticks over pretzels, in achieving better health options.

Citrus foods, such as orange slices, lemons, lemonade and juice or fruit bars are foods that encourage sucking and thus improve tongue and lip control. The cold temperature of the juice or fruit bars tends to increase oral stimulation, awareness, and sucking movements. Thickened juices, such as nectars or shakes (see our "power shake" formulas in *Chapter 11*), as well as lollipops, can also facilitate sucking. Health food stores can offer choices of naturally sweetened fruit bars or casein-free ice cream bars, and naturally sweetened lollipops can replace sugary and less healthy ones to help the child's oral motor abilities while still maintaining a child's healthy diet. Whole orange is allowed on all the diets, while only fresh orange juice that does not have sugar added is allowed on the SCD Diet. While diarrhea is active, avoid having orange juice in the morning. We use Tropicana's Original Orange Juice, because it does not have sugar added.

Children with oral hypo-sensitivity, or insufficient sensory input, may tend to crave foods that increase oral awareness, such as spicy foods or foods with a strong taste. Examples of such foods are dips such as salsa and ketchup, pickles, sour candies and lemons. Healthy versions of dips would include organic and naturally sweetened ketchup with organic chopped pickles, Vegenaise Grapeseed Oil (a healthy alternative to mayonnaise. Refer to our Casein Free Resource List).

Foods that are challenging for children who have difficulty chewing, sucking, transferring food or swallowing are whole nuts, popcorn, small pieces of cereal, and foods that stick to the roof of the mouth, such as peanut butter on soft white bread. A healthy alternative would be to use gluten-free bread, toasted, spread with a seed cream or nut butter with added healthy essential oils (such as BodyBio Balance Oil), and cut up into small bite-size pieces. Giving small pieces of food will help the child who tends to overstuff his or her mouth.

Foods with two or more textures are more advanced and can be problematic for a child with oral motor problems. For example, a chicken noodle soup will have solid pieces of chicken and soft noodles besides the chicken broth. Many times the solid food is swallowed whole, and can potentially pose a choking hazard. It is best to start with pureed soups, which allow a single consistency and can include many types of cooked vegetables that can be added by pureeing. This may be helpful in getting vegetables into children who refuse to eat them, or foods whose appearance disturbs them. This also applies to the "power shake", which is a healthy protein-and-fat shake that might include fresh or frozen fruit blended with essential oils and protein, in a casein-free base. Fruit nectars and fruit smoothies are healthier alternatives to fruit juice, and are also thickened liquids. Ideally, these should be offered in a cup with a built-in straw, or a cup with a top that has a wide lip and holes to allow the liquid to come out slowly.

Understanding Your Child's Eating Problems

There may be other factors related to a child's eating problem. The following must be considered and should be discussed with your child's therapist or a feeding specialist:

- **Medical Problems and Child's Eating:** Medical problems such as gastroesophageal reflux, food allergies/intolerances, constipation, diarrhea, delayed gastric emptying or motility problems, dysphasia (difficulty swallowing), cardiac problems, respiratory problems or metabolic disease can adversely affect children's eating.

- **Medications** can produce side effects such as nausea, irritability or gastrointestinal symptoms. It is most often best, unless otherwise recommended, to separate medications from mealtime, as your child may associate the taste of unpleasant medications with foods.

- **Sleep problems** may cause your child to be irritable during the daytime and may interfere with eating. A well rested child is much more likely to find success in having his or her eating problems treated.

- **Behavioral problems** may be exacerbated when demands such as eating are presented. It is necessary to treat behavioral problems prior to implementing an eating program.

- **Limited Food Choices or Types of Foods Consumed.** Many children with special needs eat a narrow range of foods. Some eat only foods with certain textures, brands, or foods at a certain temperature. To determine if your child has an eating problem, identifying the types of foods your child is eating can be helpful. There are several ways to evaluate a child's diet. Two of the simpler and more common ways are foods diaries and inventories.

    a) **Food preference inventory** is one way to evaluate the variety in your child's diet. It contains a lengthy list of foods from each food group. Foods eaten by everyone in the family, including the child with the eating problems, are recorded. This allows you to see how closely your child's diet matches that of your family.

b) Food Diary: Consider starting a food diary to evaluate your child's diet. Usually a three-day period is the minimum, where all foods and liquids are included.

Both Diet Quantity and Quality are Critical. It is important to consider not only what your child is eating, but also how many of the right kinds of calories are consumed. Many children with limited diets sometimes are not underweight because they are drinking large quantities of high calorie fluids such as milk, juice or formula. However, some children who are failing to grow are underweight because they are getting too few calories, and/or they may have medical conditions such as cardiac or pulmonary disease, which require them to ingest more calories than would typically be needed. Other children may have neuromotor problems which interfere with their ability to chew and swallow. In these cases it is important to seek professional help to ensure that your child gets enough calories in his or her diet.

Setting Up the Eating Environments and Behavior Guidelines

Once a child has been identified as having an eating problem, set realistic goals and determine which problems must be addressed first. Work with your child's therapists so that the same goals can be set both at home and in school or in therapy sessions. **The following are some guidelines which will help parents set up a snack and meal schedule.**

- A consistent daily schedule for meal times, snack times, bath times, and bedtime can help your child be less resistant at meal times. Most children do better with routine, and when children can predict the routine, their behavior tends to improve.

- Set approximate time for meals, snacks and other daily activities. Set up a schedule where two or three snacks and three meals can be separated evenly throughout the day. This will allow a variety of foods to be offered and ensure adequate calorie intake.

- Note fluid intake and types of fluid. It is common among children with eating problems to intake large quantities of fluids, which can interfere with hunger. Limit liquid intake between meals and snacks. The best fluid source to consider is water, as it has no calories, will keep the child hydrated, and will not interfere with hunger.

- Set the eating environment. Teach your child to sit at the table. A comfortable chair, booster seat, high chair, or adaptive equipment can be used, based on your child's individual needs. Encourage him to eat, and do not allow him to walk around the house while eating. Eating while walking, especially for a child with motor problems or with difficulty chewing and swallowing, can be a potential hazard, since a child may trip or fall with food in his or her mouth, thereby increasing the chances of aspiration or oral trauma.

- Avoid distractions while eating. Bad habits, such as eating while watching television or playing video games, must be addressed. If your child refuses to sit at the table, encourage him to be there by starting with a few minutes at a time.

- Modify the rate of eating. This will help children who eat too rapidly or who overstuff their mouths, gag, and even choke on food. You can use such strategies as cutting food into smaller pieces, encouraging smaller bites, extending intervals between bites, and having the food chewed properly.

- Avoid mealtime battles. Do not argue with your child. Calmly present foods to him. Discourage inappropriate behaviors, and praise appropriate ones. Negative reactions or statements can cause a child to eat less.

Notes:

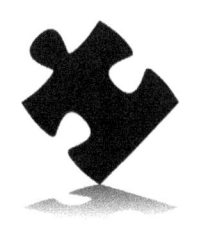

CHAPTER NINE

Getting Started in Meal Planning

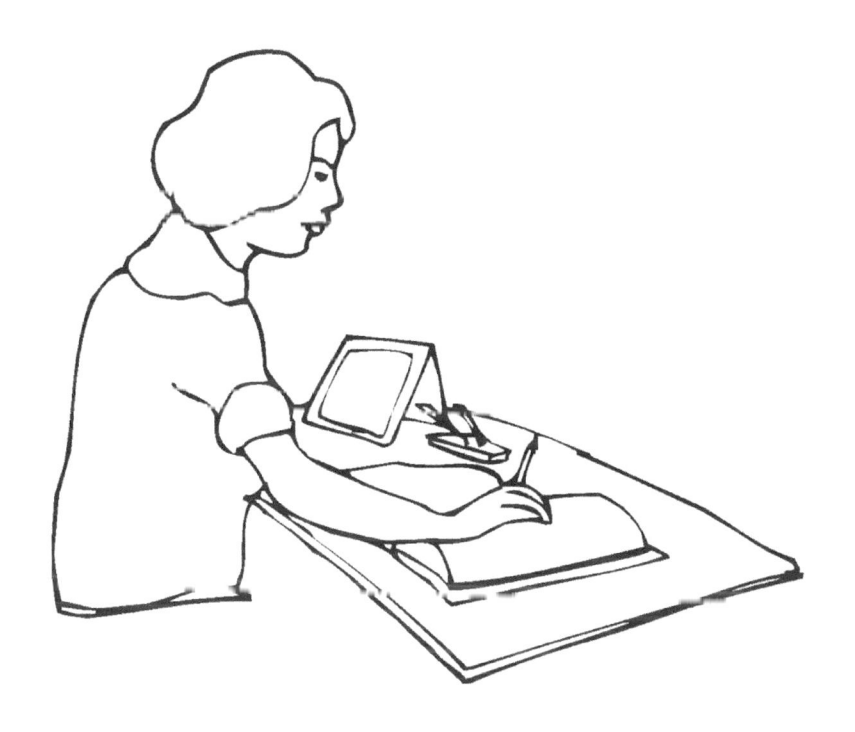

Gluten Free Cooking Flour Options

For many parents, eliminating wheat in the diet is a challenge because wheat is the grain found in many foods. Sometimes parents are not aware of other nutritious grains that can be substituted. These may even increase nutrient value. This section describes the gluten-free grains and flours that have been used in most of the recipes in breakfast, snacks, and desserts.

- **Coconut Flour:** It is gluten-free and hypoallergenic. With as much protein as wheat flour, coconut flour has none of the specific protein in wheat called "gluten." This is an advantage for the growing percentage of the population that has allergies to gluten or has wheat sensitivity.

  Coconut flour boasts the highest percentage of dietary fiber (58 percent) of any flour. Wheat bran has only 27 percent fiber. Coconut flour is ideal for baking because it has fewer digestible (net) carbs than other flours, and even some vegetables. Coconut flour can be used to make breads, cakes, pies, and other baked goods. Use 15 to 25 percent in place of other flours in most standard recipes. A variety of delicious baked goods can also be made using 100 percent coconut flour (see recipes in this book).

- **Amaranth Flour:** It contains more fiber and iron than wheat and is a good source of calcium. Amaranth flour is high in protein and, when it is combined with other flours (such as wheat), the protein value rivals that of fish or poultry. It is rich not only in protein and iron, but also in calcium and zinc. Amaranth flour is milled from the seeds of the amaranth plant. Because it lacks gluten, it must be combined with other types of flour when preparing yeast breads. A suitable mixture contains one part of amaranth flour to three or four parts of non-gluten flour. It does not have to be added to other flours when preparing pastas or flatbreads. Amaranth flour can also be used as a food extender, for making cookies and desserts, or it may be added to other foods as a means of increasing the nutrient value.

- **Buckwheat flour:** Buckwheat flour is a variety of gluten-free flour obtained by grinding the seeds of the buckwheat plant. In spite of its name, buckwheat is not a type of wheat. It is actually an herbaceous plant related to rhubarb. Buckwheat flour is an excellent substitute for people who are allergic to gluten (celiac disease). It is used in pancakes, waffles, blintzes, crepes, muffins, and soba noodles. Even when using a small quantity in yeast breads, buckwheat flour provides a distinctive flavor to the loaf. It is a good source of protein, calcium, magnesium, phosphorous, B vitamins and Iron.

- **Millet Flour:** The natural alkalinity of millet flour makes it easily digestible, so it is beneficial to people with ulcers and digestive problems. It is also believed to be one of the least allergenic varieties of flour. Millet is an excellent source of iron, magnesium, calcium, phosphorous, manganese, zinc, B vitamins and fiber.

- **Arrowroot Flour:** The fleshy round tubers of the arrowroot plant produce an edible starch after processing, which is then ground into a fine powder. The powder is used in cooking as a thickener, in much the same way as cornstarch or flour. It is often used to thicken glazes, fruit pie fillings, puddings, and sauces. It is high in fiber and is easily digestible, so it is suitable for breads and biscuits for small children. Arrowroot is a rich source of calcium and potassium.

- **Quinoa Flour:** Quinoa is produced from grinding the seeds into a powder. It may be used for making breads, biscuits, cookies, crepes, muffins, pancakes, and tortillas. Quinoa flour is rich in protein and nutrients, especially amino acids. It contains about 17 percent high-quality protein, which is more than any other grain flour, being equivalent to milk in protein quality. It is an excellent source of protein, iron, calcium, zinc, potassium, magnesium and phosphorus.

- **Rice Flour:** All types of rice flour are high in protein, but brown rice flour has a higher level of B vitamins, iron, and fiber than white rice flour because the bran is included.

- **Sorghum Flour:** It is in the corn family, but has a higher concentration of protein than corn flour. It is an excellent source of protein, calcium, iron and potassium.

- **Soy Flour:** Flour ground from soybeans is very high in protein and low in carbohydrates. It is available in full-fat, low-fat, and defatted versions. The full-fat variety contains about 20 percent fat and 35 percent protein; the low-fat variety contains about 6 percent fat and nearly 45 percent protein. The defatted variety contains less than 1 percent fat and about 50 percent protein. Soy flour can be added to wheat flour when making baked goods to boost the protein level.

- **Potato Flour/Potato Starch Flour:** Potato flour is made from cooked, dried, and ground potatoes. It is used as an ingredient in potato-based recipes to enhance the potato flavor and is often mixed with other types of flour for baking breads and rolls. It is also used as a thickener for soups, gravies, and sauces. Potato flour is often confused with potato starch, but potato flour is produced from the entire dehydrated potato, whereas potato starch is produced from the starch only.

- **Sweet Potato Flour:** Sweet potato flour is produced from white sweet potatoes, is dull white in color, stiff in texture, and has a somewhat sweet flavor. It is high in fiber and contains a higher level of carbohydrates and lower level of protein than common wheat flour. It can be used for baked goods, such as breads, cookies, muffins, pancakes, and doughnuts, and as a thickener for sauces and gravies. It is an excellent source of potassium, vitamin A, vitamin C, and fiber.

- **Water Chestnut Flour:** Flour ground from water chestnuts is used more as a thickener and a coating for foods rather than as an ingredient for baked goods. The water chestnut is the edible tuber of an aquatic plant that grows along the muddy edges of lakes, ponds, rivers, and streams and is cultivated commercially in flooded fields. Water chestnut flour is usually stirred into water before adding to hot liquids and sauces for use as a thickener. This technique reduces the formation of lumps that may otherwise occur (similar to cornstarch). Foods that are to be fried can be dredged in water chestnut flour to create a coating.

- **Yam Flour:** Yam flour is produced by grinding dried yams into a powder. A yam is a hearty tuber that does not have the sweet taste of a sweet potato, but instead may have flavors that range from bland to earthy, slightly smoky in taste, or nutty and only moderately sweet.

- **Almond Meal Flour:** Almond flour and meal are both merely ground almonds. Almond flour is most often made with blanched almonds (no skin), whereas almond meal can be made either with whole or blanched almonds. Almond flour is good in "quick-bread" type recipes, like muffins, nut breads, and pancakes.

- **Flaxseed or Flax meal:** It is an excellent source of cholesterol-reducing omega-3 fatty acids and soluble fiber. It is also one of the best sources of lignin, which may play a role in fighting certain types of cancer. Flax seed meal is coarsely ground flax seed. It can be added to many cooked and uncooked dishes, providing texture and flavor. It can be used as a fat substitute or thickening agent in some recipes, although it is not a flour.

- **Garbanzo Bean Flour:** It is a variety of flour that is most often used in East Indian and Middle Eastern cooking. Garbanzo beans, also known as chickpeas, are processed into a flour that is very similar to millet, providing a rich sweet flavor to baked foods. Since it is gluten-free, it must be combined with another flour containing gluten (such as wheat) in order to produce raised breads.

- **Mung Bean Flour:** It is a type of fine textured gluten-free flour made from ground mung beans. The flour is common in foods from India, where the bean originates. Mung bean flour contains a starch that is beneficial in making several varieties of thin, transparent noodles, referred to as bean threads or cellophane noodles. The noodles are high in calcium, magnesium, and phosphorous. Mung bean flour is also used to produce a variety of sweet pastries and breads.

Other Gluten Free Ingredients

- **Vanilla Extract.** Vanilla extract is typically in an alcohol base, which usually does contain some gluten. Some Celiac people say the amount of gluten in a recipe made with it is too small to matter, and for some it's too much. It is possible to find gluten-free vanilla made with corn alcohol (all pure Nielsen-Massey and also McCormick's vanillas are gluten-free). The vanilla paste and vanilla powder are both gluten-free. Your other option is just to use whole or ground vanilla beans, which do not contain gluten. In any recipe which has a liquid phase, simply steep the bean in the liquid, or add ground beans to the dry phase of the recipe. It is also possible to make your own gluten-free extract with vanilla beans, using a non-wheat based alcohol such as corn alcohol or very strong potato vodka.

  NOTE: Pure vanilla extract is SCD-legal; that is, vanilla extract, alcohol and water. Adulterated vanilla extract with illegal sugars [or corn syrup] are not permitted. Most supermarkets and even specialty shops carry vanilla extract with sugar or corn syrup added.

- **Vinegars.** White vinegar or just plain vinegars are typically distilled, and, if so, are gluten-free. Malted vinegars are usually not gluten-free. Red and white wine and true balsamic vinegars are gluten-free.

Quick Recipes to Speed Cooking

These quick recipes for common ingredients, which can be made prior to cooking and stored, will make cooking both easier and more fun.

Egg Replacer Recipe

    1 1/2 tablespoons water

    1 1/2 tablespoons oil

    1 teaspoon baking soda

    1/2 teaspoon vinegar (optional)

Whisk above ingredients together in a cup and pour into mixture that calls for an egg. If a recipe requires two eggs, the ingredients can be doubled, and so forth.

Chicken Broth
Yield: Scant 2 quarts

    1 tablespoon olive oil

    1 onion, medium, diced

    3 pounds chicken legs and thighs,

    (optimum skinless) trimmed of excess fat

    1 teaspoon sea salt

    2 bay leaves

    2 cups water

In a heavy bottomed soup kettle, over medium-high heat, heat the oil, add onion and chicken pieces and sauté until no longer pink, approximately 5 to 7 minutes. Add water, salt, and bay leaves. Bring to boil, reduce heat, cover and simmer until broth is rich and flavorful, 20 to 30 minutes longer. Strain and remove bones. Add chicken pieces to broth or save for other dishes. Broth is ready to use. Cool to room temperature or refrigerate for later use.

Note: Chicken Broth is used in many recipes. You can make this in advance and freeze. This will reduce your cooking time, and help you make delicious and varied recipes in no time.

Vegetable Broth

Yields 2 scant quarts

This vegetable-based stock can be used as a starter for any soups.

- 2 quarts filtered water
- 4 onions, coarsely chopped
- 4 carrots, coarsely chopped
- 1 butternut squash or 1 zucchini squash, peeled and chopped
- 4 stalks celery, coarsely chopped

Peel and add carrots, celery, butternut squash or zucchini in a pot of water. Bring to a boil, then lower heat to a simmer, cover and simmer for 45 minutes. Add fresh herbs (or if using dried herbs, placing them in a tea ball can be helpful). Simmer for 5-10 minutes. Turn off heat and cool. Strain broth and store in glass containers in the refrigerator or freezer. Drink as a tea by reheating and adding one tablespoon of whey. Add to soups as a vegetable-based broth. (Adding one tablespoon of whey upon consumption can aid mineral absorption and add probiotics).

Optional: Add a bunch of greens of your choosing: fresh nettles, parsley, or cilantro.

Homemade Specialties

Homemade SCD Yogurt
(Making SCD yogurt in a yogurt maker)

    2 liters of milk (goat's milk is the official SCD but other milks can be used according to Tolerance)
    2 packages (10 grams) of yogurt starter

Directions

1. Pour 2 liters of milk into a clean pot and heat to at least 180°F, maintaining that temperature for 2 minutes. It is okay if the milk boils. Note: whenever you measure the milk's temperature, be sure to stir the milk for 15-30 seconds to get an overall reading.

2. Allow the milk to cool to below 100°F, or to room temperature. You can speed up the cooling process by putting the pot into a bath of cool water.

3. Pour the cooled milk into the plastic batch jar/container.

4. Pour two packages (10 grams) of starter into a measuring cup, and gradually stir in 5-6 tablespoons of the cooled milk. Once the starter is completely dissolved, pour it into the remainder of the cooled milk in the batch container. Stir thoroughly. It is essential that the starter and the milk are blended evenly.

5. Cover the batch container with the snap-on lid.

6. Using the marks on the inside of the yogurt maker, pour water to the top of the taller mark ("2 liter marker"). Lower the prepared batch container into the yogurt maker. The water will come up on the outside of the batch container to the same height as the milk inside. Cover the yogurt maker and plug in the power cord. The red light will come on.

7. Allow the yogurt to ferment for 24 hours. Do not move the yogurt maker during this time.

8. Unplug the yogurt maker and remove the batch container. You are now 8 hours away from delicious yogurt.

9. Gently place the batch container into the refrigerator and chill for 8 hours.

10. The homemade SCD yogurt is ready after chilling for 8 hours. The yogurt will stay fresh for three weeks if kept cold.

Yogurt Starters Sources

- **Yogourmet Freeze-Dried Yogurt Starter:** Yogourmet yogurt starter is meticulously manufactured and scientifically balanced to ensure that you make a smooth, creamy and great tasting yogurt every time. (http://www.livingright.com/index.php)

- **GI ProStart™ Yogurt Starter** produces dairy free yogurt composed of three vital strains of probiotics which are well known for their health promoting benefits. ProStart™ can be used to culture just about any type of milk, including cow, goat, soy and nut. (http://www.livingright.com/index.php)

- Yogurt maker can be purchased at (http://www.livingright.com/index.php)

Homemade Curry Powder Recipe

    2 tablespoons cumin seeds, ground
    2 tablespoons coriander seeds, ground
    2 teaspoons turmeric, ground
    1/2 teaspoon red pepper, crushed flakes
    1/2 teaspoon mustard seed
    1/2 teaspoon ginger, ground

This mixture can be used in recipes that call for curry mixed powders. The curry mixes available in stores can sometimes have gluten in some hidden ingredients. This is a good homemade version of commercial curry powder.

Homemade Nut Milk

    1 cup raw organic nuts of your choice (almonds, pecans, walnuts, hazelnuts, cashews or macadamia)
    Filtered water to cover nuts
    1 tablespoon E-lyte electrolyte concentrate

In a large bowl, cover nuts in water and soak overnight. Soaking your nuts in warm water with neutralize these enzyme inhibitors, and also help encourage the production of beneficial enzymes. These enzymes in turn increase many vitamins, especially B vitamins. It also makes these nuts much easier to digest and the nutrients will be more easily absorbed.

Place nuts in a blender with 4 cups of filtered water, honey, stevia or xylitol. Blend for a few minutes, or until no visible nuts are seen. Strain mixture using either a fine strainer or few layers of cheese cloth.

Note: This milk can be stored in the refrigerator for 2-3 days.

* You will note that xylitol has been used in many of the following recipes as a sweetener. It can be replaced with other natural sweeteners your children like. (Refer to our "Guide to Natural Sweeteners" in *Chapter 3*.)

Homemade Seed Cream

> 1 cup organic raw seeds/nuts of choice (hemp, flax, chia, sesame, sunflower or pumpkin) (Walnuts, almonds, cashews, pecans, macadamia or hazelnuts)
>
> Filtered water to cover

Soak seeds overnight in enough water to cover them. Drain off and reserve excess water.

Blend soaked seeds, nuts in blender with water (more water can be added to get the desired consistency).

A Note about Lentil Flours

Lentil flours, which are used in many of the recipes in this book, are nutritious and a rich source of proteins. They are used in Middle Eastern and Indian Specialty Cuisines for their flavor and distinctive character. They can be used in instant dry soup mixes, rice/couscous/pasta and lentil entrees, dips, and as a thickening and binding agent in many recipes. They can also be used as broth and for making many baked goods. They are available at Indian specialty grocery stores, and also in many Oriental stores where they have a separate section for specialty foods by region.

Notes:

Oral Motor Rating Chart

The chart below shows the **Oral Motor Rating**. The recipes have been given "Oral Motor Rating" based on the food texture types and skills required by the individual child to eat.

Oral Motor Rating	Foods	Food Texture Types	Eating Skills Required by Each Child
😊	Puree	Smooth puree foods, minimal lumps and minimal "adhesiveness" (the stickiness between the food and surface of the mouth)	Sucking. May still have suckling pattern and tongue and jaw thrusts.
😊😊	Thick Puree and Wet Ground Foods	Semi-solid foods that can be compressed using force between the tongue and roof of the mouth. Thicker and lumpier purees that require a little more force to move from the mouth to the stomach.	Strong sucking. Early munching
😊😊😊	Ground, Crunchy & Chopped Foods	Foods that require munching (an up-down motion on the molars not a lateral movement). Foods with "adhesiveness" (the stickiness between the food and surfaces of the mouth).	Munching mixed with a rotary chewing pattern.
😊😊😊😊	Regular-Table Foods	Foods that require breaking and tearing to chew, such as biting off a piece of a cookie, tearing off and chewing a piece of meat or poultry.	Controlled bite and release. Rotary chewing pattern.

A Few Notes about the Recipes that Follow:

All the ingredients selected in the recipes are nutritious, and every effort has been made to select only the best ingredients to comply with the individual diets.

Some ingredients that are in the moderate to high range have been included to make the food more acceptable to children. They serve only to add taste and quality, and the ingredients comply with moderate-to-acceptable ranges in diet. If any of the ingredients are on the allergenic list for your child, they can easily be substituted with other healthy food alternatives discussed in earlier chapters.

About Herbs Used in Recipes: Unless a recipe specifically says to use fresh herbs, assume that the measurements are for the dried variety. Fresh is always better, of course, so if you wish to substitute fresh herbs for dried, the rule of thumb for most herbs is: 1 teaspoon of the dried herb = 1 tablespoon of the fresh.

Ingredient Choices: For your convenience, most recipes give you a choice between two or three kinds of healthy flours, oils, milks, and sweeteners you can use. Choose the ones that are best for your child's needs or fits ingredients you have on hand. A one to one substitution can be made for a liquid sweetener such as honey or maple syrup for a dry sweetener such as sugar or xylitol in any recipe, however, 1/4 cup more dry ingredient is needed when using a liquid sweetener. When choosing honey it is best to select raw organic honey as it is unheated, pure, unpasteurized and unprocessed. Most honeys found are "commercial" and have been filtered and heated so it looks more appealing but the aromas, yeast and enzymes which are responsible for activating vitamins and minerals in the body system are partially destroyed.

CHAPTER TEN

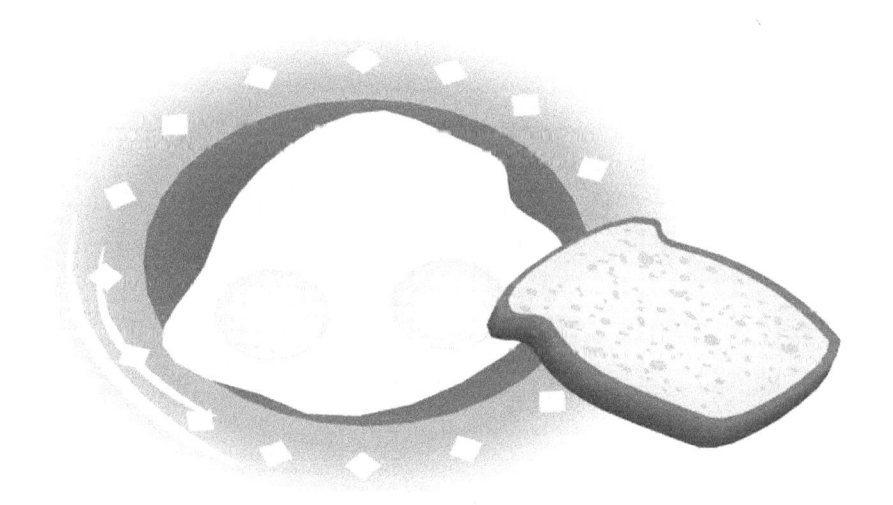

Breakfast Recipes

The Most Important Meal of the Day

BREAKFAST RECIPES
TABLE OF CONTENTS

BREADS

Sorghum Bread 183
Easy Gluten-Free Flatbread 184
Coconut Bread or Crackers 185
Pumpkinseed Fruit Bread 186
Zucchini Bread 187
Banana Bread 188
Applesauce Bread 189
Egg Bread 190

PANCAKES AND PATTIES

Carrot Pancakes 191
Almond and Coconut Pancakes 192
Lentil Cauliflower and Parsley Pancakes 193
Brown Rice Pancakes 194
Vegetable Cutlets or Pancakes 195
Golden Pancakes or Waffles 196
Fried Chicken Patties 197
Yam Latkes 198
Chopped Meat Patty 199
Easy Chicken Pancakes 200
Banana Nut Pancakes 201

BREAKFAST MUFFINS

Banana Muffins 202
Pumpkin Muffins 203
Breakfast Muffins 204
Jam Muffins 205
Brown Pear Muffins 206
Mini Squash Muffins 207
Tropical Muffins 208

EGG AND OMELET RECIPES

Soft Boiled Eggs 209
Soft Scrambled Eggs 210
Zucchini Omelet 211
Egg Rolls 212
Coconut Omelet 213

MISCELLANEOUS BREAKFAST RECIPES

Breakfast Spring Rolls 214
Hot Breakfast Porridge 215
Carrot Cutlets 216
French Toast 217
Almond Coconut Granola 218
Quick Creamy Cereal or Pudding 219
Hash Brown Casserole 220

The Importance of a Good Breakfast

The American Dietetic Association says breakfast is the most important meal of the day, because it nourishes the body and brain to help provide optimal function. When it comes to special needs children, it is critical that they be served a healthy breakfast to begin their day.

The importance of eating a healthy breakfast cannot be overemphasized. Breakfast makes a major contribution to the nutritional quality of a well-balanced diet. It provides the nutrients that are not always made up for in later meals and snacks. Breakfast should provide about one quarter of daily energy intake. Research has shown that children who skip breakfast perform less well academically, socially and emotionally. Eating breakfast improves children's problem solving abilities, memory, concentration levels, visual perception and creative thinking.

Academic performance can be boosted by a high-energy breakfast. Blood sugar levels drop overnight and can be low upon wakening. Studies have linked low blood sugar levels to difficulties with memory, concentration, and cognition. Eating a balanced, nutrient dense breakfast raises blood sugar levels and helps the body to function more effectively.

In many houses, morning is a busy time. Parents are rushing to get to work, and children with special needs take more time to get their day started. Breakfast is often the meal that is most often neglected or skipped. It is also for this reason that many children are attracted by the readymade breakfast food options, such as box cereals, breakfast bars, pastries and bottled fruit juices, all of which are loaded with sugar and lacking in good nutrition.

In our breakfast section of the cookbook that follows, we have incorporated some easy-to-make and nutritious recipes. Most of the recipes can be made ahead and frozen; some can be prepared in a matter of minutes. You will find delicious recipes for cereals, muffins, pancakes and patties, egg and omelet meals, and healthy breads. (Also refer to the smoothie recipes in Chapter 16 since a nutritious smoothie or power drink can actually take the place of a breakfast.)

BREADS

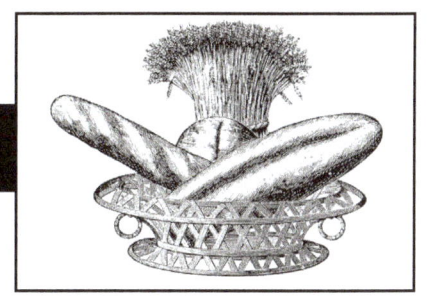

Sorghum Bread

Yields: One Loaf

Ingredients

- 2 tablespoons coconut butter or ghee
- 2 tablespoons honey or maple syrup
- 1 cup carbonated water
- 2 cups sorghum flour or coconut flour
- 1 teaspoon guar gum or xanthan gum (optional) (non aluminum)
- 1/2 teaspoon baking soda
- 1/2 teaspoon sea salt
- 2 eggs or egg replacer
- 1/2 teaspoon flaxseed meal (optional)

> **Sorghum**
>
> Sorghum is one of the five top cereal crops in the world, along with wheat, oats, corn, and barley. Sorghum is well favored by the gluten-intolerant people. The grain is fairly neutral in flavor, and sometimes slightly sweet, making it suited to a variety of dishes.

Directions

Preheat oven to 350º. Grease and flour a bread pan. In a large bowl, mix coconut butter or ghee, honey, and carbonated water. Add dry ingredients and mix well. Consistency will be like cake batter. Grease and flour a bread pan. Bake for 30 minutes, then cover with foil and bake 25 minutes longer. Remove pan from oven and cool. Also works great in a bread machine — use the one-pound loaf setting.

Ingredients to Consider on Specific Diets

Gluten & Casein Free ....Yes	Phenol Free ....Yes (if you use maple syrup)
Low Oxalate Diet........................Yes	Specific Carbohydrate Diet ....No

This recipe is also Soy free, Corn free and Rice free

Oral Motor Rating 😊 😊 😊 😊

Easy Gluten-Free Flatbread

Yields: One Loaf

Ingredients
2 cups sorghum flour or coconut flour
1/2 cup tapioca flour
1 teaspoon sea salt
1 cup rice milk
1 tablespoon coconut butter or ghee

> *Variation*
>
> *Almond milk, coconut milk, or hemp seed milk can be used as a substitute for rice milk in the recipe.*

Directions
Mix dry ingredients in a mixing bowl, then stir in milk. Add the coconut butter, mixing it in with a fork. Pat or roll into 3 to 4" flat cakes. Fry at medium heat with the oil of your choice until golden brown.

Ingredients to Consider on Specific Diets

Gluten & Casein Free ....Yes	Phenol Free ....Yes
Low Oxalate Diet.........................Yes	Specific Carbohydrate Diet ....No

This recipe is also Soy free, Corn free and Rice free (use almond milk)

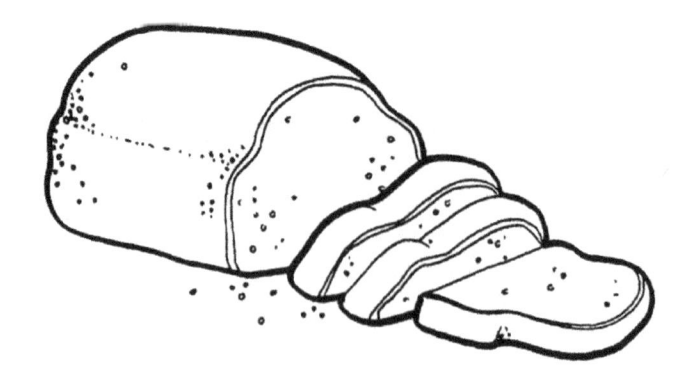

Oral Motor Rating 😊 😊 😊

Coconut Bread or Crackers

Yields: One Loaf

Ingredients
2 large eggs or 4 egg whites, or egg replacer
2 tablespoons ghee or coconut oil
1/4 cup honey or maple syrup
1 cup coconut flour
1/2 teaspoon baking soda
1 pinch sea salt
Enough water to bring to a paste-like consistency

> *Coconut Flour*
>
> *Coconut flour is made from the ground fiber of coconut meat. High in protein and dietary fiber, this non-gluten flour is an excellent choice in recipes for quick breads and muffins.*

Directions
Preheat oven to 350º, Blend the eggs in a small mixing bowl. Melt together the ghee or coconut oil and honey, and add it to the egg mixture after it has cooled a bit. Then add the dry ingredients. If the mixture is too dry, add in small amounts of water to bring it to a thick moist consistency. Place parchment paper on a cookie sheet and pour the mixture onto the center of it, spreading it out to about a half-inch thickness in a square about 8 inches in size. Bake it at 350º for 20-25 minutes until it is golden brown. This will be soft moist bread. To make it into crackers, cut up the bread into small bite-size pieces and dry them in a dehydrator or your oven at 150º for 4 to 5 hours until they are crunchy like a cracker.

Ingredients to Consider on Specific Diets

Gluten & Casein Free................ Yes
Phenol Free............................. Yes (if you use maple syrup)
Low Oxalate Diet .... Yes
Specific Carbohydrate Diet .... Yes (if you use honey)

This recipe is also Soy free, Corn free and Rice free

Oral Motor Rating 😊 😊 😊

Pumpkinseed Fruit Bread

Yields: One Loaf

Ingredients

2 1/2 cups pumpkin seeds
2 bananas, mashed
1/4 cup coconut, sunflower or safflower oil
1/4 cup honey
1/4 teaspoon sea salt
1 teaspoon baking soda
1 teaspoon apple cider vinegar
1/2 – 3/4 cup finely chopped dried fruit of your choice, (cranberries, mango, or blueberries)

> **Pumpkin seeds**
>
> *Pumpkin seeds help stimulate appetite, and are beneficial for the teeth, gums, nerves, hair and nails. They relieve constipation and also contain anti-inflammatory properties, making them a healthy food choice for children with ASD.*

Directions

Preheat oven to 350º. Grind the pumpkin seeds in a blender to make the flour. In a mixing bowl, mash bananas. Add oil, honey, salt and baking soda, and mix well. Blend in pumpkinseed flour and vinegar. Add dried fruit; mash to make a dough. Put the dough into parchment-lined or oiled and flour-dusted loaf/cake pan(s). Bake for 50-55 minutes. (Time will vary depending on pan size. Bread is done when a toothpick comes out clean). Leave in pan(s) 10 minutes before removing.

Ingredients to Consider on Specific Diets

Gluten & Casein Free .... Yes
Phenol Free .... No
Low Oxalate Diet .... Yes
Specific Carbohydrate Diet .... Yes

This recipe is also Soy free, Corn free and Rice free

Oral Motor Rating 😊 😊 😊

Note: You can purchase pumpkin seed flour from
http://www.naturalhub.com/go/Bayoils.htm

Zucchini Bread

Yields: Two Loaves

Ingredients
1/2 cup honey
3 eggs or egg replacer, lightly beaten
1 cup grape seed oil or sunflower oil
2 teaspoons gluten-free vanilla extract
2 cups zucchini, shredded
1 1/2 cup almond flour or rice flour
1 1/2 cup coconut flour
1 teaspoon baking soda
1/2 teaspoon sea salt
1 cup walnuts or pecans,
   finely chopped (optional)

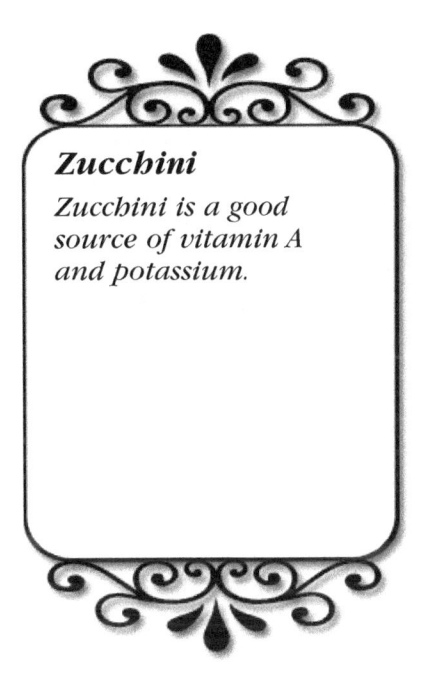

Zucchini
Zucchini is a good source of vitamin A and potassium.

Directions
Preheat oven to 350º. In a large bowl, combine xylitol or honey with eggs, oil and vanilla. Stir in zucchini. Add flour, baking soda, and salt. Add nuts if desired. Blend well and pour into two lightly greased loaf pans dusted with flour. Bake for approximately 60 minutes.

Ingredients to Consider on Specific Diets

Gluten & Casein Free............... Yes
Phenol Free............................ No
Low Oxalate Diet .... Yes (if you use rice and coconut flour)
Specific Carbohydrate Diet .... Yes (if you use almond and coconut flour and avoid rice flour)
This recipe is also Soy free, Corn free and Rice free (use almond and coconut flour)

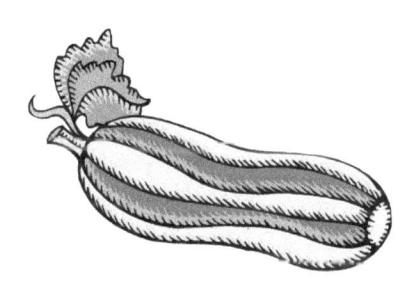

Oral Motor Rating 😊 😊 😊

CHAPTER 10: BREAKFAST RECIPES

Banana Bread

Yields: One Regular Loaf or Four Mini Loaves

Ingredients
1 1/2 cups ripe banana, mashed
1/3 cup grape seed oil or sesame oil
2 eggs lightly beaten or egg replacer
3/4 cup honey
2 cups almond or coconut flour
1 teaspoon baking soda
1 teaspoon cinnamon (optional)
1/4 teaspoon sea salt
2/3 cup walnuts or almonds (optional), finely chopped

Banana
Banana is a good source of dietary fiber, potassium, vitamin B6 and iron. Caution: banana is a high sugar fruit.

Directions
Preheat oven to 350º. Mix mashed bananas, oil, and eggs together in a large bowl and beat well. Add brown sugar (or honey). In a separate bowl, mix flour, cinnamon, and salt, then stir into banana mixture. Add finely chopped nuts if desired. Pour into oil-greased loaf pan (or four 2x5-inch mini loaf pans). Bake for 45 to 60 minutes or until a toothpick inserted in the center comes out clean.

Ingredients to Consider on Specific Diets

Gluten & Casein Free................. Yes
Phenol Free............................. No
Low Oxalate Diet .... Yes (if you use coconut flour)
Specific Carbohydrate Diet .... Yes

This recipe is also Soy free, Corn free and Rice free

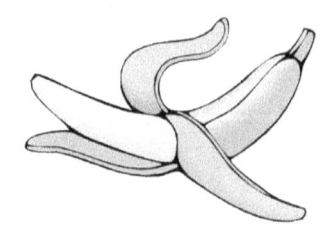

Oral Motor Rating 😊 😊 😊

Applesauce Bread

Yields: One Loaf

Ingredients
2 cups quinoa flour
1/2 cup rice flour
2 teaspoons baking soda
2 teaspoons cinnamon (optional)
1/2 teaspoon xanthan gum
1/4 cup rice bran oil or sunflower oil
1 cup applesauce, unsweetened
3/4 cup apple juice, concentrated

> *Apples*
>
> *Apples are low on the glycemic index, which means they do not cause a steep rise in blood sugar levels. Eating a lot of raw apples can cause digestive problems, so use caution for children with ASD, as many have digestive issues.*

Directions
Preheat oven to 350º. Combine the flours, baking soda and cinnamon in a large bowl. Add the xanthan gum, honey (if desired), oil, applesauce, and juice. Stir together until well mixed to form a batter. If batter is too dry, a little water can be added to make a good consistency. Pour the batter into an oiled and floured 8x4-inch loaf pan and bake for 45 to 55 minutes, or until the bread is brown and toothpick inserted into the center of the loaf comes out dry. Cool the loaf in a pan for about 10 minutes, and then remove it from the pan to cool it down before slicing.

Ingredients to Consider on Specific Diets

Gluten & Casein Free	Yes	Phenol Free	Yes
Low Oxalate Diet	Yes	Specific Carbohydrate Diet	No

This recipe is also Soy free, Corn free but is not Rice free

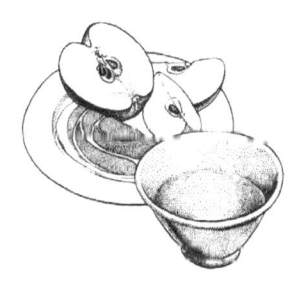

Oral Motor Rating 😊 😊 😊

Egg Bread

Yields: One Loaf

Ingredients
5 eggs
1/2 cup vegetables
   (carrot, cauliflower, red pepper, or cabbage)
1/4 teaspoon sea salt

> **Eggs**
> *An egg is the most complete protein source in a single food. Choose free range organic eggs, as they are the highest source of vitamins, minerals and important amino acids. If egg allergy is suspected, then start with egg yolks.*

Directions
Cook vegetables of your choice in water until tender. Separate the egg whites into large bowl and put the yolks into a small bowl. Beat egg whites with salt until fluffy. Squeeze water out of cooked vegetables with a paper towel, and blend in a blender. Add them to small bowl with the egg yolks and mix well. Fold in egg whites. Preheat oven to 350º. Line a cookie sheet with parchment paper and spread mixture evenly over the entire pan. Bake 40 to 50 minutes; carefully flip over and bake on the other side for another ten minutes. Cut into square pieces and sprinkle with sea salt.

Ingredients to Consider on Specific Diets

Gluten & Casein Free ....Yes	Phenol Free ....Yes
Low Oxalate Diet ....Yes	Specific Carbohydrate Diet ....Yes

This recipe is also Soy free, Corn free and Rice free

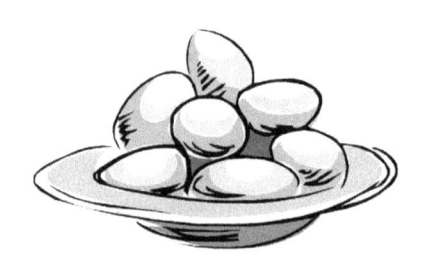

Oral Motor Rating 🙂 🙂

PANCAKES AND PATTIES

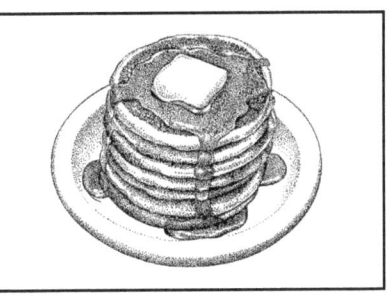

Carrot Pancakes

Yields: 6 Medium Pancakes

Ingredients
1 1/2 cup carrots or shredded vegetables, cooked and drained
4 eggs or egg replacer
1 teaspoon SCD legal vanilla
1 teaspoon cinnamon (optional)
4 teaspoons honey or maple syrup
1/2 cup almond flour or rice flour
4 tablespoons olive oil, ghee, or grape seed oil
1/4 teaspoon sea salt

> **Carrots**
> *Carrots are high in betacarotenes, but they are high on the glycemic index, and can raise blood sugar levels. Other vegetables can be added to the recipe, replacing some of the carrots.*

Directions
Mash cooked carrots and add other ingredients, mixing thoroughly until smooth. Heat the oil in an iron or steel frying pan, and fry medium-sized pancakes until brown.

Ingredients to Consider on Specific Diets

Gluten & Casein Free	Yes
Phenol Free	No
Low Oxalate Diet	Yes (if you use rice flour)
Specific Carbohydrate Diet	Yes (if you use almond flour)

This recipe is also Soy free, Corn free and Rice free (use almond flour)

Oral Motor Rating 😊 😊 😊

Almond and Coconut Pancakes

Yields: 6 Medium Pancakes

Ingredients
- 1 egg or 2 egg whites lightly beaten (optional), or egg replacer
- 3 tablespoons honey or maple syrup
- 1 cup almond or rice flour, or ground pumpkin seeds
- 1/2 cup shredded coconut
- 1/2 teaspoon baking soda
- 1/2 cup water
- 4 tablespoons ghee, coconut or grape seed oil

Coconut

Coconut has been classified as a "functional food." It is high in fiber and easy to digest medium chain fatty acids.

Directions
Lightly beat egg and honey till blended and frothy. Add flour, coconut, and baking soda and mix till all blend together. Add 1/2 cup water and stir. If mixture is too thick, add small amounts of water until you get a consistency that is slightly runny. Preheat frying pan over medium high heat. When pan is hot, melt ghee/oil. Spoon batter onto the pan. Flip after 2-3 minutes and brown the other side.

Ingredients to Consider on Specific Diets

Gluten & Casein Free	Yes
Phenol Free	Yes (if you use rice or pumpkin seed flour)
Low Oxalate Diet	Yes (if you use rice flour or ground pumpkin seeds
Specific Carbohydrate Diet	Yes (if you use almond flour or ground pumpkin seeds)

This recipe is also Soy free, Corn free and Rice free (use almond or ground pumpkin seeds)

Oral Motor Rating 😊 😊

Lentil Cauliflower and Parsley Pancakes

Yields: 6 Medium Pancakes

Ingredients
1 cup lentil flour
2 garlic cloves, chopped
2 tablespoons basil, parsley, or oregano (dried leaves)
Pinch of sea salt, vary with taste
2 heads cauliflower, grated by hand or in food processor
1 tablespoon sesame, coconut, or grape seed oil
Water to make batter

Lentils

Lentils are a good source of protein. They cook easily and are very well tolerated by people with digestive problems. They are a rich source of many nutrients.

Directions
In a bowl, mix lentil flour, garlic, salt and dried herb leaves of your choice. Stir in grated cauliflower. Add water to make a spreadable batter. Heat frying pan, add oil, and spoon the batter into small pancakes. Brown on both sides and serve.

Ingredients to Consider on Specific Diets

Gluten & Casein Free .... Yes
Phenol Free.................................. Yes (if you use parsley and avoid basil)
Low Oxalate Diet......................... Yes (if you use basil or oregano and avoid parsley)
Specific Carbohydrate Diet .... Yes
This recipe is also Soy free, Corn free and Rice free

Oral Motor Rating ☺ ☺

Brown Rice Pancakes

Yields: 6 Pancakes

Ingredients

1 egg or egg replacer
2 tablespoons sunflower, grape seed, or coconut oil
1 cup brown rice flour
1 tablespoon maple syrup
2 teaspoons baking powder
1/4 teaspoon sea salt
1/2 cup rice or hemp seed milk

Brown Rice

Brown Rice contains no gluten, so is well tolerated by those with gluten allergies.

Directions

In a bowl, blend egg and oil. Add flour, honey, baking powder, and salt. Mix well. For each pancake, spoon 2 tablespoons of batter onto a hot greased griddle. When edges are dry and bubbles form in the center, turn pancakes and finish cooking.

Note: Batter should just be thin enough to pour, but thick enough that the pancakes hold the shape of a perfect circle. If the batter is too thick, add more water.

Ingredients to Consider on Specific Diets

Gluten & Casein Free ....Yes	Phenol Free ....Yes
Low Oxalate Diet..Yes	Specific Carbohydrate Diet .... No

This recipe is also Soy free, and Corn free but is not Rice free

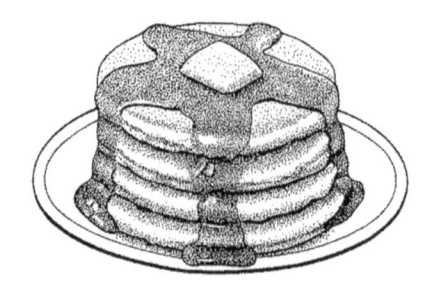

Oral Motor Rating 😊 😊

HEALING AUTISM IN THE KITCHEN

Vegetable Cutlets or Pancakes

Yields: 6 Cutlets or Pancakes

Ingredients
2 cups red lentils
1 red pepper
1 onion
2 garlic cloves, chopped
1 cup cauliflower
1 cup cabbage
1/2 cup mushrooms
6 tablespoons grape seed oil or olive oil
1/2 teaspoon sea salt
1/2 teaspoon cumin seeds (optional)

> **Flourless Recipe**
> *A great flourless recipe made from lentils, which offers vegetables to kids who do not eat raw vegetables. Lentils readily absorb a variety of wonderful flavors from other foods and seasonings, are high in nutritional value.*

Directions
Soak lentils overnight, drain excess water and set aside. In a blender, combine lentils, red pepper, onion, garlic, cauliflower, cabbage, mushrooms, and cumin seeds, if desired. Blend until smooth. Pour all out in a large bowl; add the salt and a little water from the lentils if batter mixture is too dry. Use flour as necessary to form and hold cutlets together. Make six small cutlets and set aside. In a frying pan, heat the oil and "deep fry" the cutlets, turning to brown both sides.

Variation: The batter used to make the deep fried cutlets can also be made into small six inch pancakes. Use a little of the water from the lentils as needed to make a nice spoonable batter. Heat frying pan and add only as much oil as needed to fry the pancakes on both sides.

Ingredients to Consider on Specific Diets

Gluten & Casein Free................ Yes
Phenol Free............................ Yes (if you use rice flour if needed)
Low Oxalate Diet .... Yes (If you use rice flour if needed)
Specific Carbohydrate Diet .... Yes (if you use almond flour if needed)
This recipe is also Soy free, Corn free and Rice free (use almond flour if needed)

Oral Motor Rating 😊 😊

Golden Pancakes or Waffles

Yields: 4 Pancakes

Ingredients
4 eggs or egg replacer
2 tablespoons honey or maple syrup
1 teaspoon vanilla (optional)
1/4 teaspoon sea salt
1 cup almond, rice, or chick pea flour
1/4 teaspoon baking soda
1 tablespoon ghee or grape seed oil

> **Almonds**
> *Almonds are rich in magnesium, an important mineral in which children with ASD can be deficient. Caution: Almonds are a high phenol food.*

Directions
Beat eggs; add honey, vanilla, and salt. Add flour and baking soda. Use batter to cook as pancakes or make waffles by pouring the batter in waffle maker.

Ingredients to Consider on Specific Diets

Gluten & Casein Free................ Yes
Phenol Free............................ Yes (if you use rice or chick pea flour and omit honey)
Low Oxalate Diet .... Yes (if you use rice or chick pea flour)
Specific Carbohydrate Diet .... Yes (if you use almond flour)
This recipe is also Soy free, Corn free and Rice free (use almond or chick pea flour)

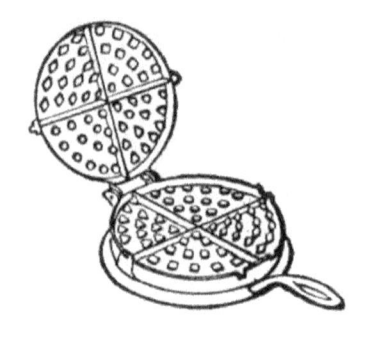

Oral Motor Rating 😊 😊

HEALING AUTISM IN THE KITCHEN

Fried Chicken Patties

Yields: 2 Patties

Ingredients
4 to 6 ounce boned chicken breast
1 teaspoon sea salt
1 cup vegetables (carrot, cauliflower, red pepper or cabbage)
6 tablespoons coconut oil, olive oil or grape seed oil

> ### *Chicken*
> *Chicken can be roasted, broiled, grilled or poached, and combined with a wide range of herbs and spices, making it a delicious, flavorful and nutritious meal option.*

Directions
Cook chicken in a small amount of water (about 1/2 inch high) in a covered frying pan for 15 minutes. Transfer chicken, salt, and vegetables to a food processor and pulse until completely chopped and mixed evenly. Form into two patties and fry in a frying pan, spread with a small amount of olive oil or coconut oil. Brown and turn over to brown the other side. Serve.

Ingredients to Consider on Specific Diets

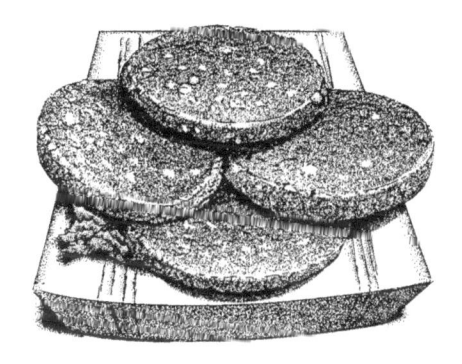

Gluten & Casein Free ....Yes	Phenol Free ....Yes
Low Oxalate Diet ....Yes	Specific Carbohydrate Diet ....Yes

This recipe is also Soy free, Corn free and Rice free

Oral Motor Rating 😊 😊 😊

Yam Latkes

Yields: 6 Latkes

Ingredients

2 cups yams, coarsely grated
1 cup butternut squash, peeled and coarsely grated
1/2 cup red bell pepper, chopped fine
1 apple, peeled and grated
15 ounce can garbanzo beans (chickpeas) drained
1 egg or egg replacer
1 teaspoon sea salt
1/4 cup parsley or cilantro
1/2 cup brown rice flour
8 tablespoons coconut or grape seed oil

> **Yams**
>
> *Creamy or firm when cooked, yams have an earthy taste. There is great confusion between yams and sweet potatoes. Most of the vegetables labeled "yams" in the market are really orange-colored sweet potatoes.*

Directions

Preheat oven to 350º. Line a cookie sheet with parchment paper. Combine yams, squash, bell pepper and apple in a large bowl. Puree garbanzo beans in a processor; add egg and salt and blend. Transfer to a small bowl and mix in cilantro/parsley and add to yam mixture along with the brown rice flour. Mix well. Heat skillet with 8 tablespoons of oil and drop one heaping tablespoon of batter into the hot oil, spread to a 3-inch round, cook until brown, turn over and cook the other side. Repeat till all batter has been used. Place browned latkes on a parchment-lined cookie sheet and bake for 15 minutes.

Ingredients to Consider on Specific Diets

Gluten & Casein Free	Yes	Phenol Free	Yes
Low Oxalate Diet	Yes	Specific Carbohydrate Diet	No

This recipe is also Soy free, Corn free, but is not Rice free

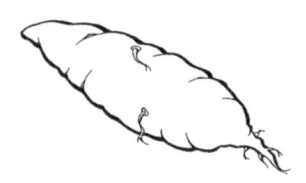

Oral Motor Rating 😊 😊

Chopped Meat Patties

Yields: 4 Medium Patties

Ingredients
- 1 pound chopped meat (use only free-range beef, bison or buffalo meat)
- 1 teaspoon sea salt
- 6 tablespoons coconut, olive, or grape seed oil

> ### *Free Range Meats*
> *Free range meats are cuts of meat from animals that are allowed unlimited access to pastures. They have plenty of room to roam and eat their natural diets and grow and live free of stress.*

Directions
Preheat oven to 350º. Mix meat and sea salt together in a bowl; divide evenly into 4 amounts. Form 4 patties and place on ungreased cookie sheet lined with parchment paper. Bake approximately 10 to 15 minutes. Cool and serve. Paties may also be sauteed in a pan with a little oil. Cook over medium heat for 2-3 minutes per side.

Ingredients to Consider on Specific Diets

Gluten & Casein Free .... Yes	Phenol Free .... Yes
Low Oxalate Diet .... Yes	Specific Carbohydrate Diet .... Yes

This recipe is also Soy free, Corn free and Rice free

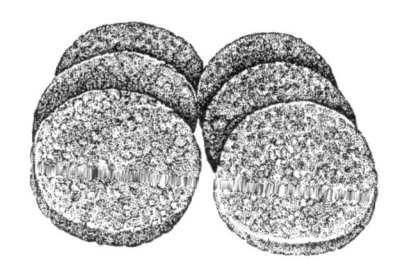

Oral Motor Rating 😊 😊 😊

Easy Chicken Pancakes

Yields: 2 Pancakes

Ingredients
1 boneless chicken breast
3 eggs or egg replacer
1/2 cup coconut or almond flour

> *Coconut Flour*
>
> *Coconut flour is gluten-free and hypoallergenic; it consists of the highest percentage of dietary fiber found in any flour. Coconut flour is ideal for baking. Almonds are one of the most nutritious nuts and are a rich source of magnesium. The texture of either flour makes it a good choice in a variety of baking recipes.*

Directions
Boil chicken breast in water until done, season as desired. Using a food processor, blend the chicken, eggs, and flour and process until completely smooth. Mixture will look just like thick pancake batter. Use 1/4 cup of the mixture and cook on hot greased skillet like a pancake. Batter may need to be spread out a bit so that it is not too thick. These cook much faster than flour pancakes. Flip them fast and cook both sides and enjoy.

Ingredients to Consider on Specific Diets

Gluten & Casein Free	Yes
Phenol Free	Yes (if you use coconut flour)
Low Oxalate Diet	Yes (if you use coconut flour)
Specific Carbohydrate Diet	Yes

This recipe is also Soy free, Corn free and Rice free

Oral Motor Rating 😊 😊 😊

HEALING AUTISM IN THE KITCHEN

Banana Nut Pancakes

Yields: 6 Pancakes

Ingredients
1 1/2 cups rice or coconut flour
2 tablespoons baking powder (aluminum free)
1 teaspoon sea salt
1/2 teaspoon xanthan gum
2 large ripe bananas, mashed
3 eggs or egg replacer
1 1/2 cups water
3 tablespoons safflower or grape seed oil
2 tablespoons honey or maple syrup
1/2 cup walnuts, finely chopped

> **Xanthan Gum**
> *Xanthan gum can also be used as a replacement for gluten in gluten free bread. It helps bind bread dough together so that it can trap gas from yeast, allowing bread dough to rise.*

Directions
In a large bowl, combine flour, baking powder, salt and xanthan gum. In a small bowl, mash bananas with a fork and set aside. In another small bowl, beat eggs, water, oil and honey until completely mixed. To this small bowl, add mashed bananas and beat until completely mixed. Add all this to the flour mixture in large bowl. Blend all together to form a batter and make small pancakes from it. Heat frying pan spread with some grape seed oil, and cook pancakes on both sides until light brown.

Ingredients to Consider on Specific Diets

Gluten & Casein Free ....Yes	Phenol Free ....Yes (if you use maple syrup)
Low Oxalate Diet.............................Yes	Specific Carbohydrate Diet ....No

This recipe is also Soy free, Corn free and Rice free (use coconut flour)

Oral Motor Rating :) :) :)

BREAKFAST MUFFINS

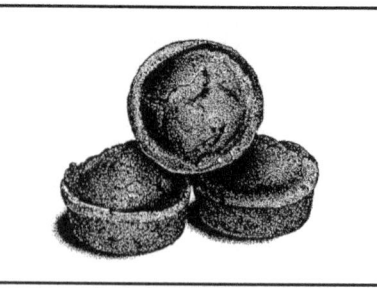

Banana Muffins

Yields: 12 Muffins

Ingredients
1 ripe banana
2 eggs, lightly beaten, or egg replacer
1/4 cup sunflower, grape seed, or coconut oil
1/2 cup almond or rice milk
1/2 cup honey
1 1/2 cups almond or coconut flour
2 teaspoons baking soda
1 teaspoon cinnamon (optional)
1/4 teaspoon sea salt
1/2 cup walnuts (optional), finely chopped

> **Rice Milk**
> *Compared with cow's milk, rice milk contains more carbohydrates. Many people are allergic to dairy and soy, so rice, nut, or seed milk remains an alternative.*

Directions
Preheat oven to 350º. In a small bowl, mash banana and set aside. In a large bowl, blend together the eggs, oil, and milk, and then add xylitol or honey and bananas. Stir in all dry ingredients. Mix well and add chopped walnuts, if desired. Spoon into oil-sprayed muffin pan or into paper muffin cups and bake 40 to 45 minutes, or until a toothpick inserted in the center comes out clean.

Ingredients to Consider on Specific Diets

Gluten & Casein Free	Yes
Phenol Free	No
Low Oxalate Diet	Yes (if you use coconut flour and rice milk)
Specific Carbohydrate Diet	Yes (if you use almond milk)

This recipe is also Soy free, Corn free and Rice free (use almond milk)

Oral Motor Rating 😊 😊

Pumpkin Muffins

Yields: 12 Muffins

Ingredients
1 cup pumpkin or butternut squash (fresh or canned)
1 1/2 cups almond or coconut flour
2 teaspoons baking soda
1 teaspoon cinnamon
1/4 teaspoon sea salt
2 eggs, lightly beaten, or egg replacer
1/2 cup honey
1/3 cup almond, rice, or hemp milk
1/4 cup grape seed, safflower, or sunflower oil

> *Cinnamon*
>
> Cinnamon's essential oils qualify it as an "anti-microbial" food, and cinnamon has been studied for its ability to help stop the growth of bacteria as well as fungi, including the commonly problematic yeast Candida. When added to food it is a natural preservative.

Directions
Preheat oven to 350º. If using fresh pumpkin/squash, cut up and cook for 15 minutes in a covered pot with a little water, then blend in a blender until smooth. Set aside. In a large bowl, mix eggs, honey, milk, oil, water, and pumpkin. Combine flour, baking soda, salt and cinnamon in a bowl and then stir into the egg-pumpkin mixture. With a hand mixer, beat for 3 minutes. Spoon into an oil-sprayed muffin pan or into paper muffin cups. Bake 40 to 45 minutes or until a toothpick inserted in the center comes out clean.

Ingredients to Consider on Specific Diets

Gluten & Casein Free............... Yes
Phenol Free............................ No
Low Oxalate Diet .... Yes (if you use coconut flour, hemp or rice milk)
Specific Carbohydrate Diet .... Yes (if you use almond milk)
This recipe is also Soy free, Corn free and Rice free (use hemp or almond milk)

Oral Motor Rating 😊 😊

Breakfast Muffins

Yields: 12 Muffins

Ingredients

1 1/4 cups brown rice flour
1 cup coconut flour
1/2 cup ground flax seed (flax meal)
 or hemp seeds
1 1/2 teaspoons xanthan gum
1 1/2 teaspoons baking soda
1 teaspoon sea salt
1/2 cup honey or maple syrup
1 1/4 cups rice milk
1/4 cup safflower, coconut, or grape seed oil
1 teaspoon gluten-free vanilla extract
1 lemon, grated lemon peel
1 1/4 cups mashed banana, or finely
 chopped pear or apple

> *Hemp Seeds*
>
> *Hemp seeds contain all the essential amino acids and a balanced ratio of omega 6 to omega 3. They can be eaten raw, sprouted, made into hemp milk, and used in baking. Flaxseed has ample amounts of omega 3 essential fatty acids, amino acids, and high dietary fiber.*

Directions

Preheat oven to 325º. Use a standard 12-cup muffin tin and line with paper liners or oil. In large bowl, combine flours, flax meal, xanthan gum, baking soda, salt, and honey. Mix well, and set aside. In medium bowl, add together milk, oil, vanilla, and lemon peel. Stir liquid mixture into dry ingredients. Gently fold fruit into batter, which will be the consistency of thick cake batter. Distribute batter evenly among tins. Bake for 35 minutes or until toothpick inserted in center comes out clean. Remove from oven. While muffins are still warm, brush with a mixture of honey and lemon juice.

Ingredients to Consider on Specific Diets

Gluten & Casein Free ....Yes	Phenol Free ....Yes (if you use maple syrup)
Low Oxalate Diet..Yes	Specific Carbohydrate Diet ....No

This recipe is also Soy free, Corn free, but is not Rice free

Oral Motor Rating 😊 😊

Jam Muffins

Yields: 6 Muffins

Ingredients
1 cup rice, almond, or hemp seed flour
1/2 cup ground flax seed
2 tablespoons honey or maple syrup
2 tablespoons baking soda
1 teaspoon sea salt
1 egg or egg replacer
6 tablespoons coconut oil
5 tablespoons no-sugar fruit jam (All Fruit)

> **All Fruit**
>
> *Jelly, jam and preserves are all made from fruit mixed with sugar and pectin. Instead use All-Fruit jams as they are sweetened only with fruit and fruit juice and they are 100% all natural.*

Directions
Preheat oven to 400º. Oil muffin tin, or use liners In a large bowl, blend flour, baking soda and salt. In a small bowl, mix egg, oil, honey, and fruit jam and add to the flour mixture in large bowl to make a batter. Fill a muffin tin with batter and bake for 25 minutes or until toothpick comes out clean.

Ingredients to Consider on Specific Diets

Gluten & Casein Free .... Yes
Phenol Free .... Yes (if you use hemp seed flour and maple syrup as sweetener)
Low Oxalate Diet .... Yes (if you use rice flour or hemp seed flour)
Specific Carbohydrate Diet .... No

This recipe is also Soy free, Corn free and Rice free (use almond flour hemp seed flour)

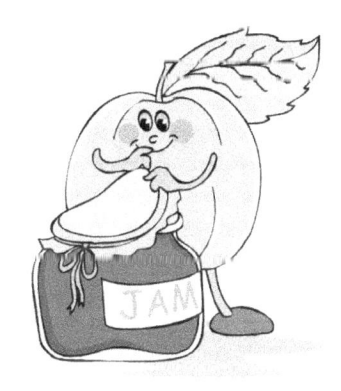

Oral Motor Rating 😊 😊

Brown Pear Muffins

Yields: 6 Muffins

Ingredients
1 cup brown rice flour
1/4 cup honey or maple syrup
1 1/2 teaspoons sea salt
1 teaspoon ground flaxseed
2 teaspoons baking powder
1 teaspoon xanthan gum
2 eggs or egg replacer
1 3/4 cup water
1/2 cup safflower, coconut, or rice bran oil
8 ounces canned pear sauce

> ***Ground Flaxseed***
> *Flaxseed can be used for its fiber content as well as a source of omega 3 fatty acids.*

Directions
Preheat oven to 400º. Oil muffin tin or use liners. In a small bowl, mix all dry ingredients. In another small bowl, blend eggs, water, honey, oil, and pear sauce. Mix with dry ingredients to form a batter. Pour batter into muffin tin. Bake for 25 minutes. Remove the muffins from tray when cool.

Ingredients to Consider on Specific Diets

Gluten & Casein Free ....Yes	Phenol Free ....Yes (if you use maple syrup)
Low Oxalate Diet..Yes	Specific Carbohydrate Diet ....No

This recipe is also Soy free, Corn free, but is not Rice free

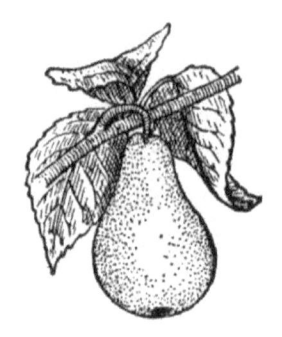

Oral Motor Rating 😊 😊

Mini Squash Muffins

Yields: 6 Mini Muffins

Ingredients
- 1 cup acorn or butternut squash, peeled and chopped in large chunks
- 1 cup almond or coconut flour, or a combination of both
- 3 eggs or egg replacer
- 1/2 cup coconut milk
- 2 tablespoons coconut, safflower, or sunflower oil
- 2 tablespoons honey or maple syrup
- 1/4 teaspoon cinnamon or nutmeg

> *Nutmeg*
> Nutmeg is used in small amounts. It can reduce flatulence, aid digestion, improve the appetite and treat diarrhea, vomiting and nausea.

Directions
Preheat oven to 300º. Grease a mini-muffin tin. Combine all ingredients in a food processor or blender and process just until smooth. Spoon batter into the muffin cups, filling cups only halfway. Bake 30 to 40 minutes until muffins rise from the sides of the pan and appear dry and browned around the edges. Carefully cut around the edges and lift out. (This is a good snack option for school.)

Ingredients to Consider on Specific Diets

Gluten & Casein Free	Yes
Phenol Free	Yes (if you use coconut flour and maple syrup as sweetner)
Low Oxalate Diet	Yes (if you use coconut flour)
Specific Carbohydrate Diet	Yes (if you use honey as a sweetener)

This recipe is also Soy free, Sugar free, Corn free and Rice free

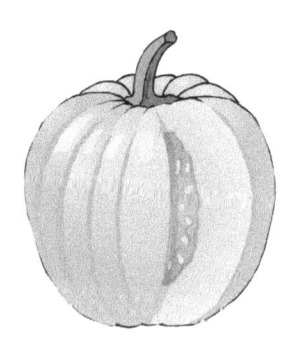

Oral Motor Rating ☺ ☺

Tropical Muffins

Yields: 6 Mini Muffins

Ingredients

3 eggs (egg substitute) or egg replacer
4 tablespoons coconut oil
6 tablespoons pineapple or orange juice
4 tablespoons honey
1/2 teaspoon sea salt
1/2 teaspoon vanilla (optional)
1/2 cup coconut flour
1 tablespoon baking soda
1/2 teaspoon xanthan gum (optional)
1 cup pineapple, blueberries, mango, or cranberries, chopped

Fruits in the Recipe

In this recipe, dried fruits have been used for convenience. Fresh fruits can also be used if available. Choose the fruit your child can best tolerate.

Directions

Preheat oven to 400º. Mix first six ingredients in a bowl. Combine flour, baking soda, and xanthan gum (if using), and add to bowl. Mix thoroughly, and then add fruit of choice. Pour into lined muffin cups and bake for 15 minutes.

Ingredients to Consider on Specific Diets

Gluten & Casein Free .... Yes
Phenol Free .... No
Low Oxalate Diet .... Yes (moderate, as fruits are all in moderate range)
Specific Carbohydrate Diet .... Yes (omit xanthum gum)
This recipe is also Soy free, Corn free and Rice free

Oral Motor Rating 😊 😊 😊

EGG OR OMELET RECIPES

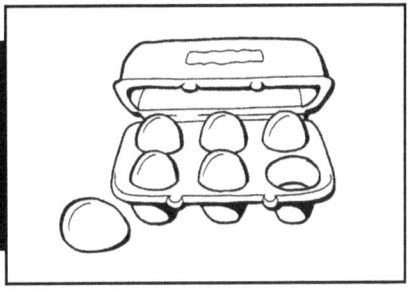

Soft Boiled Eggs

Yields: 2 Servings

Ingredients
2 eggs, free range organic
1/2 teaspoon apple cider vinegar
2 cups water
Salt to taste

> **Eggs**
> *Choose fresh, free-range eggs as they have up to 5 times more vitamin D than caged commercial eggs. They also have 2/3 more vitamin A, 2 times more omega-3 fatty acids, 3 times more vitamin E, and 7 times more beta carotene.*

Directions
Bring two eggs to room temperature. Fill a small saucepan with water at least three inches deep in order to cover the eggs. Add a little salt and vinegar to the water, which will help the eggs to hold their shape. Heat until boiling, and then reduce to simmer. Crack the eggs into a small cup or bowl and gently lower them into the water. Immediately cover and turn off the heat. For a medium firm yolk, allow eggs to stand for 3 minutes. Remove with a slotted spoon and serve. Add salt to taste and serve.

Ingredients to Consider on Specific Diets

Gluten & Casein Free ....Yes	Phenol Free ....Yes
Low Oxalate Diet ....Yes	Specific Carbohydrate Diet ....Yes

This recipe is also Soy free, Corn free and Rice free

Oral Motor Rating 😊 😊 😊 😊

Soft Scrambled Eggs

Yield: 2 Servings

Ingredients
1 onion, chopped
1 tablespoon olive oil, ghee or coconut oil
4 eggs
1/2 cup almond or hemp seed milk
1 teaspoon sea salt or pepper

Optional Variations: Add any vegetables, soy cheese, rice cheese, or meats.

> ### Casein-Free Cheese
> *There are dairy free cheeses that are rice and soy based, available in a variety of flavors. They can be found in the dairy section or the Kosher sections at natural foods stores. Caution: These cheeses can have casein in the ingredients. Read the label carefully.*

Directions
In a medium sized bowl, mix eggs, seasonings, and almond, rice or hemp seed milk. Melt oil/ghee in a frying pan, over medium low heat. Add chopped onion, and saute until soft. Pour egg mixture into the pan. Using a flexible spatula, scrape eggs toward the center as they begin to stick. When eggs are not quite done, remove the pan from the heat, and return to the bowl, letting them cook in their own heat for a minute or two.

Note: This low-heat method and taking care not to overcook the eggs will ensure that the protein will be digested. Served with cultured veggies, they digest even better.

Ingredients to Consider on Specific Diets

Gluten & Casein Free	Yes
Phenol Free	Yes (if you use hemp or rice milk)
Low Oxalate Diet	Yes (if you use hemp or rice milk)
Specific Carbohydrate Diet	Yes (if you use almond milk)

This recipe is also Soy free, Corn free and Rice free (if you do not use any cheese)

Oral Motor Rating 🙂 🙂

Zucchini Omelet

Yields: 2 Servings

Ingredients
1 zucchini, small
1 tablespoon coconut or grape seed oil
2 eggs
1/2 cup goat cheese, grated

> ### *Goat's Milk*
> *When individuals have sensitivity to cow's milk, goat's milk can sometimes be used as an alternative.*
>
> *Goats' milk does have casein, but still it is the easiest for humans to digest because goat milk proteins are most similar to the protein found in human milk.*

Directions
Peel and finely grate a small zucchini. In a small frying pan, saute grated zucchini in oil for a few minutes. Lightly beat 2 eggs and add to pan. Cook and stir till done and then pat down in pan and top with grated goat cheese. Turn off heat and cover pan for a minute so that cheese can melt well. Salt to taste and enjoy.

Ingredients to Consider on Specific Diets

Gluten & Casein Free	No
Phenol Free	No
Low Oxalate Diet	Yes
Specific Carbohydrate Diet	Yes

This recipe is also Soy free, Corn free and Rice free

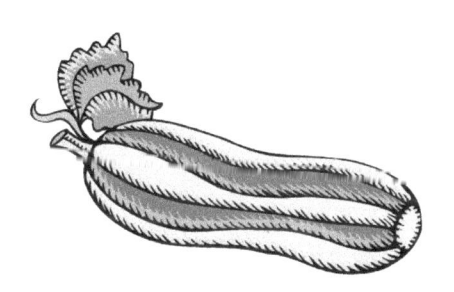

Oral Motor Rating ☺ ☺ ☺ ☺

Egg Rolls

Yields: 6 Small Rolls

Ingredients
4 tablespoons grape seed oil or olive oil
4 eggs
1/2 cup rice or almond milk
1/2 teaspoon sea salt
1 onion, chopped in small pieces
1/4 cup cauliflower, grated 1 small red pepper, diced
1/4 cup mung bean sprouts (optional)

> **Sprouts**
>
> *Sprouts contain a high source of fiber, are easily digestible and contain a high concentration of enzymes facilitating the digestive process, so they can prove beneficial for children with ASD.*

Directions
In a small bowl, combine eggs, milk and salt. Beat well. Heat 1-2 tablespoons of oil in a medium sized frying pan. Pour eggs into pan, making six small omelets. When just beginning to set, flip and cook for another minute. Set aside. In another frying pan, heat 1-2 tablespoons of oil and saute the chopped vegetables until soft. Spoon the vegetables onto the center of each omelet and carefully roll up. Cut and serve.

Ingredients to Consider on Specific Diets

Gluten & Casein Free .... Yes
Phenol Free .... Yes (if you use rice milk)
Low Oxalate Diet .... Yes (if you use rice milk)
Specific Carbohydrate Diet .... Yes (if you use almond milk)
This recipe is also Soy free, Corn free and Rice free (use almond milk)
Oral Motor Rating 😊 😊 😊

Coconut Omelet

Yields: 1 Serving

Ingredients
1 egg, free range organic
1 teaspoon honey or maple syrup
2 tablespoons coconut flakes

> ### *Coconut Flakes*
> *Freeze-dried coconut flakes should be the choice in this recipe as they have a very sweet taste and contain no preservatives or chemical additives.*

Directions
Beat egg and honey together, add coconut flakes and mix well. Prepare as pancakes.

Ingredients to Consider on Specific Diets

Gluten & Casein Free .... Yes
Phenol Free .... Yes (if you omit honey)
Low Oxalate Diet .... Yes
Specific Carbohydrate Diet .... Yes

This recipe is also Soy free, Corn free and Rice free

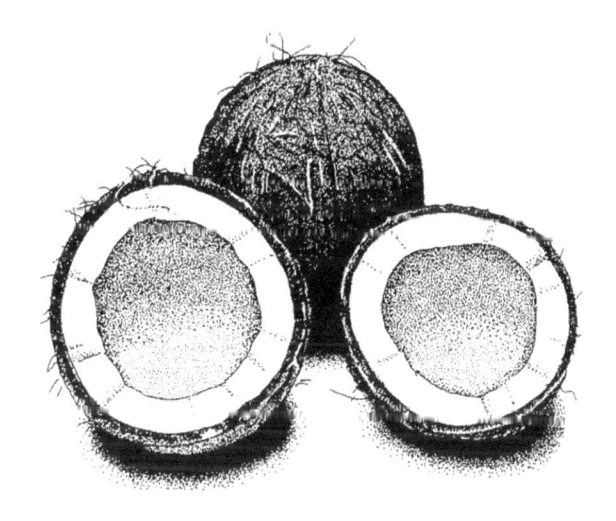

Oral Motor Rating 😊 😊 😊

CHAPTER 10: BREAKFAST RECIPES

MISCELLANEOUS

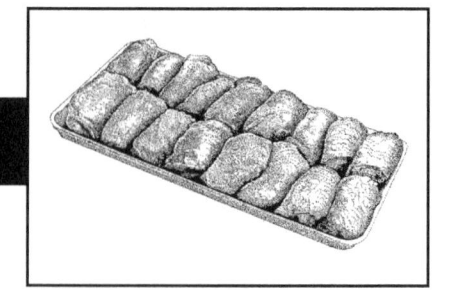

Breakfast Spring Rolls

Yields: 4 Servings

Ingredients
- 1 packet rice stick noodles
- 1/2 pound chicken breast, turkey, bacon or other breakfast meat
- 2 tablespoons sesame oil
- 1 small bunch of parsley
- 1 small bunch cilantro
- 1/2 teaspoon sea salt
- 1 packet rice paper spring roll wrappers (check to make sure they are rice flour only)

> ### Rice Paper
> *Rice paper usually refers to paper made from parts of the rice plant, like rice straw or rice flour. Edible rice paper is used for making fried spring rolls. Ingredients of the food rice paper include white rice flour, tapioca flour, salt, and water.*

Directions
Cook the rice noodles in a large pot of salted boiling water for 3-4 minutes until tender but not mushy (add a little oil). Rinse with cold water and set aside. To prepare chicken or other meat of choice, heat a skillet and cook in sesame oil for 5 to 10 minutes, and then dice into small cubes. Pick the leaves off the parsley and cilantro and discard stems. Chop into medium sized pieces, sprinkle with a little salt, and set aside. Spread about 1/4 cup of noodles across the bottom third of each wrapper, leaving a little space empty at each end. Spread small amount of salted parsley and cilantro mixture on top of the noodles and lay several small cubes of meat on top of that. Roll the wrapper firmly over the chicken and noodles and tuck in the ends as you continue to roll it up. The roll should be tight — you will be cutting them in half to serve and you do not want your filling to fall out. Cover your finished rolls with a towel while you continue to roll more. These should not be made too far in advance — a couple of hours at most. Just before serving, fry briefly in skillet with oil to make them crispy. Drain on paper towels.

Ingredients to Consider on Specific Diets

Gluten & Casein Free .... Yes	Phenol Free .... Yes
Low Oxalate Diet .... Yes (if you use basil instead of parsley)	Specific Carbohydrate Diet ...... No

This recipe is also Soy free, and Corn free, but is not Rice free

Oral Motor Rating 😊 😊 😊 😊

Hot Breakfast Porridge

Yields: 4 Smaller Servings

Ingredients
2 cups water
1 cup amaranth, quinoa, or millet
1/4 teaspoon sea salt
1 teaspoon honey or maple syrup
1/2 teaspoon cinnamon powder (optional)
2 teaspoons vanilla flavoring (optional)
1 tablespoon of BodyBio Balance Oil

> **Amaranth**
> *Amaranth is high in protein, particularly in the amino acid, lysine, which is low in the cereal grains. In fact, amaranth has the highest lysine content of all the grains in one study, with quinoa coming in a close second.*

Directions
Bring water to boil in a one quart saucepan over medium-high heat. Add the grain, sea salt, xylitol and cinnamon, if desired. Cover and reduce heat to very low. Simmer for 10 minutes. Remove from heat and allow to cool slightly before adding vanilla flavor (optional), BodyBio Balance Oil. Serve at once.

Ingredients to Consider on Specific Diets

Gluten & Casein Free	Yes	Phenol Free	Yes (omit honey)
Low Oxalate Diet	Yes	Specific Carbohydrate Diet	No

This recipe is also Soy free, Corn free and Rice free

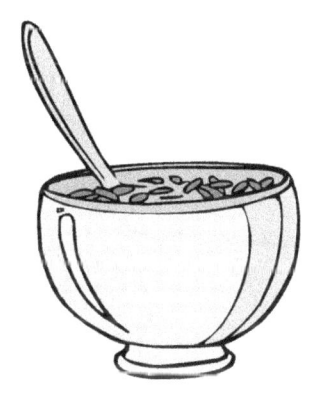

Oral Motor Rating 🙂 🙂

CHAPTER 10: BREAKFAST RECIPES

Carrot Cutlets

Yields: 4 Small Cutlets

Ingredients
1 1/2 cups baby carrots
1/2 cup chickpea, almond or other nut flour
4 eggs or egg replacer
1 teaspoon vanilla
1 teaspoon cinnamon (optional)
1/4 teaspoon sea salt

> **Nutritious Tip**
> *The water drained from carrots can be used in soups and stews, as it retains important nutrients.*

Directions
Cook carrots until well done, drain (reserving water), and then squeeze out as much water as possible. Mash carrots; add all other ingredients and mix until smooth. Form mixture into four cutlets and fry in a skillet using a small amount of oil. Drain on paper towels and serve.

Ingredients to Consider on Specific Diets

Gluten & Casein Free	Yes
Phenol Free	Yes (if you use chickpea flour)
Low Oxalate Diet	Yes (if you use chickpea flour)
Specific Carbohydrate Diet	Yes (if you use almond flour)

This recipe is also Soy free, Corn free and Rice free

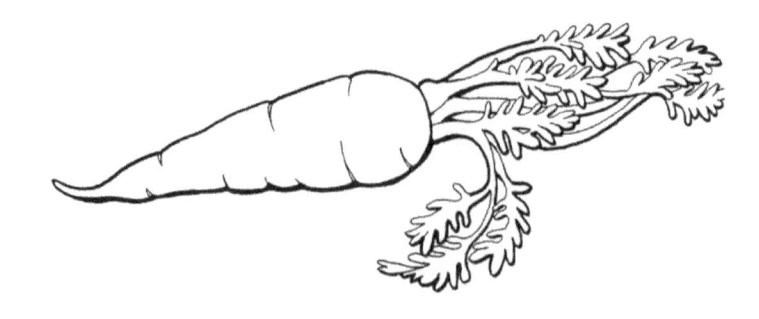

Oral Motor Rating 😊 😊

HEALING AUTISM IN THE KITCHEN

French Toast

Yields: 6 Slices Of Toast

Ingredients
2 large eggs, beaten
1/2 cup almond milk or rice milk
6 slices gluten and casein free bread
2 tablespoons coconut oil/ghee

> **Gluten-Free Breads**
> *There are many healthy GFCF breads available; opt for breads that have no yeast or any other allergens in the loaf.*

Directions
Combine eggs and milk. Dip each piece of bread in egg mixture to coat both sides. Sauté in oil/ghee coated pan over medium heat until golden brown on both sides. Note: As an alternative to overly sweet syrups, try any of the following on top of pancakes, waffles and French toast: naturally sweetened apple sauce, natural maple syrup, agave syrup, or All Fruit spreads.

Ingredients to Consider on Specific Diets

Gluten & Casein Free .... Yes
Phenol Free .... Yes (if you use rice milk)
Low Oxalate Diet .... Yes (if you use rice milk)
Specific Carbohydrate Diet .... Yes (if you use almond milk)
This recipe is also Soy free, Corn free and Rice free (use almond milk)

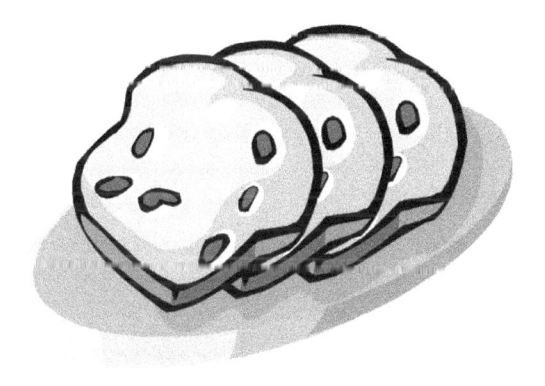

Oral Motor Rating :) :) :)

Almond Coconut Granola

Yields: 6 Granola Bars

Ingredients

3 cups puffed rice or millet cereal
1 cup coconut, shredded
1 cup almonds, sliced or finely chopped
2 tablespoons coconut oil
1/3 cup honey
1 cup dried cranberries or blueberries
1 teaspoon gluten-free and casein-free vanilla (optional)

> *Coconut Oil*
>
> *Flavorful and easy to digest, coconut oil and shredded coconut are pleasant additives to cereal.*

Directions

In a large bowl, combine all ingredients and store in the refrigerator.

Fat-Free: Replace oil and honey mixture with 2/3 cup defrosted frozen organic apple juice concentrate and 2 teaspoons of vanilla.

Ingredients to Consider on Specific Diets

Gluten & Casein Free .... Yes
Phenol Free .... No
Low Oxalate Diet .... Yes (moderate to high due to almonds)
Specific Carbohydrate Diet .... No

This recipe is also Soy free, Corn free and Rice free (if you use millet cereal)

Oral Motor Rating 😊 😊 😊 😊

Quick Creamy Cereal or Pudding

Yields: 1 Serving

Ingredients
3/4 cup water
1/4 cup rice, quinoa or millet cereal
1/8 teaspoon sea salt
2 tablespoons protein powder
1 tablespoon BodyBio Balance oil,
   (4:1 ratio of omega-6 and 3)

> ### *Rise and Shine*
> *Rise and Shine is cereal made with organic brown rice grits. Organic Quinoa Flakes cereal can also be used.*

Directions
Bring water to a boil in a saucepan. Add cereal and salt, stirring constantly. Reduce heat, cover and simmer for about 2 minutes. Serve in a bowl, let it cool down, add oil and protein powder and serve.

Ingredients to Consider on Specific Diets

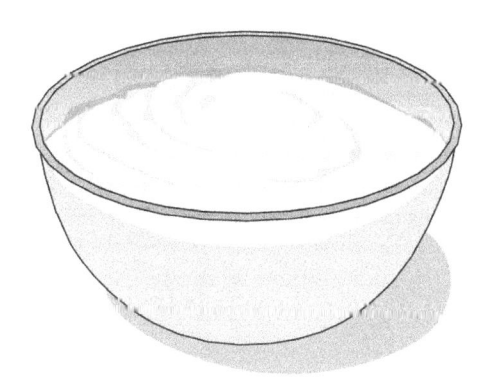

Gluten & Casein Free ....Yes	Phenol Free ....Yes
Low Oxalate Diet ....Yes	Specific Carbohydrate Diet .... No

This recipe is also Soy free, and Corn free and Rice free (if you use quinoa or millet cereal)

Oral Motor Rating 😊 😊

Hash Brown Casserole

Yields: 4 to 6 Servings

Ingredients

- 4 cups gluten-free and casein-free organic frozen hash browns, thawed, (shredded or cubed)
- 1 pound gluten-free and casein-free bacon, chopped into 1-inch pieces
- 2 small onions, chopped
- 1 cup fresh mushrooms, sliced
- 1 teaspoon sea salt
- 1/4 teaspoon garlic salt
- 1/2 teaspoon pepper
- 4 eggs or egg replacer
- 1 1/2 cups hemp seed or nut milk
- Grated cheese (optional)

> ### Bacon
> *When bacon is cooked, its fat naturally melts, releasing highly flavorful grease. Bacon grease is traditionally used as an all-purpose flavoring for everything from gravy to cornbread to salad dressing. Bacon should be a no nitrate variety from a free range source.*

Directions

Preheat oven to 375º. Grease a 9x13" baking dish or pan. Place potatoes in the prepared dish. Cook bacon until brown and drain. Set aside. In 1 tablespoon bacon fat, fry onions and mushrooms until tender. Sprinkle with the seasonings. Top potatoes with the fried onions, mushrooms, bacon and spread well. Beat eggs and milk and pour over casserole. Top with cheese if desired, or sprinkle with paprika. Bake uncovered for 45 minutes or until middle is set.

Ingredients to Consider on Specific Diets

Gluten & Casein Free ....Yes	Phenol Free ....Yes
Low Oxalate Diet..................Yes	Specific Carbohydrate Diet ....No

This recipe is also Soy free, Corn free and Rice free

Oral Motor Rating 😊 😊 😊 😊

Chapter Eleven

The Main Course

Lunch and Dinner Recipes

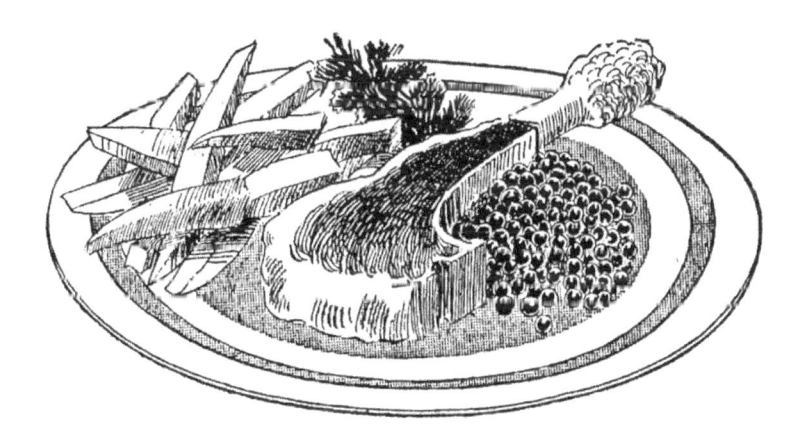

PARENTS STRIVE TO KEEP THEIR CHILDREN healthy. As their school-aged children go through remarkable physical and mental changes, food intake is the most critical aspect to their growth and development. Research shows that nutritious foods make children healthier, more emotionally stable, and improves their school performance. This is especially true of special needs children who have sometimes tremendous stress placed in their everyday living.

The time-honored tradition of breakfast, lunch, and dinner seems to be the best way to ensure a balanced diet. Lunch is typically not eaten at home during the week in the U.S., so it is important to pack a lunch that your child will enjoy eating while also providing a variety of different nutritious foods.

For many families, eating dinner together has become a lost art. The family dinner is a crucial time for for reconnecting with those we love. Over a simple dinner of scrambled eggs or a more elaborate meal, important things happen. Relationships are strengthened, news of the day is exchanged and upcoming events are planned and discussed. This all takes place in the kitchen where meals are prepared.

Many children prefer to do their homework in the kitchen while dinner is being prepared, just so they can be around their parents at this time of day. The kitchen is often the hub of the entire household. Thus we titled this book *Healing Autism in the Kitchen,* as healing and nourishment take on many forms, the most important of which is food.

THE MAIN COURSE –
LUNCH AND DINNER RECIPES
TABLE OF CONTENTS

VEGETARIAN MEALS

Stuffed Acorn Squash 225
Pizza Crust 226
Brussels Sprouts 227
Sautéed Broccoli 228
Alkaline Coleslaw 229
Dutch Style Red Cabbage 230
Sautéed Kale with Garlic 231
Baked Butternut Squash 232
Spaghetti Squash 233
Cinnamon Baby Carrots with Roasted Sesame Seeds 234
Quinoa Pilaf 235
Simmered Greens 236
Sautéed Snow Peas with Ginger and Onion 237
Roasted Potatoes with Garlic and Rosemary 238
Easy Pressure-Cooked Vegetables 239
Creamed Peas and Potatoes 240
Red Bell Peppers Stuffed With Millet 241
Creamy Macaroni (Mac & Cheese) 242
Hummus-Stuffed Portobello Caps 243
Roasted Mixed Vegetables 244
Artichoke Pate Roll-Ups 245
Vegetable Fried Rice 246

NON-VEGETARIAN MEALS

Beefy Spinach with Mushrooms 247
Meat Loaf 248
Turkey Meatballs 249

Baked Turkey Patties	250
Turkey Burgers with Sweet Mustard Sauce	251
Spinach Tofu or Chicken Curry	252
Chicken Patties	253
Salmon Patties	254
Chicken Teriyaki with Broccoli	255
Spaghetti Carbonara	256
Chicken Nuggets	257
Turkey or Chicken Lettuce Wraps	258
Chicken Breasts Roasted in Fresh Garden Herbs	259
Broccoli Beef	260
Quick Chicken Vegetable Stir-Fry	261
Spaghetti with Meat Sauce	262
Sesame Chicken Wings	263
Avocado Meatloaf	264
Chicken Chow Mein	265
Deep-Fried Shrimp	266
Tandoori Chicken	267

VEGETARIAN MEALS

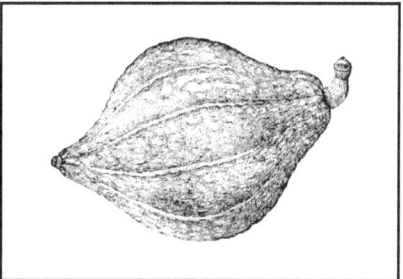

Stuffed Acorn Squash

Yields: 2 Servings

Ingredients
2 acorn squash (1 to 1 1/2 lbs. each)
1 large tart red apple, diced
2 tablespoons pine nuts, water chestnuts or walnuts, finely chopped
2 tablespoons maple sugar or honey
1 tablespoon ghee, sunflower oil or melted coconut butter

> *Acorn squash*
>
> *Acorn is a winter squash. It can be baked, stuffed and baked, or steamed, and the flesh can easily be pureed for adding to soups, making it a healthy addition to a child's diet.*

Directions
Preheat oven to 350º. Cut each squash in half lengthwise. Remove the seeds and fibers. Place the squash with the cut side up in an ungreased pan. Bake for 30 minutes. In a small mixing bowl, combine the apple, pine nuts, maple sugar or honey and melted butter or oil. Spoon this mixture into the squash halves. Return the squash to the oven and continue baking for 30 minutes longer or until the squash is tender.

Ingredients to Consider on Specific Diets

Gluten & Casein Free .... Yes
Phenol Free .... Yes (you use pine nuts or walnuts & maple sugar)
Low Oxalate Diet .... Yes (use pine nuts or walnuts)
Specific Carbohydrate Diet .... Yes (use honey as sweetener)
This recipe is also Soy free, Corn free and Rice free

Oral Motor Rating 😊 😊 😊 😊

CHAPTER 11: THE MAIN COURSE

Pizza Crust

Yields: 3 to 4 Servings

Ingredients
1 cup garbanzo bean flour
1 cup brown rice flour
2 teaspoons baking soda
2 teaspoons sea salt
1 teaspoon oregano
1 teaspoon xanthan gum
1/2 cup water
3 teaspoons olive oil

> ### *Pizza Topping*
> *Vegetables or meat can be added as topping. For extra protein, add a beaten egg on top and bake until pizza is set. (This looks like cheese.) You can also add casein-free cheese.*

Directions
Combine water and oil, and mix in all dry ingredients to make soft dough. Knead in bowl 12 times. Grease a cookie sheet with olive oil, and roll or pat out the dough into a thin 11 or 12-inch circle or rectangle. Turn up edges of dough to form a little rim. Bake in a 425º oven for 8 to 10 minutes or until partially baked and starting to brown. Remove from oven and lower oven temperature to 350º. Add your choice of toppings.

Topping Ideas
Pizza is a good way to sneak in vegetables. Shred or puree just about anything into GFCF sauce and kids won't notice. Use plain tomato sauce and a few seasonings children can tolerate. Top with veggies sauce and cooked meat; then add the secret ingredient to the top (a beaten egg — just pour it on top of everything). Bake the pizza at 350º until the egg is set. It sounds weird, but it keeps the toppings on and looks a lot like cheese.

Ingredients to Consider on Specific Diets

Gluten & Casein Free ....Yes	Phenol Free ....Yes
Low Oxalate Diet..........................Yes	Specific Carbohydrate Diet ....No

This recipe is also Soy free, and Corn free, but is not Rice free

Oral Motor Rating 😊 😊 😊 😊

Brussels Sprouts

Yields: 3 to 4 Servings

Ingredients
1-2 tablespoons coconut, olive, or grape seed oil
1 onion, sliced thin slices
3 garlic cloves, chopped
1 pound fresh brussels sprouts
1/3 cup walnuts or pecans, finely chopped

> **Brussels sprouts**
> *Brussels sprouts are a rich source of vitamins and minerals. Cooked brussels sprouts go well with a little olive oil, walnuts, and black pepper.*

Directions
In a frying pan, add oil and sauté onion and garlic. Wash and cut brussels sprouts (in half or pieces). After onion begins to brown and caramelize, add brussels sprouts and nuts and cook until brussels sprouts have browned a bit. Add 1/8 cup of water and cook for 20 to 30 minutes on low heat till sprouts are tender.

Ingredients to Consider on Specific Diets

Gluten & Casein Free .... Yes
Phenol Free .... Yes (if you use pecans)
Low Oxalate Diet .... Yes (if you use pecans)
Specific Carbohydrate Diet .... Yes
This recipe is also Soy free, Corn free and Rice free

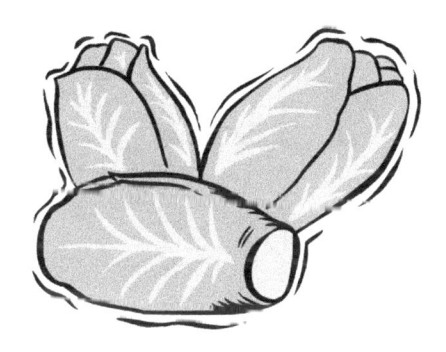

Oral Motor Rating 😊 😊 😊 😊

Sautéed Broccoli

Yields: 2 Servings

Ingredients
1 cup fresh broccoli
1 teaspoon sesame or olive oil
2 garlic cloves, minced
1/4 cup water
1 tablespoon BodyBio Balance Oil
   or tamari 1 teaspoon sesame seeds
   (optional)

Quick Recipe
This is a simple and quick recipe. You can also substitute broccoli with any vegetables kids like.

Directions
Cut off the broccoli heads and then cut the stems to make small pieces for stir-frying. Heat a fry pan, add oil, garlic, and vegetables and quickly stir-fry till done. Add water and tamari, mix well, and serve with a topping of sesame seeds, if desired.

Ingredients to Consider on Specific Diets

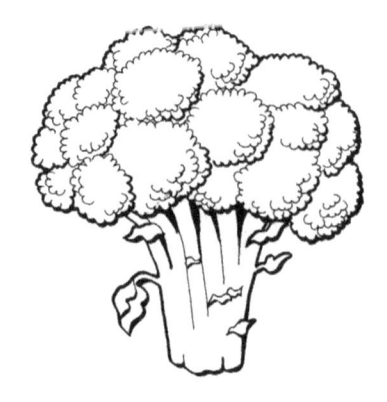

Gluten & Casein Free ....Yes	Phenol Free ....Yes
Low Oxalate Diet ....Yes	Specific Carbohydrate Diet ....Yes

This recipe is also Soy free, Corn free and Rice free

Oral Motor Rating 😊 😊 😊 😊

Alkaline Coleslaw

Yields: 4 Servings

Ingredients
1 small head of green cabbage, shredded
2 medium-size carrots, shredded
1/2 small red onion, sliced thinly
1/2 cup parsley or basil, chopped
1/2 teaspoon sea salt
Dash cayenne pepper
1/4 teaspoon celery seeds
1/2 tablespoon lime juice, fresh
2 tablespoons olive oil, cold pressed
1 cup coconut milk
   (fresh coconut blended together with water from the coconut)

> *Coconut Milk*
>
> *Coconut milk is a blend of coconut water and coconut cream resulting in a wonderful milk emulsion.*
>
> ***Caution:*** *Look for canned coconut milk that does not contain some kind of binder, such as carrageen.*

Directions
Combine all ingredients in a bowl except the coconut milk. Mix well, then pour coconut milk over the salad and mix again. Let it sit for a while. It will taste even better after all the flavors blend together by sitting overnight in the refrigerator.

Ingredients to Consider on Specific Diets

Gluten & Casein Free .... Yes
Phenol Free .... Yes (if use parsley and avoid basil)
Low Oxalate Diet .... Yes (if use basil and avoid parsley)
Specific Carbohydrate Diet .... Yes
This recipe is also Soy free, Corn free and Rice free

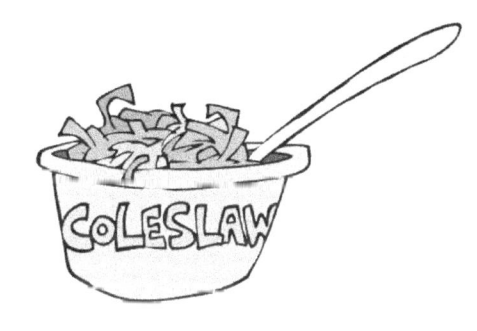

Oral Motor Rating ☺ ☺ ☺ ☺

Dutch Style Red Cabbage

Yields: 4 Servings

Ingredients
1 red cabbage, medium size
1 small onion, chopped
1 teaspoon orange zest (orange rind grated)
4 ounces orange juice
1 garlic clove, finely chopped
1 teaspoon sea salt
1 tablespoon raw honey or maple syrup
3 tablespoons apple cider vinegar
4 tablespoons ghee, olive oil, or grape seed oil

Red Cabbage
Red cabbage has a slightly stronger flavor than green cabbage and takes longer to cook. It is very appetizing in salads. Raw cabbage is rich in vitamin C.

Directions
Shred cabbage and set aside. Combine onion, orange zest, orange juice, chopped garlic, salt, honey and vinegar. Pour over cabbage and mix well. Marinate overnight and toss occasionally. Melt butter or oil in a frying pan, add marinated cabbage mixture, and bring to a low boil. Reduce heat and simmer uncovered for about an hour, or until liquid has evaporated and cabbage is tender.

Ingredients to Consider on Specific Diets

Gluten & Casein Free	Yes
Phenol Free	No
Low Oxalate Diet	Yes
Specific Carbohydrate Diet	Yes

This recipe is also Soy free, Corn free and Rice free

Oral Motor Rating ☺ ☺ ☺ ☺

Sautéed Kale with Garlic

Yields: 4 Servings

Ingredients
2 tablespoons coconut oil or olive oil
1 large bunch of organic kale, coarsely chopped
3 or 4 cloves garlic, coarsely chopped
Sea salt to taste

> ### Kale
> *Kale is a dark green leafy vegetable, rich in calcium, iron and carotenoids. It has a milder flavor than mustard greens, so can be easily shredded and added to soups or a meatball mix.*

Directions
Heat oil in large skillet and add kale, garlic and sea salt. Sauté on low heat until kale is wilted. Reduce heat even further, cover skillet, and continue to let kale "sweat" in its own juice until it is tender (about 25 minutes). Serve hot.

Ingredients to Consider on Specific Diets

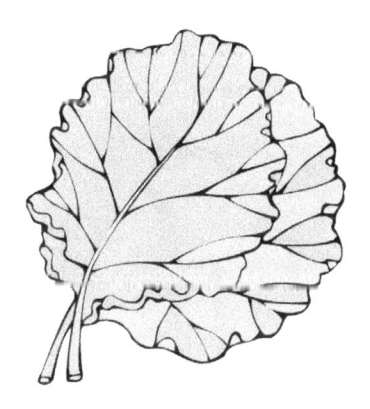

Gluten & Casein Free ....Yes	Phenol Free ....Yes
Low Oxalate Diet ....No	Specific Carbohydrate Diet ....Yes

This recipe is also Soy free, Corn free and Rice free

Oral Motor Rating 😊 😊 😊 😊

Baked Butternut Squash

Yields: 4 to 6 Servings

Ingredients
3 butternut squash
3 eggs, lightly beaten, or egg replacer
1/4 teaspoon nutmeg
3/4 cup pecans, finely chopped
1 teaspoon sea salt
1/2 teaspoon cracked pepper
2 tablespoons butter, ghee, or coconut oil

> **Nutmeg**
> *Nutmeg used in small amounts aids in digestion and improves appetite.*

Directions
Preheat oven to 350º. Cut squash in half; remove the seeds, and place cut side down in a baking pan with one-half inch of water added to the pan. Bake until tender (approx one hour). Scoop out squash and add to a food processor along with the eggs, nutmeg, pecans and seasonings and blend until smooth. Pour puree in an oven-proof serving dish and drizzle the ghee or oil over the top. Bake for about 30 minutes. Serve warm.

Ingredients to Consider on Specific Diets

Gluten & Casein Free ....Yes	Phenol Free ....Yes
Low Oxalate Diet........................Yes	Specific Carbohydrate Diet ....Yes

This recipe is also Soy free, Corn free and Rice free

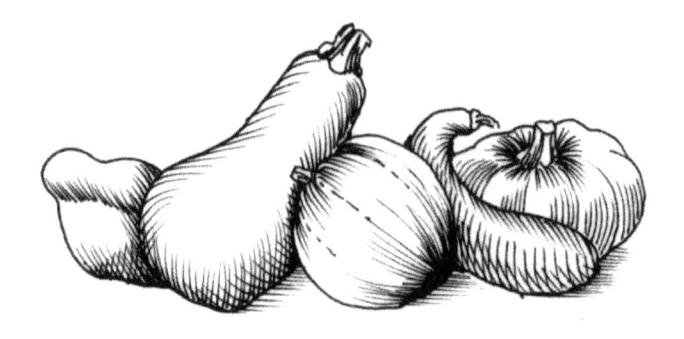

Oral Motor Rating 😊 😊

Spaghetti Squash

Yields: 4 Servings

Ingredients
1 large spaghetti squash, cooked
2 medium onions, chopped
4 tablespoons olive oil
1/2 cup chopped canned tomatoes
1 clove minced garlic
1/2 teaspoon thyme
2 teaspoons dried basil
  (or 2 tablespoons fresh, finely chopped)
1 teaspoon dried oregano
1/4 cup parsley, finely chopped
1 tablespoon ghee, melted
1 cup ground flax seeds

> **Spaghetti Squash**
> Spaghetti squash can be baked, boiled or steamed, and served with sauce in place of pasta, or used as a vegetable base for macaroni and cheese. It contains many nutrients including potassium, vitamin A, and beta carotene.

Directions
Preheat oven to 350º. Cut squash in half, remove seeds, and place cut side down in a baking pan filled with 1/2 inch of water. Bake for about 1 hour or until tender. Let cool and remove the strands with a fork. In a pan, sauté onion in olive oil until light brown. Add chopped tomatoes, garlic and herbs, and cook until most of the liquid is absorbed. Mix with the squash and place in a lightly oiled Pyrex dish. In a small bowl, mix melted ghee and ground flax seed and pour over the top. This will give it a cheesy look. Bake uncovered for about 1/2 hour.

Ingredients to Consider on Specific Diets

Gluten & Casein Free .... Yes
Phenol Free .... Yes (if you use parsley avoid basil)
Low Oxalate Diet .... Yes (if you use basil avoid parsley)
Specific Carbohydrate Diet .... No
This recipe is also Soy free, Corn free and Rice free

Oral Motor Rating 😊 😊 😊

Cinnamon Baby Carrots with Roasted Sesame Seeds

Yields: 4 Servings

Ingredients

1/2 cup sesame seeds
1 tablespoon coconut butter
1 medium red onion, chopped
2 cups carrots or butternut squash, chopped, medium chunks
1 teaspoon cinnamon

> **Sesame Seeds**
> Sesame seeds are the oldest condiment known to man. They add a nutty and a delicate taste to dishes and are highly nutritious.

Directions

Dry roast sesame seeds in pan and set aside. Over medium heat, sauté onion in coconut butter, then add chopped carrots or squash. Add cinnamon and stir well. Reduce heat, cover and cook for 20 to 30 minutes until carrots or squash are moist and cooked well. Add roasted sesame seeds on top and serve.

Ingredients to Consider on Specific Diets

Gluten & Casein Free ....Yes	Phenol Free ....Yes
Low Oxalate Diet..Yes	Specific Carbohydrate Diet ....No

This recipe is also Soy free, Corn free and Rice free

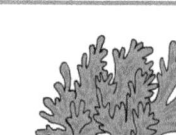

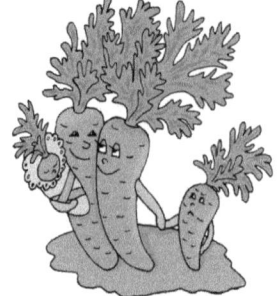

Oral Motor Rating 😊 😊 😊

Quinoa Pilaf

Yields: 4 Servings

Ingredients
3 tablespoons coconut oil
2 small shallots or 1 onion, finely minced
1/2 cup carrots, finely chopped
1 cup quinoa, rinsed and soaked
4 cups organic vegetable stock
1 bunch parsley, finely chopped

> *Quinoa*
>
> *Quinoa is a protein rich vegetable that has a fluffy, slightly crunchy texture and a somewhat nutty flavor when cooked.*

Directions
In a pan, sauté onion or shallots with coconut oil over medium heat, until golden brown. Add minced carrots and sauté for 3 minutes. In a separate pan, heat broth and add quinoa and stir for 30 more seconds to almost boiling. Add this broth into the sautéed vegetables, simmer, and cook 20 minutes. Remove from heat, add chopped parsley, and serve.

Ingredients to Consider on Specific Diets

Gluten & Casein Free ....Yes	Phenol Free ....Yes
Low Oxalate Diet ....Yes	Specific Carbohydrate Diet ....No

This recipe is also Soy free, Corn free and Rice free

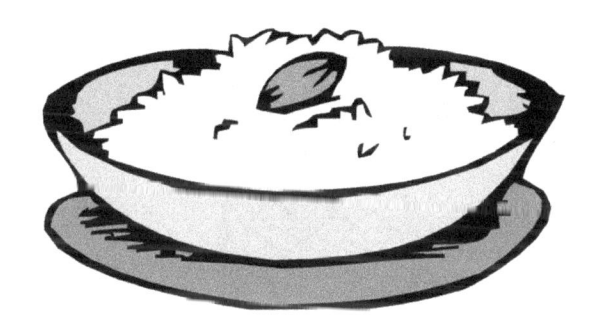

Oral Motor Rating 😊 😊 😊

Simmered Greens

Yields: 4 Servings

Ingredients
1 tablespoon ghee, olive oil, or coconut oil
1 large red onion, chopped
2 garlic cloves, finely chopped
1 ounce piece of ginger, finely chopped
2 bunch of collard greens, roughly chopped
1 medium head cabbage, thinly sliced
2 teaspoons sea salt 2 cups water

Collard Greens
Collard greens, unlike their cousins, kale and mustard, have a very mild, almost smoky flavor. Very high in oxalates.

Directions
In large stockpot, melt ghee and sauté onions until soft. Add garlic, ginger and greens, cook for 3-5 minutes. To the pot add cabbage, salt, and water to cover, and simmer for 20 minutes.

Ingredients to Consider on Specific Diets

Gluten & Casein Free	Yes
Phenol Free	Yes (moderate to high)
Low Oxalate Diet	Yes (moderate to high)
Specific Carbohydrate Diet	Yes

This recipe is also Soy free, Corn free and Rice free

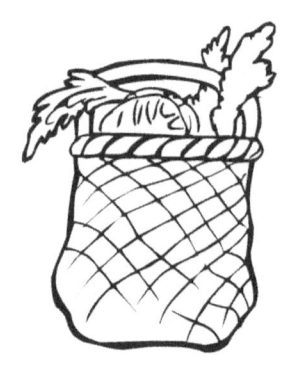

Oral Motor Rating 😊 😊 😊 😊

Sautéed Snow Peas with Ginger and Onion

Yields: 4 Servings

Ingredients
2 tablespoons olive oil or grape seed oil
1 tablespoon fresh ginger, minced
1/2 red onion, finely chopped
3 cups snow peas, fresh or frozen
1/2 cup red bell pepper, finely chopped
2 garlic cloves, finely chopped
1/4 cup parsley or basil
1 teaspoon sea salt

> ### Snow Peas
> *Snow peas, often confused with snap peas, are in the legume family. They are flat with tiny seeds that are barely visible through the pods. They are high in vitamins A and C — a great addition to a healthy diet.*

Directions
In a pan, sauté ginger, red onion, snow peas and red bell pepper in oil over medium high heat for 2 to 3 minutes. Add the rest of the ingredients and sauté for another 2 to 3 minutes. Serve at once.

Ingredients to Consider on Specific Diets

Gluten & Casein Free	Yes
Phenol Free	Yes (if you use parsley and avoid basil)
Low Oxalate Diet	Yes (if you use basil and avoid parsley)
Specific Carbohydrate Diet	Yes

This recipe is also Soy free, Corn free and Rice free

Oral Motor Rating ☺ ☺ ☺ ☺

Roasted Potatoes with Garlic and Rosemary

Yields: 6 Servings

Ingredients
6 cups potatoes, peeled and diced
2 medium red onions, finely chopped
2 sprigs fresh rosemary
1/4 cup olive oil
1 teaspoon sea salt
2 tablespoons garlic, finely diced

Variation

If you are avoiding potatoes in your child's diet, zucchini or cauliflower can be used instead. This will give the recipe an oral motor rating of 3.

Directions
Preheat oven to 375º. In a large bowl, add all the ingredients and toss until all mixed together. Place in ovenproof pan, cover with parchment paper, and top with aluminum foil. Bake for approximately 45 minutes or until potatoes are tender. Remove the parchment paper and foil and let it brown for another 15 minutes.

Ingredients to Consider on Specific Diets

Gluten & Casein Free .... Yes
Phenol Free .... Yes
Low Oxalate Diet .... Yes (if you use zucchini instead of potatoes)
Specific Carbohydrate Diet .... Yes (if you use zucchini instead of potatoes)
This recipe is also Soy free, Corn free and Rice free

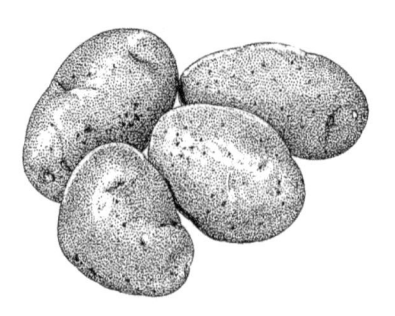

Oral Motor Rating 😊 😊 😊 😊

Easy Pressure-Cooked Vegetables

Yields: 6 Servings

Ingredients
1/2 cup cabbage, diced in small pieces
2 cups turnips, diced
2 cups carrots, sliced in small chunks
1/2 onion, finely chopped
2 cups mustard greens or collards, chopped
2 to 3 cloves of garlic, finely chopped
1/2 teaspoon lemon juice
1/4 cup chopped parsley or basil
1 teaspoon sea salt
1 cup water

> **Pressure Cooker**
> *The pressure cooker is a convenient way of cooking food, as it makes the food cook faster and seals in the juices.*

Directions
Combine all ingredients in pressure cooker. Bring to full hard steam for approximately 15 minutes. Reduce heat and simmer for 15 to 20 minutes. Remove from heat and cool for 15 to 20 minutes before opening. Add parsley or basil to taste.

Ingredients to Consider on Specific Diets

Gluten & Casein Free .... Yes
Phenol Free .... Yes (if you use parsley and avoid basil)
Low Oxalate Diet .... Yes (if you use basil and avoid collards and parsley)
Specific Carbohydrate Diet .... Yes
This recipe is also Soy free, Corn free and Rice free

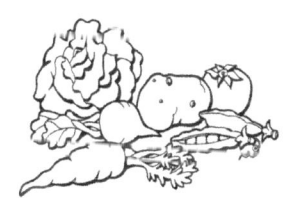

Oral Motor Rating ☺ ☺ ☺ ☺

CHAPTER 11: THE MAIN COURSE

Creamed Peas and Potatoes

Yields: 6 Servings

Ingredients
4 or 5 medium potatoes, diced
1 small onion, finely diced
1 tablespoon olive oil
16 ounce package of frozen peas
14-ounce can of coconut milk
1 teaspoon sea salt
1/2 teaspoon pepper

> *Potatoes*
>
> *People often consider potatoes a comfort food. Mashed, baked or roasted, they are an important food staple and the number one vegetable crop in the world. Potatoes are a good source of Vitamin C and potassium*

Directions
Boil diced potatoes in a pot of boiling water over medium heat for 10 minutes or until tender. Drain and set aside. Sauté diced onion with oil in a pan, add peas and simmer covered for 5 minutes. Add potatoes to the pan. Stir in coconut milk, add salt and pepper to taste. Continue cooking until all ingredients are hot, then serve.

Ingredients to Consider on Specific Diets

Gluten & Casein Free ....Yes	Phenol Free ....Yes
Low Oxalate Diet ....No	Specific Carbohydrate Diet ....No

This recipe is also Soy free, Corn free and Rice free

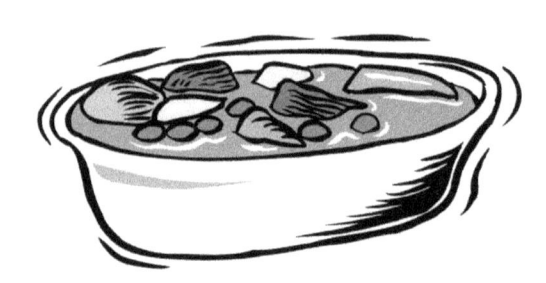

Oral Motor Rating 🙂 🙂 🙂

Red Bell Peppers Stuffed with Millet

Yields: 4 Servings

Ingredients
4 large red bell peppers, halved and seeded
3 tablespoons olive oil
1 medium onion, finely chopped
2 celery stalks, finely chopped
1 1/2 teaspoons sea salt
Pepper to taste
3 cups millet, cooked
2 tablespoons flat-leaf parsley, finely chopped
3 tablespoons fresh lemon juice
   (about 1 lemon)

> *Non Vegetarian Variation*
>
> Stuff bell peppers with a combination of 1 cup ground beef or turkey to 2 cups of millet.
>
> This recipe is also Soy free, Sugar free, Corn free, and Rice free.

Directions
Preheat the oven to 350º. Sprinkle a little salt inside the peppers and set aside. Heat the oil in a large skillet; add the onion, celery, salt and pepper. Cover and cook over medium heat for approximately 4 minutes. Add the cooked millet, parsley and lemon juice, stir to mix well. Add more salt and pepper if desired. Stuff the millet mixture into the pepper halves. Arrange the peppers in a glass baking dish large enough to hold them in one layer. Pour 1 cup of water around, not over, the peppers. Cover the pan tightly with parchment paper and foil. Bake for about one hour, or until the peppers are fork-tender.

Ingredients to Consider on Specific Diets

Gluten & Casein Free ....Yes	Phenol Free ....Yes
Low Oxalate Diet ....Yes	Specific Carbohydrate Diet ....No

This recipe is also Soy free, Corn free and Rice free

Oral Motor Rating 😊 😊 😊 😊

Creamy Macaroni (Mac & Cheese)

Yields: 4 Servings

Ingredients
- 12-ounce package macaroni elbows, gluten free
- 3-ounce jar of baby carrot puree
- 2 slices rice cheese (Tofuti) or goat cheese
- 1 teaspoon sea salt

Variation to the Recipe

Instead of carrot puree, a homemade version of puree can be made with any orange or yellow vegetables like butternut squash. These can be cooked fresh and pureed for a smooth texture.

Directions
Bring a large pot of water to a boil. Add pasta and cook until tender. Drain. In a frying pan, add cooked pasta and carrot puree, rice cheese, and salt. Mix till cheese melts. For extra flavor add ketchup.

Ingredients to Consider on Specific Diets

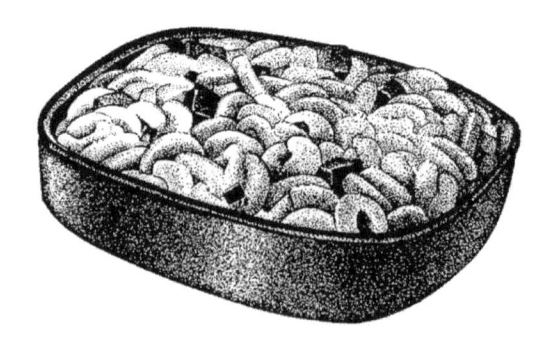

Gluten & Casein Free ....Yes	Phenol Free ....Yes
Low Oxalate Diet ....Yes	Specific Carbohydrate Diet ....No

This recipe is also Soy free and Corn free

Oral Motor Rating 😊 😊

Hummus-Stuffed Portobello Caps

Yields: 4 Servings

Ingredients
- 2 tablespoons olive oil
- 6 portobello mushroom caps, stems and ribs removed
- 1/2 green bell pepper, diced
- 1/2 cup coconut or almond flour
- 3/4 cup hummus or homemade yogurt
- 1 teaspoon sea salt
- 1/4 teaspoon pepper
- 1 teaspoon lemon pepper seasoning

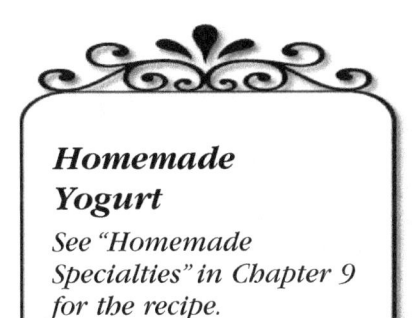

> ***Homemade Yogurt***
> *See "Homemade Specialties" in Chapter 9 for the recipe.*

Directions
Preheat oven to 375º. Grease a baking sheet large enough to hold the mushroom caps. Heat olive oil in a large skillet over medium-high heat. Sear the portobello mushrooms for 3 minutes on each side until browned, remove and place on the baking sheet. In the same pan, add the diced green pepper and sauté until softened. In a separate bowl, blend the hummus/yogurt and coconut/almond flour. Add some pepper to the mixture. Season the mushroom caps with salt and pepper on each side, and, with the stem-side facing up, fill with the hummus mixture. Bake for 15 minutes or until the filling is hot.

Ingredients to Consider on Specific Diets

Gluten & Casein Free	Yes
Phenol Free	Yes (if you use coconut flour)
Low Oxalate Diet	Yes (if you use coconut flour)
Specific Carbohydrate Diet	Yes (if you use homemade yogurt)

This recipe is also Soy free, Corn free and Rice free

Oral Motor Rating ☺ ☺ ☺ ☺

Roasted Mixed Vegetables

Yields: 10 Servings

Ingredients
1 medium yellow onion cut into 1-1/2" wedges
1 medium red onion cut into 1-1/2" wedges
1 rutabaga, peeled and cut into 1-inch pieces
4 small turnips, peeled and cut in half
3 medium carrots, peeled and cut in half lengthwise
1 pound butternut or acorn squash, peeled and cut into 2-inch pieces
12 ounces brussels sprouts, cleaned and trimmed
2 tablespoons olive oil
1 teaspoon sea salt
1/2 teaspoon black pepper, freshly ground
1 tablespoon fresh rosemary, chopped
2 teaspoons fresh thyme, chopped

> *Variation to the Recipe*
>
> *This is a wonderful roasted vegetable recipe which offers a variety of vegetables. If your child does not like any vegetable in the recipe, omit them and replace with favorites.*

Directions
Preheat oven to 450º with two racks centered. Coat a large roasting pan with oil; arrange onions, rutabaga, turnips, carrots, squash, and brussels sprouts evenly in the pan. Drizzle all with olive oil, and toss lightly to coat vegetables. Sprinkle with salt and pepper, then sprinkle rosemary and thyme evenly over the vegetables and roast on center oven rack for 35 to 40 minutes. In between you may turn for even browning. Vegetables are ready when tender when pierced with a knife.

Ingredients to Consider on Specific Diets

Gluten & Casein Free .... Yes
Phenol Free .... Yes (moderate)
Low Oxalate Diet .... Yes (moderate)
Specific Carbohydrate Diet .... Yes
This recipe is also Soy free, Corn free and Rice free

Oral Motor Rating 😊 😊 😊

Artichoke Pate Roll-Ups

Yields: 6 to 8 Rolls

Ingredients
1 14-ounce can of artichokes
1/4 cup water
1/4 cup extra virgin olive oil
1/4 cup lemon juice, fresh organic
1 cup almonds or walnuts, finely chopped (optional)
1/4 red onion, coarsely chopped
2 tablespoons capers, (optional), soaked to help remove citric acid
1/2 teaspoon sea salt
1/2 teaspoon garlic powder
Romaine lettuce leaves (use small ones and leave whole)

> **Artichoke**
>
> *Artichokes are an excellent source of fiber, and a good source of folate and magnesium. Artichokes also are a great source of powerful disease-fighting antioxidants.*

Directions
Put all ingredients except the Romaine lettuce leaves into blender and puree at high speed until creamy and smooth. Taste and adjust sea salt if needed. Place a spoonful of mixture into each lettuce leaf and roll up. This quick and delicious side dish can be added to any meal.

Ingredients to Consider on Specific Diets

Gluten & Casein Free ....Yes	Phenol Free ....Yes
Low Oxalate Diet ....Yes	Specific Carbohydrate Diet ....Yes

This recipe is also Soy free, Corn free and Rice free

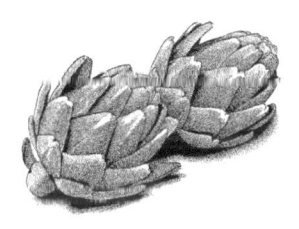

Oral Motor Rating 😊 😊 😊

Vegetable Fried Rice

Yields: 4 Servings

Ingredients
2 cups cooked rice
4 tablespoons sesame or olive oil
1 cup frozen green peas
2 medium carrots, cut lengthwise into strips
14-15 green beans, chopped
3-4 green scallion sticks, chopped
1 red onion, finely chopped
1 teaspoon sea salt

> ### Variation to the Recipe
> *To make this a main dish, add pork or chicken cut into small bite-sized pieces while sautéing vegetables. Then add rice and cook.*

Directions
Cook rice to half-done stage and set aside. In a deep sauté pan, heat oil, add all vegetables, sprinkle with the sea salt, and sauté until tender. Add rice, cover and cook for 10 minutes until all is well cooked.

Ingredients to Consider on Specific Diets

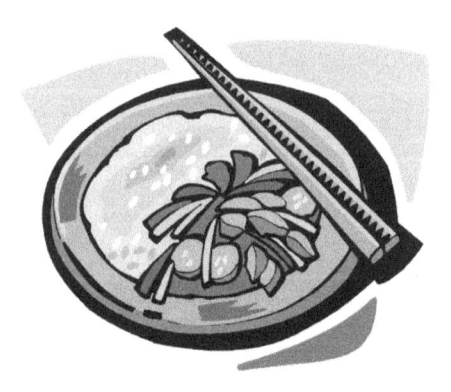

Gluten & Casein Free ....Yes	Phenol Free ....Yes
Low Oxalate Diet ....Yes	Specific Carbohydrate Diet ....No

This recipe is also Soy free, Corn free and is not Rice free

Oral Motor Rating 😊 😊 😊 😊

NON-VEGETARIAN MEALS

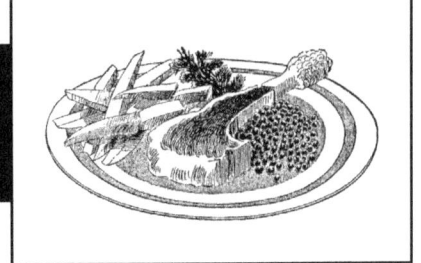

Beefy Spinach with Mushrooms

Yields: 4 Servings

Ingredients
1 pound frozen spinach, thawed and drained
8 ounces fresh mushrooms, sliced
1 onion, sliced
3 garlic cloves, crushed
1 teaspoon ghee, or coconut or olive oil
1 pound ground beef
1 cup SCD ketchup

> *Green Leafy Vegetables and Calories*
>
> Calorie for calorie, leafy green vegetables like spinach, with its delicate texture and jade green color, provide a rich source of potassium, iron and folic acid.

Directions
Heat an iron skillet, add oil and sauté spinach, mushrooms, onion, and garlic. Add a little water if needed, cover and cook until vegetables are soft. Meanwhile, brown the ground beef in another skillet, drain fat, and add to the vegetables. Allow to cook until liquid reduces somewhat. Add ketchup and serve.

Ingredients to Consider on Specific Diets

Gluten & Casein Free .... Yes
Phenol Free .... Yes (moderate)
Low Oxalate Diet .... Yes (if you use zucchini and avoid spinach)
Specific Carbohydrate Diet .... Yes
This recipe is also Soy free, Corn free and Rice free

Oral Motor Rating 😊 😊 😊 😊

Meat Loaf

Yields: 15 to 20 Meatballs

Ingredients
2 pounds ground beef or buffalo
1 1/2 cups flax meal
2 eggs or egg replacer
1 teaspoon oregano
1 teaspoon basil or parsley
1 teaspoon sea salt
1 teaspoon peppercorns, freshly ground
1 onion, quartered
1 carrot, chunked
1 celery stalk, cut in sections

> *Peppercorns*
>
> *The flavor of peppercorn has been described as being a rich combination of cloves, ginger, black pepper, nutmeg, and cinnamon. This makes it an ideal spice for a number of applications. Beef roasts especially benefit from the presence of the peppercorns as part of the roasting process.*

Directions
Preheat oven to 350º. In a food processor, add the vegetables and pulse until finely chopped. Add ground beef, flax meal, spices, and eggs and mix well. Form into a loaf pan or shape into individual meat balls about 2 inches round. For meatballs: Place on a cookie sheet and bake about 30 minutes, or until browned. For meatloaf: Bake for about 1 1/2 hours.

Ingredients to Consider on Specific Diets

Gluten & Casein Free .... Yes
Phenol Free .... Yes (moderate — all spices are moderate to high)
Low Oxalate Diet .... Yes (if you use basil and avoid parsley)
Specific Carbohydrate Diet .... No
This recipe is also Soy free, Corn free and Rice free
Oral Motor Rating 😊 😊 😊

Turkey Meatballs

Yields: 15 to 20 Meatballs

Ingredients
2 pounds ground turkey
1 onion, finely chopped
1 teaspoon basil or parsley
1 teaspoon sea salt
1 teaspoon fresh ground peppercorns
1 1/2 cups flax meal
2 eggs or egg replacer

> *Turkey*
>
> *Turkey is a very good source of protein and the trace mineral selenium, which is of fundamental importance to human health.*
>
> *This recipe will yield 15-20 meat balls. They can be made and frozen, then defrosted to be used to make quick meals.*

Directions
Preheat oven to 350º. In a food processor add ground turkey, onion, spices, flax meal and eggs and mix well. Form into a loaf pan or shape into individual small meat balls about 2 inches round. Place meat balls on a cookie sheet and bake for 25 minutes or until browned. If a loaf is desired, bake about 1 1/2 hours.

Ingredients to Consider on Specific Diets

Gluten & Casein Free .... Yes
Phenol Free .... Yes (if you use parsley and avoid basil)
Low Oxalate Diet .... Yes (if you use basil and avoid parsley)
Specific Carbohydrate Diet .... No

This recipe is also Soy free, Corn free and Rice free

Oral Motor Rating 😃 😃 😃

Baked Turkey Patties

Yields: 12 Small Patties

Ingredients
2 pounds ground turkey
2 garlic cloves, finely chopped
1 celery stalk, finely chopped
1 small onion, finely chopped
1/3 cup fresh mushrooms, chopped
1/4 teaspoon sea salt
1/4 teaspoon pepper

Celery
Celery has a crunchy texture and distinctive flavor which makes it a popular addition to stocks, soups, and stews. Especially nice when paired with a roasted or braised meat dish.

Directions
Preheat oven to 350º. Combine all ingredients and mix well. Form into approximately 12 small patties and bake until browned (approximately 20 minutes).

Ingredients to Consider on Specific Diets

Gluten & Casein Free ....Yes	Phenol Free ....Yes
Low Oxalate Diet ....Yes	Specific Carbohydrate Diet ....Yes

This recipe is also Soy free, Corn free and Rice free

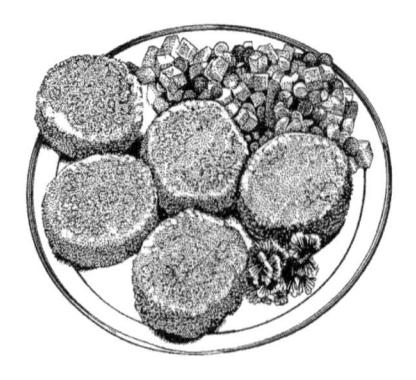

Oral Motor Rating 😊 😊 😊

HEALING AUTISM IN THE KITCHEN

Turkey Burgers with Sweet Mustard Sauce

Yields: 4 Patties

Ingredients
1 pound ground turkey
2 teaspoons sea salt
1 tablespoon coconut oil

Mustard Sauce
4 tablespoons Dijon mustard
1 teaspoon dry mustard
1/2 cup honey
2 tablespoons apple cider vinegar
1/2 cup olive oil
1/2 cup dill chopped fresh, or 1 teaspoon dried

> *Essential oils*
>
> Essential oils like flax, sunflower, safflower or BodyBio balance oil (4:1 ratio) can be added to the mustard sauce. It is a good way to add essential fats (oil) in children's diets.
>
> **Caution: Do not heat these essential oils.**

Directions
Prepare sauce ahead of time, as it needs to chill for at least an hour before serving. Whisk the Dijon mustard, dry mustard, honey and vinegar together in a medium-size bowl. Slowly add the oil, continuing to whisk the mixture until it is thick and well blended. Stir in the dill. Cover and refrigerate at least one hour. Mix turkey and salt in a medium-size bowl, then divide the mixture into four equal size patties. Heat the coconut oil in a large skillet over medium heat. Add the patties and cook for five to seven minutes. Turn the burgers over and continue to cook another five minutes, or until they are no longer pink inside when cut with a knife. Serve the burgers hot, topped with chilled sweet mustard sauce.

Ingredients to Consider on Specific Diets

Gluten & Casein Free	Yes
Phenol Free	No
Low Oxalate Diet	Yes
Specific Carbohydrate Diet	Yes

This recipe is also Soy free, Corn free and Rice free

Oral Motor Rating ☺ ☺ ☺ ☺

Spinach Tofu or Chicken Curry

Yields: 2 to 4 Servings

Ingredients
2 garlic cloves, finely chopped
1 onion, small finely chopped
6 tablespoons of olive oil
2 teaspoons ground cumin
1 teaspoon ground turmeric
3 pounds fresh spinach, torn
1 large tomato, quartered
1/2 cup organic tofu, sliced, or chicken cubes
1/2 teaspoon sea salt Pepper to taste

> *Tofu*
>
> *Tofu is an easy-to-digest and somewhat bland food with a texture similar to cheese. It is made from soybean curd and is often substituted for meats, cheeses, and certain dairy products because of its healthful properties. It has high concentrations of B-vitamins.*

Directions
In a large saucepan heat half the olive oil and sauté garlic and onion until brown. Mix in the cumin and turmeric. Add the spinach, handfuls at a time, until it is cooked down, about 15 minutes total. Remove from heat and allow cooling slightly. Pour spinach mixture into a blender or food processor, add the tomato, and blend for 15 to 30 seconds, or until the spinach is finely chopped. Pour back into the saucepan and keep warm over low heat. In a medium frying pan heat the remaining olive oil over medium heat, and fry tofu or chicken cubes until browned; drain and add to spinach. Cook for 10 minutes on low heat. Season with salt and pepper to taste. Serve with rice.

Ingredients to Consider on Specific Diets

Gluten & Casein Free	Yes
Phenol Free	Yes (moderate)
Low Oxalate Diet	No
Specific Carbohydrate Diet	Yes (if you use chicken cubes instead of tofu)

This recipe is not Soy free, but is Corn free and Rice free

Oral Motor Rating 😊 😊 😊

Chicken Patties

Yields: 8 to 12 Patties

Ingredients
2 pounds ground chicken
2 cups flax meal, ground almonds or pecans
3/4 cup frozen or cooked fresh spinach, drained, chopped
1 medium onion, finely chopped
2 eggs or egg replacer
1 teaspoon sea salt
1 teaspoon thyme

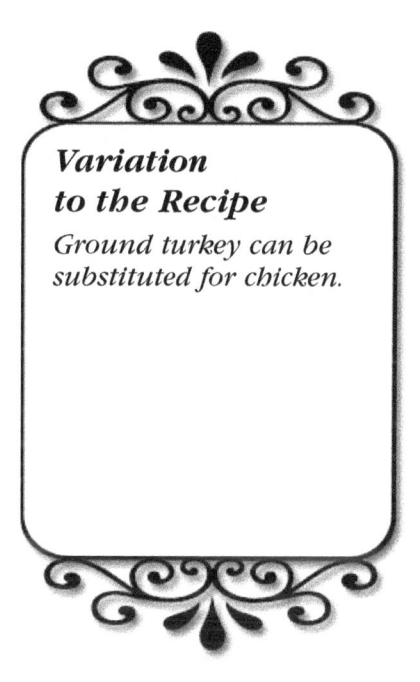

> *Variation to the Recipe*
> Ground turkey can be substituted for chicken.

Directions
Mix all ingredients together, and form into patties about 3 to 4 inches in diameter. Heat a skillet, add olive oil and fry patties for five to seven minutes. Turn and continue to cook another five minutes, or until they are no longer pink inside when cut with a knife.

Ingredients to Consider on Specific Diets

Gluten & Casein Free .... Yes
Phenol Free .... Yes
Low Oxalate Diet .... Yes
Specific Carbohydrate Diet .... Yes (if you use ground nuts and avoid flax meal)
This recipe is also Soy free, Corn free and Rice free

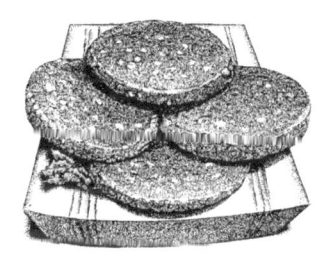

Oral Motor Rating 😊 😊 😊

Salmon Patties

Yields: 2 to 4 Patties

Ingredients
6-7 ounce can wild salmon, drained
2 eggs or egg replacer
1 teaspoon apple cider vinegar
1/2 cup gluten- and casein-free bread crumbs or almond flour
1/2 teaspoon sea salt
1/8 teaspoon paprika

> ### *Wild Salmon*
> *Wild salmon is a delicious fish with exceptional nutritional value found in few other foods (omega-3 fatty acids). Use wild salmon whenever possible.*

Directions
Mix all ingredients together, form into patties, and either fry in a skillet or bake at 350º for 20 minutes on a cookie sheet lined with parchment paper.

Ingredients to Consider on Specific Diets

Gluten & Casein Free .... Yes
Phenol Free .... Yes
Low Oxalate Diet .... Yes
Specific Carbohydrate Diet .... Yes (if you use almond flour and avoid gluten and casein free breads)

This recipe is also Soy free, Corn free and Rice Free (if you use almond flour and avoid gluten and casein free breads)

Oral Motor Rating 😊 😊 😊

Chicken Teriyaki with Broccoli

Yields: 4 to 6 Servings

Ingredients
4 tablespoons olive oil, coconut oil, or ghee
2 garlic cloves, minced
1 pound chicken breast
4 medium scallions, chopped (green and white parts)
1/2 cup chicken broth (homemade or packaged organic)
2 tablespoons gluten-free teriyaki sauce
2 cups brown rice, cooked (regular or instant), and kept hot
4 cups fresh broccoli florcts, steamed

> **Chicken Breast**
> Use skinless, boneless chicken breast in this recipe. To lower the fat content, opt for fat free, gluten free chicken broth.

Directions
Cut chicken into one-inch cubes. In a pan over medium-high heat, add olive oil and garlic, then the chicken. Cook until chicken is golden brown on all sides, stirring often for about 5 minutes. Add scallions and cook until soft, stirring, another 2 minutes. Add broth and teriyaki sauce; simmer until chicken is cooked through and sauce reduces slightly. While chicken is cooking, steam the broccoli florets. When chicken is done, spoon 1/2 cup of cooked rice into each of 4 bowls; add about 1 cup of chicken mixture and 1/2 cup of broccoli over each serving of rice.

Ingredients to Consider on Specific Diets

Gluten & Casein Free ....Yes	Phenol Free ....Yoc
Low Oxalate Diet ....Yes	Specific Carbohydrate Diet .... No

This recipe is also Corn free but is not Soy free or Rice free

Oral Motor Rating 😊 😊 😊 😊

Spaghetti Carbonara

Yields: 4 to 6 Servings

Ingredients

16-ounce package of brown rice or legume spaghetti
2 tablespoons olive oil
4 garlic cloves, minced
8 strips bacon, cooked and crumbled
4 eggs, beaten, or egg replacer

> *Caution for Parents*
> *Nitrates are often used to preserve meats. Select bacon that is both nitrate and gluten free.*

Directions

Cook spaghetti in a large pot, drain and set aside. Fry bacon, drain on paper towels, and crumble. Set aside. Heat oil in pot, and add garlic and cook briefly. Reduce heat to low. Return spaghetti to pot with bacon and stir in beaten eggs. Cook stirring frequently, until eggs are heated through.

Ingredients to Consider on Specific Diets

Gluten & Casein Free ....Yes	Phenol Free ....Yes
Low Oxalate Diet ....Yes	Specific Carbohydrate Diet .... No

This recipe is also Soy free, and Corn free but is not Rice free

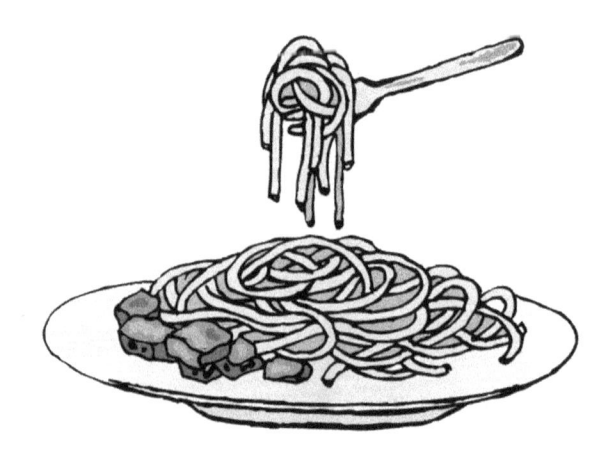

Oral Motor Rating 😊 😊 😊

Chicken Nuggets

Yields: 4 Servings

Ingredients
1 pound boneless chicken breast, cubed
2 eggs, beaten, or egg replacer
1 cup almond or coconut flour
1 teaspoon sea salt
Grapeseed or coconut oil for frying

> ### *Almond Flour*
> *Almond flour is an excellent substitute for regular flour. It's all natural and loaded with nutrients; in particular, magnesium.*

Directions
Beat eggs in medium sized bowl. In a second bowl, mix flour with salt, and pour in a gallon-sized plastic bag. Heat 1/2" oil in large skilled. Toss chicken cubes in the seasoned flour mix and then dip in the egg. Drop in skillet, turning to cook on all sides.

Note: To make oven-baked chicken nuggets, spread 2 tablespoons of oil in the bottom of a 9"x13" baking dish. Arrange coated chicken nuggets in a single layer. Bake in 375º oven for 30 minutes, turning a couple of times during baking to brown evenly.

Ingredients to Consider on Specific Diets

Gluten & Casein Free .... Yes
Phenol Free .... Yes (if you use coconut flour)
Low Oxalate Diet .... Yes (if you use coconut flour)
Specific Carbohydrate Diet .... Yes
This recipe is also Soy free, Corn free and Rice free

Oral Motor Rating 😊 😊 😊

Turkey or Chicken Lettuce Wraps

Yields: 6 to 8 Servings

Ingredients
2 cups cooked turkey or chicken, finely diced
1/2 cup onion, chopped
1/4 cup celery, chopped
2 teaspoons fresh tarragon, chopped
BodyBio Balance Oil and apple cider vinegar oil dressing
Romaine lettuce leaves

Mix and add to each wrap:
1 tablespoon BodyBio Balanced oil

1 tablespoon apple cider vinegar

Directions
Sauté the onion and celery in a fry pan with a little oil until tender. Cool, then add the cooked meat of choice, mix well, and spread on Romaine lettuce leaves. Drizzle oil and vinegar over ingredients and then roll up. Drizzle a little more oil on top of the wraps if desired.

Ingredients to Consider on Specific Diets

Gluten & Casein Free ....Yes	Phenol Free ....Yes
Low Oxalate Diet....................................Yes	Specific Carbohydrate Diet ....Yes

This recipe is also Soy free, Corn free and Rice free

Oral Motor Rating 😊 😊 😊 😊

Chicken Breasts Roasted in Fresh Garden Herbs

Yields: 4 Servings

Ingredients
4 chicken breasts (with bone), free-range organic
1 cup fresh oregano leaves
1 cup green onions, coarsely chopped
4 tablespoons fresh cilantro
2 small garlic cloves
1/4 cup lemon juice (juice of two lemons)
3/4 tablespoon coconut oil, ghee, or extra virgin olive oil
1 teaspoon sea salt

> *Advice for Parents*
>
> *It is best to use fresh lemon while cooking, as most commercial and citrus fruits are treated with cholinesterase inhibitors to prevent spoilage.*

Directions
Combine all ingredients except chicken in a food processor, and process until minced. Place chicken breasts in a casserole dish and spread fresh herb mixture over them. Marinate chicken at least one hour in refrigerator, then roast very slowly in a 325-350º oven for one hour, or until the breasts are done.

Ingredients to Consider on Specific Diets

Gluten & Casein Free ......Yes	Phenol Free ......Yes
Low Oxalate Diet ......Yes	Specific Carbohydrate Diet ......Yes

This recipe is also Soy free, Corn free and Rice free

Oral Motor Rating ☺ ☺ ☺ ☺

Broccoli Beef

Yields: 4 Servings

Ingredients
1 pound beef sirloin cut in thin strips
2 tablespoons sesame or olive oil
4 cups broccoli cut in small cubes

Marinade/gravy
1 tablespoon gluten-free soy sauce (tamari)
2 tablespoons almond nut butter or tahini
1/2 cup water or broth

> *Gluten-Free Soy Sauce*
>
> *Parents often report that children eat vegetables only from Chinese foods. This may be due to the salty soy sauce. Our version of this healthy recipe uses GF soy sauce (tamari).*

Directions
Mix gravy ingredients in a medium bowl, and set aside. Heat a large skillet or wok, add oil, and then stir-fry beef strips for a few minutes until they are nearly done. Remove and set aside. Add broccoli to the skillet with 1/4 cup of water/broth, and cook, stirring often, until tender crisp (about 6 minutes). Return meat to skillet with vegetables. Stir in gravy and cook until it thickens (about 1 minute). Serve with rice or quinoa.

Ingredients to Consider on Specific Diets

Gluten & Casein Free ....Yes	Phenol Free ....Yes
Low Oxalate Diet ....Yes	Specific Carbohydrate Diet ....No

This recipe is also Corn free and Rice free but is not Soy free

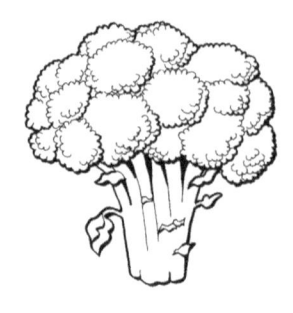

Oral Motor Rating ☺ ☺ ☺ ☺

Quick Chicken Vegetable Stir-Fry

Yields: 4 Servings

Ingredients
- 1 pound boneless chicken breast cut in 1-inch cubes
- 2 tablespoons olive oil
- 1 pound bag frozen oriental vegetables
- 4 cups rice, rice noodles or quinoa cooked

Gravy
- 1/2 cup water
- 2 tablespoons gluten-free soy sauce (or tamari)
- 1/2 tablespoon minced ginger or
- 1/2 teaspoon ground ginger

> *Variation to the Recipe*
>
> *Fresh vegetables are ideal for this recipe. You can also use oriental vegetables, which provide a healthy meal that can be prepared in minutes.*

Directions
Mix gravy in a small bowl and set aside. Heat oil in a large skillet or wok. Stir-fry chicken 3 minutes or until chicken is thoroughly cooked (no longer pink). Remove from skillet and set aside while you prepare the vegetables. In the same skillet, add oriental vegetables and stir-fry till almost done (check cooking instructions on bag.). Add chicken pieces back to the skillet and pour gravy mixture over chicken and vegetables. Bring to a boil and cook one minute to thicken sauce. Serve over cooked rice, quinoa or rice nooodles.

Ingredients to Consider on Specific Diets

Gluten & Casein Free ....Yes	Phenol Free ....Yes
Low Oxalate Diet ....Yes	Specific Carbohydrate Diet ....No

This recipe is Corn free, Rice free (use quinoa noodles) but is not Soy free

Oral Motor Rating ☺ ☺ ☺ ☺

Spaghetti with Meat Sauce

Yields: 6 Servings

Ingredients
16 ounce package of brown rice or legume spaghetti
1 pound ground beef or buffalo
2 tablespoons olive oil
1 cup onion, chopped
2 garlic cloves, minced
1 can tomatoes, crushed
1 bay leaf
2 teaspoons oregano
2 teaspoons basil or parsley
1/4 teaspoon sea salt

> *Ground Turkey*
> Ground turkey can be substituted for ground beef in this recipe.

Directions
Bring a large pot of water to a boil. Cook the spaghetti according to package instructions. Drain and keep warm. In a large saucepan, heat olive oil and brown beef with onion and garlic. Stir in crushed tomatoes and seasonings; simmer for 15 minutes or more, stirring occasionally. Serve over spaghetti.

Ingredients to Consider on Specific Diets

Gluten & Casein Free .... Yes
Phenol Free .... Yes (if you use parsley and avoid basil)
Low Oxalate Diet .... Yes (if you use basil and avoid parsley)
Specific Carbohydrate Diet .... No

This recipe is also Soy free, and Corn free, but is not Rice free

Oral Motor Rating 😊 😊 😊

HEALING AUTISM IN THE KITCHEN

Sesame Chicken Wings

Servings: 40 Chicken Wing Pieces

Ingredients
20 chicken wings (about 4 pounds)
1 tablespoon ghee, melted

Dipping Mixture:
2 eggs or egg replacer
2 tablespoons rice milk
1/2 cup coconut or almond flour

Coating Mixture:
1/2 cup sesame seeds
2 teaspoons paprika
1 1/2 teaspoons crushed sesame seeds
1/2 teaspoon sea salt
1/4 cup ghee, melted (for drizzling over all)

> **Sesame Seeds**
> Sesame seeds are used whole, ground into pastes such as tahini, or pressed for their rich, nutty oil. Toasted, the whole seeds can be sprinkled on a variety of dishes for extra crunch and flavor.

Directions
Preheat oven to 425º. Spread 1 tablespoon ghee in a baking pan large enough to hold all the chicken pieces. Separate chicken wings at joints; discard tips. In one bowl, beat eggs, rice milk and flour with fork. In another bowl mix sesame seeds, paprika, mustard, and sea salt. Dip chicken wings first in egg mixture and then coat with sesame seed mixture. Arrange pieces close together in pan. Drizzle 1/4 cup ghee over chicken. Bake uncovered 35 to 40 minutes or until brown and crisp.

Ingredients to Consider on Specific Diets

Gluten & Casein Free	Yes
Phenol Free	Yes (moderate all spices are moderate to high)
Low Oxalate Diet	Yes
Specific Carbohydrate Diet	No

This recipe is also Soy free, Corn free and Rice free (use almond milk)

Oral Motor Rating ☺ ☺ ☺ ☺

CHAPTER 11: THE MAIN COURSE

Avocado Meatloaf

Yields: 4 Servings

Ingredients
1 egg or egg replacer
1 avocado, peeled and pit removed
1/4 cup butternut squash, already cooked
1 pound ground beef, turkey or buffalo

Avocado
An avocado is considered a fruit, but is closer to a berry. It is used as a meat substitute in sandwiches due to its high fat content. In some respects, an avocado is a tropical fruit akin to a banana, but its oily content and nutty flavor are reminiscent of an olive.

Directions
Preheat oven to 350º, Grease a loaf pan. Put egg, avocado and butternut squash in a food processor. Mix completely until totally blended. Add ground meat and blend again. Put the mixture in a loaf pan and bake for 45 minutes.

Ingredients to Consider on Specific Diets

Gluten & Casein Free ....Yes	Phenol Free ....Yes
Low Oxalate Diet ....Yes	Specific Carbohydrate Diet ....Yes

This recipe is also Soy free, Corn free and Rice free

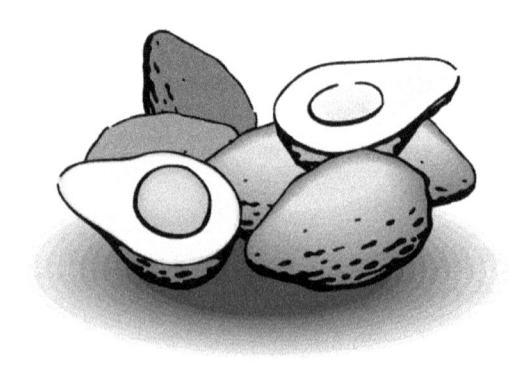

Oral Motor Rating 😊 😊 😊

Chicken Chow Mein

Yields: 4 Servings

Ingredients
4 ounces rice or quinoa noodles
1 teaspoon oil
1 boneless, skinless chicken breast
2 tablespoons olive oil
1 clove garlic, minced
1/3 cup mushrooms
1/3 cup red pepper, cut in small cubes
1/3 cup chopped green scallions
1 cup cabbage, chopped
1/4 cup bean sprouts
1 teaspoon sea salt
1 cup chicken stock

Quinoa

Quinoa is a good source of protein.

Caution: *Quinoa noodles can sometimes have corn in the ingredients.*

Directions
Cook noodles in boiling water, with 1 teaspoon oil added to it, for 3 to 4 minutes. Drain and set aside. Cut chicken into thin strips. Heat oil in a frying pan, add garlic, chicken, vegetables and salt, and sauté for 5 minutes. Add chicken stock, reduce heat and simmer for 15 minutes. When liquid is semi-thick, add noodles and cook for another 10 minutes and serve.

Ingredients to Consider on Specific Diets

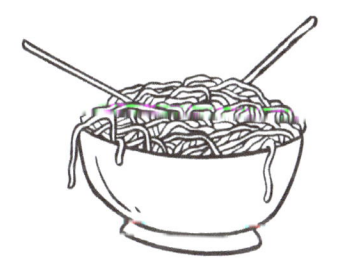

Gluten & Casein Free	Yes	Phenol Free	Yes
Low Oxalate Diet	Yes	Specific Carbohydrate Diet	No

This recipe is also Soy free, Corn free and Rice free (use quinoa noodles)

Oral Motor Rating 😊 😊 😊 😊

CHAPTER 11: THE MAIN COURSE

Deep-Fried Shrimp

Yields: 2 Servings

Ingredients

2 cups raw shrimp, large to jumbo size, cleaned and deveined
1/2 cup almond, chickpea, or rice flour
1 teaspoon baking soda
1 teaspoon sea salt
1 egg or egg replacer
1 cup water
1/2 cup coconut oil

> ### Dried Shrimp
> *Dried shrimp makes an excellent addition to soups, stews and vegetable dishes. It is a rich source of vitamin D and it contains a least eight times more vitamin D than liver.*

Directions

In a small bowl, mix flour, baking powder and salt. In another small bowl, beat egg and water until mixed. Add this to the flour mixture to make a batter. Squeeze excess water from the shrimp and add to the batter. In a frying pan, heat the oil. Dip shrimp in the batter and drop in the hot oil. Deep fry until golden brown(3-4 minutes). Drain and serve.

Ingredients to Consider on Specific Diets

Gluten & Casein Free .... Yes
Phenol Free .... Yes (if you use rice or chick pea flour)
Low Oxalate Diet .... Yes (if you use rice or chick pea flour)
Specific Carbohydrate Diet .... Yes (if you use almond flour)
This recipe is also Soy free, Corn free and Rice free (use almond or chick pea flour)

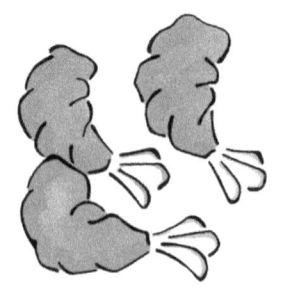

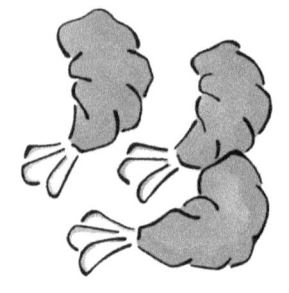

Oral Motor Rating 😊 😊 😊 😊

Tandoori Chicken

Yields: 2 Servings

Ingredients
2 boneless chicken breasts

Marinade:
2 tablespoons coconut butter
1 teaspoon garlic, crushed
1/2 teaspoon ginger powder
1 tablespoon cilantro, chopped
1 teaspoon sea salt
1 teaspoon black pepper
1/2 cup orange juice

> **Coconut Butter**
> *Coconut butter is also known as coconut oil. It is used commonly in cooking, specifically frying and sautéing. It is also used as a healthy substitute for shortening, butter, or margarine in cooking and baking.*

Directions
Remove and discard the skin from chicken and cut it into serving-size pieces. Prick pieces with a fork to allow marinade to penetrate the meat. In a bowl, mix coconut butter, garlic, ginger, cilantro, salt, black pepper and orange juice. Put the chicken in the mix and let it marinate for 6 hours in the refrigerator. Place the chicken on a greased tray and grill at 425º for 15 minutes on each side. (When done, juices should run clear when a piece is pierced with a fork.) Brush ghee on each side, and serve with onion slices on side. The chicken can also be roasted in the oven at 425º for 20 to 25 minutes.

Ingredients to Consider on Specific Diets

Gluten & Casein Free ....Yes	Phenol Free ....Yes
Low Oxalate Diet........................Yes	Specific Carbohydrate Diet ....Yes

This recipe is also Soy free, Corn free and Rice free

Oral Motor Rating 😊 😊 😊 😊

Notes:

CHAPTER TWELVE

Tasty Meal Companions

Soups and Salads

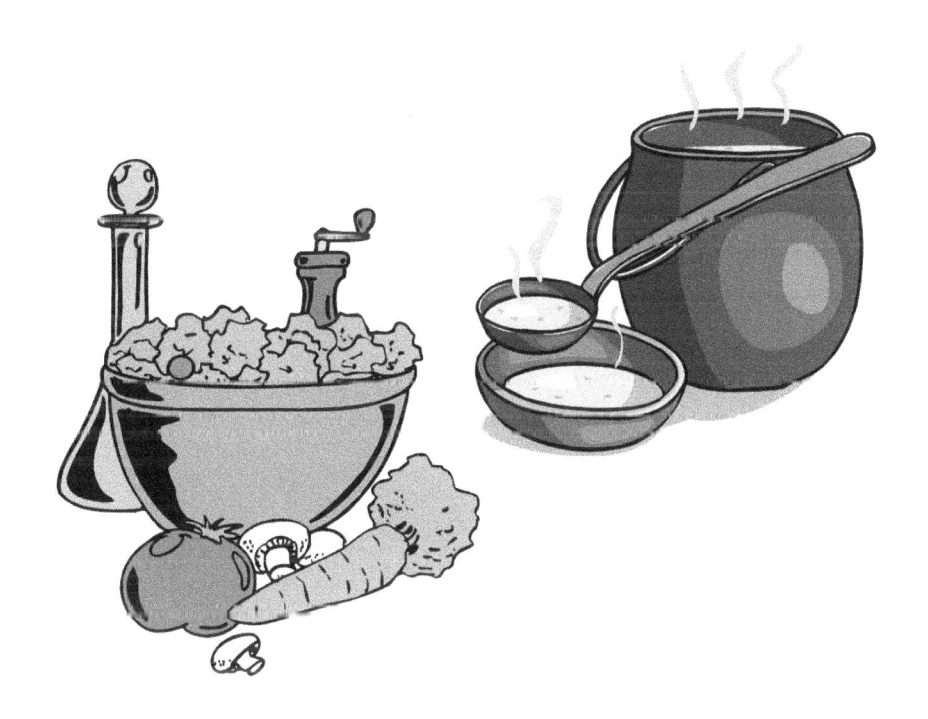

Tasty Meal Companions – Soups and Salads
Table of Contents

SOUP RECIPES

VEGETARIAN SOUPS

Potato Celery Soup	272
Basil Veggie Stew	273
Water Chestnut Soup	274
Watercress Soup	275
Butternut Squash Soup	276
Asparagus Soup	277
Red Pepper and Mushroom Soup	278
Avocado Summer Soup	279
Cauliflower, Carrot and Celery Soup	280
Easy English Pea Soup	281
Curried Celery and Lima Bean Soup	282
Red Lentil Soup	283
Quick Black Bean Soup	284
Sephardic Leek Soup	285
Split Pea Soup	286
Oriental Cabbage Soup	287
French Onion Soup	288
Beet and Carrot Soup	289

NON-VEGETARIAN SOUPS

Coconut Chicken Broth	290
Beef Stew	291
Hearty German Soup	292
Chicken Rice Soup	293
Mulligatawny Soup	294
Turkey or Chicken Soup	295
Two-Bean Chili Soup	296

SALAD RECIPES

VEGETARIAN SALADS

Spinach Pear or Guava Salad	300
Tomato, Cucumber and Avocado Salad	301
Bean Sprout Spinach Pine Nut Salad	302
Lentil Salad	303
Quinoa & Cilantro Salad with Lemon & Garlic	304
Broccoli Salad	305
Potato Salad	306
Three-Bean Salad	307
Cucumber Pressed Salad	308
Bok Choy Salad	309
Tempeh Salad	310

NON-VEGETARIAN SALADS

Hard-Boiled Egg Salad	311
Hamburger Salad	312
Turkey Salad	313
Ham and Fresh Asparagus Salad	314

VEGETARIAN SOUPS

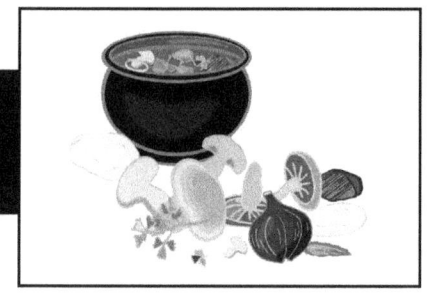

Potato Celery Soup

Yields: 4 Servings

Ingredients
4-5 medium size potatoes
1 medium onion, peeled and chopped
1 teaspoon olive oil or coconut butter
2 carrots, peeled and chopped
1 celery root, diced
2 garlic cloves, chopped
2 cups vegetable stock
2 cups water
1 teaspoon sea salt
Freshly ground pepper to taste
1 tablespoon fresh parsley chopped

Variation
To vary this stock, add chicken stock instead of water. If your child is very sensitive, you can pass the soup through a strainer for a smoother consistency.

Directions
Peel and dice the potatoes and set aside. Heat the oil in a heavy bottomed soup pot over medium heat. Add the onions, and sauté until brown. Add chopped vegetables and garlic, and sauté for another 3 minutes. Add the potatoes to soup pot with the chicken/vegetable stock and water. Bring to a boil, and then simmer over medium heat for 20 to 25 minutes until vegetables are all very soft. Let the soup cool down, and then puree it in a blender. Bring the soup back to the stockpot, and boil for another 10 minutes. Add salt, pepper, parsley or basil and serve.

Ingredients to Consider on Specific Diets

Gluten & Casein Free......................Yes	Phenol Free................................Yes (moderate to high)
Low Oxalate Diet............................No	Specific Carbohydrate Diet........................No

This recipe is also Soy free, Corn free and Rice free

Oral Motor Rating 😊 😊 😊 😊

HEALING AUTISM IN THE KITCHEN

Basil Veggie Stew

Yields: 4 Servings

Ingredients
1 large onion, chopped
3 tablespoons basil (or to taste)
2 tablespoons coconut or olive oil
3 large carrots, diced
3 potatoes or 1 large butternut squash, peeled and cut in small pieces
1 cup water
1/2 teaspoon sea salt
1 small head cauliflower, chopped into small florets

> *Dried Basil Leaf*
>
> *It is found in the mixed spice called "Italian seasoning" and used in desserts like basil ice cream and sorbet and custards. Basil seeds are used to thicken the consistency of certain Thai foods. Also used as a seasoning in tomato sauce, pizza, salad dressing, and cooked vegetable dishes.*

Directions
In a deep skillet, heat oil and sauté the onion with the basil until translucent. Add carrots and potatoes or butternut squash, continuing to cook on very low heat for five minutes. Add water and sea salt. Stir well. Cover and cook on low heat for 20 minutes, until vegetables are almost tender. For the last 7 to 10 minutes, drop in cauliflower on top of the other vegetables. Cover again. Cook until cauliflower is tender. Taste and add more sea salt or basil if desired before serving.

Ingredients to Consider on Specific Diets

Gluten & Casein Free	Yes
Phenol Free	Yes (use parsley and avoid basil)
Low Oxalate Diet	Yes (use butternut squash and avoid potatoes)
Specific Carbohydrate Diet	Yes (use butternut squash)

This recipe is also Soy free, Corn free and Rice free

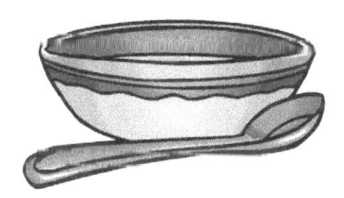

Oral Motor Rating ☺ ☺

Water Chestnut Soup

Yields: 6 Servings

Ingredients
2 carrots, peeled and chopped
2 medium onions, chopped
4 tablespoons coconut butter
6 cups vegetable or chicken stock
4 cups of water chestnuts
   (fresh or canned and drained)
Pinch nutmeg
1/2 cup fresh basil or parsley
1/2 teaspoon sea salt
1/4 teaspoon cayenne (optional)

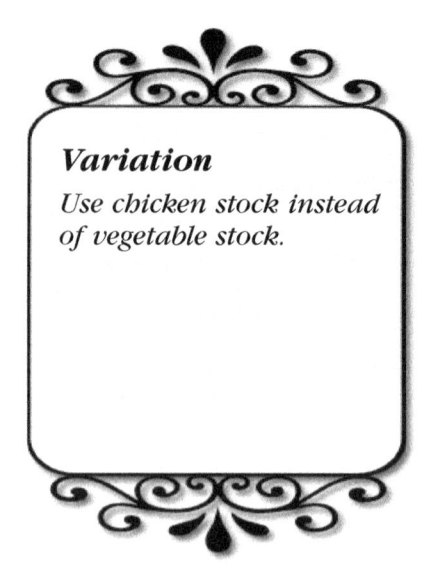

Variation
Use chicken stock instead of vegetable stock.

Directions
Sauté carrots and onion in coconut butter until soft. Add stock and chestnuts. Bring to boil and skim until clear. Add nutmeg, basil or parsley, salt and cayenne, if desired. Simmer covered, for about 15 minutes. Set aside to cool a little. Puree soup with an immersion blender. Adjust seasonings as desired, and serve.

Ingredients to Consider on Specific Diets

Gluten & Casein Free .... Yes
Phenol Free .... No
Low Oxalate Diet .... Yes (if you use basil and avoid parsley)
Specific Carbohydrate Diet .... Yes
This recipe is also Soy free, Corn free and Rice free

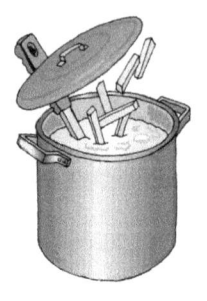

Oral Motor Rating

HEALING AUTISM IN THE KITCHEN

Watercress Soup

Yields: 6 Servings

Ingredients
2 medium onions, chopped
3 tablespoons ghee or coconut butter
1 quart vegetable/chicken stock
1 medium butternut squash, peeled and cut in small pieces
2 large bunches of watercress leaves, rinsed
1/2 teaspoon sea salt
Pinch pepper (optional)

> *Watercress*
>
> *Watercress is known for its peppery taste and is used as a green and garnish. It is often used to spice up sandwiches and used frequently in salads, in combination with greens or citrus fruits due to its milder flavor.*

Directions
In a stock pot, add ghee or butter and onion and sauté until golden brown. Add stock and butternut squash, bring to boil and skim. Simmer for about 20 minutes or until squash is soft. Add watercress and simmer another 5 minutes. Let it cool a bit. Puree soup with handheld blender. Season to taste and serve.

Ingredients to Consider on Specific Diets

Gluten & Casein Free .... Yes
Phenol Free .... Yes (moderate, watercress is moderate to high)
Low Oxalate Diet .... Yes
Specific Carbohydrate Diet .... Yes

This recipe is also Soy free, Corn free and Rice free

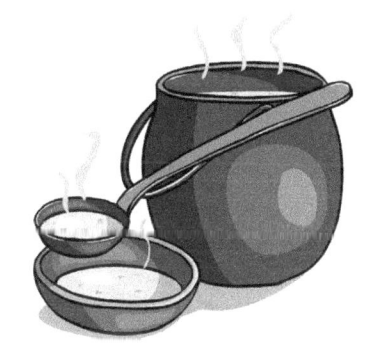

Oral Motor Rating 😊 😊 😊 😊

CHAPTER 12: TASTY MEAL COMPANIONS 275

Butternut Squash Soup

Yields: 4 Servings

Ingredients
3 large onions, halved and sliced
2 tablespoons coconut or grape seed oil
5 cups vegetable/chicken stock
1 cup hot water
1 medium butternut squash, peeled and cubed
1 teaspoon sea salt
3 teaspoons dill, parsley, or basil
Pinch pepper

> **Dill**
> *Dill is best known as the prime flavoring ingredient in dill pickles and other pickled vegetables, but it is also popular for flavoring vinegars. It is used as a garnish and seasoning in onion dill bread, dips, salad dressings, and potato salad.*

Directions
Heat oil in a heavy bottomed soup pot over medium heat. Add onion and sauté until golden brown. Add broth, water, and squash cubes to the stew pot. Simmer and cook for 20 minutes. Add salt, and continue to cook for 7 to 10 minutes until soft. Puree with hand blender, and add dill, parsley or basil and serve hot.

Ingredients to Consider on Specific Diets

Gluten & Casein Free	Yes
Phenol Free	Yes (if you use parsley and avoid dill and basil)
Low Oxalate Diet	Yes (if you use basil and avoid dill and parsley)
Specific Carbohydrate Diet	Yes

This recipe is also Soy free, Corn free and Rice free

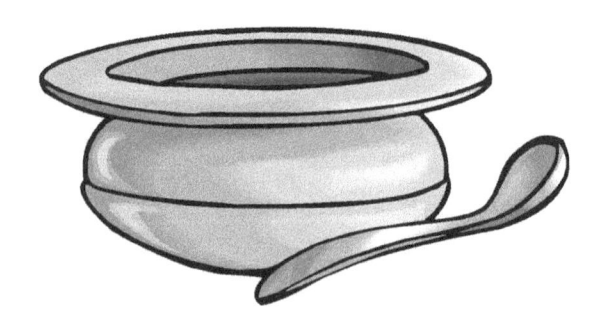

Oral Motor Rating ☺ ☺ ☺ ☺

HEALING AUTISM IN THE KITCHEN

Asparagus Soup

Yields: 6 Servings

Ingredients
2 medium onions, chopped
3 tablespoons ghee, coconut butter, or grape seed oil
2 garlic cloves, coarsely chopped
1 1/2 quarts vegetable/chicken stock
2 cups red potatoes or butternut squash, peeled and diced
2 bunches of asparagus
1/4 teaspoon sea salt

Note:
Discard the tough ends of asparagus and cut into 1/4 inch pieces. Strain the finished soup to remove any pieces of asparagus. This will make the soup more acceptable to children.

Directions
In a stock pan; add ghee or oil and sauté onion until golden brown. Add garlic, stock and potatoes or butternut squash. Bring to boil and skim. Simmer for 15 minutes. Add asparagus and simmer for another 15 minutes. Let it cool down a little. Puree the soup in blender, until it has a creamy consistency. Add seasoning to taste, and serve hot.

Ingredients to Consider on Specific Diets

Gluten & Casein Free .... Yes
Phenol Free .... Yes
Low Oxalate Diet .... Yes (if you use butternut squash and avoid potatoes)
Specific Carbohydrate Diet .... Yes (if you use only butternut squash)
This recipe is also Soy free, Corn free and Rice free

Oral Motor Rating

Red Pepper and Mushroom Soup

Yields: 6 Servings

Ingredients
- 2 medium onions, chopped
- 1 pound (16 oz.) fresh mushrooms cut in thin slices
- 2 red peppers, seeded and chopped
- 3 tablespoons coconut butter, ghee, or grape seed oil
- 1 1/2 quarts vegetable/chicken stock
- 1 small bunch fresh basil or parsley, finely chopped
- 1/2 teaspoon sea salt
- 1/4 teaspoon pepper (optional)

> ### Mushrooms
> Buy mushrooms that are firm, plump and clean. Those that are wrinkled or have wet slimy spots should be avoided. The best way to store loose mushrooms is to keep them in the refrigerator in a loosely closed paper bag. They will keep fresh for about one week.

Directions
In a large skillet, heat coconut butter or ghee over medium heat and sauté onion, pepper and mushrooms until tender. Add stock of choice, bring to boil and skim. Add basil or parsley and simmer for 15 minutes. Let it cool down a little, then puree in blender until it has a creamy consistency. Add salt and pepper to taste and serve hot.

Ingredients to Consider on Specific Diets

Gluten & Casein Free .... Yes
Phenol Free .... Yes (if you use parsley and avoid basil)
Low Oxalate Diet .... Yes (if you use basil and avoid parsley)
Specific Carbohydrate Diet .... Yes
This recipe is also Soy free, Corn free and Rice free

Oral Motor Rating 🙂

Avocado Summer Soup

Yields: 2 Servings

Ingredients
2 cups vegetable/chicken stock
2 cucumbers, peeled and cubed
2 avocados, peeled and cubed
1 teaspoon dill leaves
1 teaspoon sea salt
Few sprigs mints leaves (optional)

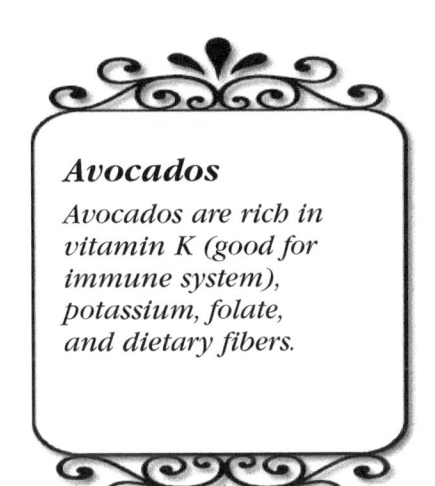

> ### *Avocados*
> *Avocados are rich in vitamin K (good for immune system), potassium, folate, and dietary fibers.*

Directions
Place all ingredients in food processor or a blender. Mix until smooth. Garnish with mint leaves and serve. You can eat this soup hot or cold. It's good either way.

Ingredients to Consider on Specific Diets

Gluten & Casein Free ....Yes	Phenol Free ....No
Low Oxalate Diet ....Yes	Specific Carbohydrate Diet ....Yes

This recipe is also Soy free, Corn free and Rice free

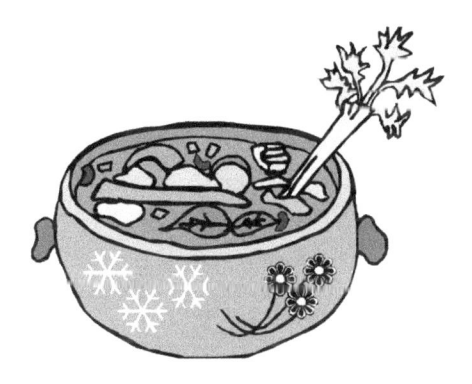

Oral Motor Rating 🙂 🙂

Cauliflower, Carrot and Celery Soup

Yields: 4 Servings

Ingredients
1 cauliflower, heads chopped
4 cups water
6 medium baby carrots, diced
2 celery stalks, diced
2 garlic cloves, left whole
1 medium onion, chopped
2 teaspoons sea salt
1 tablespoon dried parsley or basil leaves
1 teaspoon dried dill leaves (optional)

> *Cauliflower*
>
> *Cauliflower is high in biotin, a B vitamin that plays an important role in the body's fat metabolism. It is rich in fiber and mineral content, but lower in nutrient content than its close relative, broccoli.*

Directions
In a large stockpot heat water. Add salt, cauliflower, carrots, celery, and chopped onion. Cook for 15 minutes and then puree the soup in blender until creamy. Season with herbs and serve.

Ingredients to Consider on Specific Diets

Gluten & Casein Free .... Yes
Phenol Free .... Yes (if you use parsley and avoid dill and basil)
Low Oxalate Diet .... Yes (if you use basil and avoid parsley and dill)
Specific Carbohydrate Diet .... Yes
This recipe is also Soy free, Corn free and Rice free

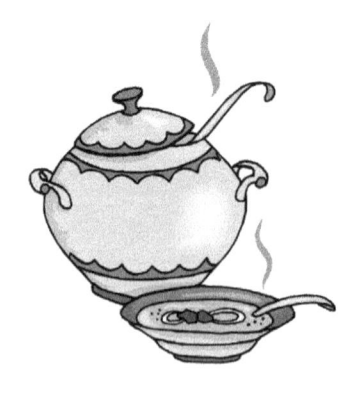

Oral Motor Rating 😊 😊 😊 😊

HEALING AUTISM IN THE KITCHEN

Easy English Pea Soup

Yields: 4 Servings

Ingredients
1 medium onion, diced
2 tablespoons coconut oil, butter, or grape seed oil
1 bay leaf (optional)
3 leeks (white part only), diced
2 celery stalks (including leaves), diced
1 small head lettuce (Boston or leafy), chopped
2 sprigs parsley or basil
4 cups water
3 cups frozen peas
1 teaspoon sea salt

> **Winter Soup**
> *This is good soup for winter. If fresh peas are used instead of frozen, you may have to cook a little longer.*

Directions
In a soup pan add oil and sauté onion until brown. Add bay leaf if desired. Add leeks, celery, lettuce, and parsley or basil, and sauté until tender. Add water, peas, and salt; cover and simmer until peas are very soft. Puree the soup in blender until it has a creamy consistency. Simmer 10 minutes and serve.

Ingredients to Consider on Specific Diets

Gluten & Casein Free	Yes
Phenol Free	Yes (if you use parsley and avoid basil and bay leaf)
Low Oxalate Diet	Yes (if you use basil and avoid parsley and bay leaf)
Specific Carbohydrate Diet	Yes

This recipe is also Soy free, Corn free and Rice free

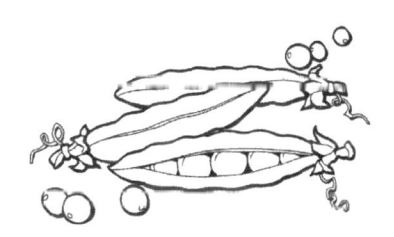

Oral Motor Rating :)

CHAPTER 12: TASTY MEAL COMPANIONS

Curried Celery and Lima Bean Soup

Yields: 4 to 6 Servings

> **Lima Beans**
> Lima beans are sometimes called "butter beans" because they are starchy and yet have a buttery texture. They have a delicate flavor and are an excellent source of molybdenum.

Ingredients
- 3 cups cooked lima beans (leftovers, or 1 can)
- 2 tablespoons ghee, coconut butter, or grape seed oil
- 1 medium onion, chopped
- 1 bunch of celery, chopped
- 1 teaspoon sea salt
- 2 tablespoons parsley

Directions
Heat the ghee or oil in a large saucepan; add onion and celery, and sauté until brown. Add water or stock, beans, salt, parsley or basil. Simmer for 20 minutes, or until tender. Puree the soup in blender until it has a creamy consistency. Strain the soup (optional) if you see any celery threads. Return to the saucepan and reheat gently until piping hot. Serve in bowls.

Ingredients to Consider on Specific Diets

Gluten & Casein Free .... Yes	Phenol Free .... Yes
Low Oxalate Diet .... No	Specific Carbohydrate Diet .... Yes

This recipe is also Soy free, Corn free and Rice free

Oral Motor Rating 😊 😊

Red Lentil Soup

Yields: 4 to 6 Servings

Ingredients
1 1/2 cups red lentils
1 small onion, finely chopped
1 tablespoon coconut oil, olive oil,
   or grape seed oil
3 cups zucchini or butternut squash, grated
2 garlic cloves, minced
1 1/2 teaspoons sea salt
1/4 teaspoon dried rosemary
2 teaspoons ginger, grated
4 cups vegetable/chicken stock

> *Rosemary*
>
> Rosemary has a pine-like fragrance, and its pungent flavor goes a long way in flavoring chicken, lamb, pork, salmon and tuna dishes, as well as soups and sauces.

Directions
In a soup pan, soak lentils for 7 hours, then drain. In a fry pan, heat oil and sauté chopped onion, shredded zucchini and garlic until glazed. Add to lentils along with the vegetable or chicken stock and cook over low heat for 25 minutes. Add salt, rosemary powder and grated ginger. Cook for an additional 10 minutes until all flavors are blended. Add extra water if needed and adjust seasonings to taste.

Ingredients to Consider on Specific Diets

Gluten & Casein Free	Yes
Phenol Free	Yes (moderate) (if you use butternut squash and avoid zucchini)
Low Oxalate Diet	Yes
Specific Carbohydrate Diet	Yes

This recipe is also Soy free, Corn free and Rice free

Oral Motor Rating 😊 😊

Quick Black Bean Soup

Yields: 4 Servings

Ingredients
- 1 medium onion, chopped
- 3 garlic cloves, minced
- 1 celery stalk, chopped
- 2 tablespoons olive oil, coconut butter, or grape seed oil
- 2 (15 ounce) cans black beans, drained and rinsed
- 2 cups vegetable/chicken stock
- 1/2 cup water
- 1/2 teaspoon sea salt
- 1/4 teaspoon cayenne pepper (optional)
- 1/4 cup cilantro, finely chopped

Black Beans
Black beans can be enjoyed "as is." For children with oral motor issues, it is good to puree them before serving. The consistency of the soup can be decided based on your child's needs.

Directions
In a large saucepan, heat oil and sauté onion, garlic, and celery until tender. Add beans, broth, water and salt and simmer for 15 minutes. Puree all in blender. Return soup to pot. Add cilantro and cayenne pepper if desired. Bring soup to a boil, stirring frequently. Simmer on low until ready to serve.

Ingredients to Consider on Specific Diets

Gluten & Casein Free ....Yes	Phenol Free ....Yes
Low Oxalate Diet ....Yes	Specific Carbohydrate Diet ....Yes

This recipe is also Soy free, Corn free and Rice free

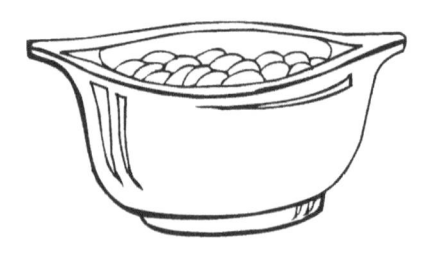

Oral Motor Rating 😊 😊

Sephardic Leek Soup

Yields: 6 Servings

Ingredients
1/4 cup olive oil or ghee
10 medium size leeks, trimmed, sliced, and well-washed
2 large baking potatoes or butternut squash, peeled and grated
3 medium carrots, peeled and grated
1 bunch parsley, chopped
8 cups vegetable/chicken stock
1/4 teaspoon freshly ground pepper
Pinch grated nutmeg (optional)

> *Leek*
> With a more delicate and sweeter flavor than onions, leeks add a subtle touch to recipes without overpowering the other flavors that are present.

Directions
Heat the oil in a 6-quart pot over medium heat. Add the leeks, potatoes and carrots. Sauté until softened, about 5 to 10 minutes. Add the parsley, broth, salt and pepper, and nutmeg (optional). Bring to a boil. Reduce the heat to low and simmer the contents, covered, 40 minutes, until tender. Serve the soup as is or process in a blender.

Ingredients to Consider on Specific Diets

Gluten & Casein Free .... Yes
Phenol Free .... Yes (if you avoid potatoes and substitute with butternut squash)
Low Oxalate Diet .... No
Specific Carbohydrate Diet .... Yes (if you avoid potatoes substitute with butternut squash)
This recipe is also Soy free, Corn free and Rice free

Oral Motor Rating :) :)

Split Pea Soup

Yields: 4 Servings

Ingredients
1 large onion, peeled and chopped
2 garlic cloves, minced
1 tablespoon coconut butter, grape seed oil, or olive oil
2 cups green split peas
3 celery stalks, chopped
1 teaspoon sea salt
8 cups water

> *Variation*
> Other traditional versions of split pea soups have ham or ham bone for stock; they can be easily added to the recipe with the vegetables.

Directions
In a large stockpot, heat oil and sauté onion and garlic until light brown. Add peas, celery, salt and water. Bring to boil, reduce heat and simmer for 2 hours, or until peas are soft and soup is thick.

Ingredients to Consider on Specific Diets

Gluten & Casein Free .... Yes
Phenol Free .... Yes
Low Oxalate Diet .... Yes (if you avoid celery)
Specific Carbohydrate Diet .... Yes
This recipe is also Soy free, Corn free and Rice free

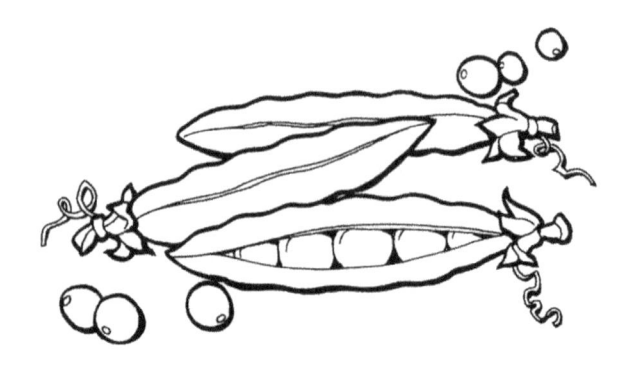

Oral Motor Rating 😊 😊 😊 😊

Oriental Cabbage Soup

Yields: 4 Servings

Ingredients
1 large head of Chinese cabbage
4 ounces lean pork tenderloin
3 cups water
1 teaspoon sea salt
1 teaspoon gluten free soy sauce/tamari (optional)

Pork tenderloin
Pork tenderloin is one of the leanest meats. It is particularly suited to stir fry dishes, or sliced and flattened for medallions.

Directions
Wash and chop cabbage into small pieces. Slice pork into small shreds. Bring water to boil and add salt and pork, and simmer for 5 minutes. Add cabbage and soy sauce (optional) and simmer for another 10 minutes. Keep pot covered and hot until ready to serve.

Ingredients to Consider on Specific Diets

Gluten & Casein Free .... Yes
Phenol Free .... Yes
Low Oxalate Diet .... Yes
Specific Carbohydrate Diet ..... Yes (omit soy sauce)

This recipe is also Corn free, Rice free, but is not Soy free

Oral Motor Rating :) :) :) :)

French Onion Soup

Yields: 4 Servings

Ingredients
4 large onions, thinly sliced
2 tablespoons sesame or olive oil
2 medium dried shiitake mushrooms, stems removed
5 cups vegetable stock, chicken stock or water
1/2 bunch parsley, chopped
1 teaspoon tamari sauce
1/4 cup scallions, finely chopped

> **Shiitake mushrooms**
> *Shiitake mushrooms are very porous, so if they are exposed to too much water they will quickly absorb it and become soggy. So simply wipe them with a slightly damp paper towel or kitchen cloth to clean.*

Directions
In a frying pan, heat oil, add onions, and sauté till light brown. Add thinly sliced shiitake mushrooms, and sauté for another 2 or 3 minutes. Add stock or water and bring to boil. Add tamari, scallions and parsley. Simmer for 30 minutes.

Ingredients to Consider on Specific Diets

Gluten & Casein Free .... Yes
Phenol Free .... Yes
Low Oxalate Diet .... Yes (if you use basil instead of parsley)
Specific Carbohydrate Diet .... Yes (if you avoid tamari sauce)
This recipe is also Corn free, Rice free, but is not Soy free

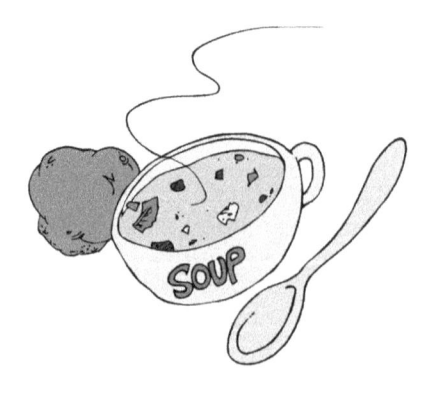

Oral Motor Rating 😊 😊 😊 😊

Beet and Carrot Soup

Yields: 4 Servings

Ingredients
4 medium beets, peeled and sliced
2 medium onions, chopped
4 tablespoons grape seed oil
4 cups vegetable/chicken stock
1 cup water
1/2 teaspoon lemon rind, freshly grated
1/2 teaspoon ginger, freshly grated
1/2 teaspoon basil or parsley leaves
1/2 teaspoon sea salt
1/4 teaspoon pepper (optional)

> **Beets**
> *Choose small or medium-sized beets whose roots are firm, smooth-skinned and deep in color. Avoid beets that have spots, bruises or soft, wet areas, all indicators of spoilage.*

Directions
In a soup pot with lid, sauté onion and beets in oil for 15 minutes or until tender. Add water and stock, bring to boil and skim. Add lemon rind and ginger. Cover and simmer for about 15 minutes. Set aside to cool. Puree the soup in blender, until it has a creamy consistency. Strain the soup (optional) if needed. Add herbs and seasonings to taste and serve.

Ingredients to Consider on Specific Diets

Gluten & Casein Free ....Yes	Phenol Free ....No
Low Oxalate Diet ....No	Specific Carbohydrate Diet ....Yes

This recipe is also Soy free, Corn free and Rice free

Oral Motor Rating 😊 😊

NON-VEGETARIAN SOUPS

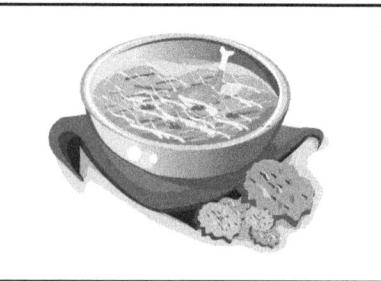

Coconut Chicken Broth

Yields: 4 Servings

Ingredients
1 quart chicken stock or vegetable broth
1 1/2 cups whole coconut milk
1 tablespoon lemon juice
1 teaspoon ginger, fresh grated,
    or 1/2 teaspoon ginger powder
1/2 teaspoon sea salt
1 tablespoon basil or parsley, finely chopped

> **Chicken Stock**
>
> Chicken stock can be homemade or commercial. Consider adding cubed chicken or turkey, and/or finely chopped vegetables.
> **Note:** Puree to a soup-like consistency, or else the oral-motor rating will go higher.

Directions
Bring the stock to boil, skimming any foam on top. Add coconut milk, lemon juice and ginger. Simmer for 15 minutes. Season to taste with salt, basil or parsley, and serve hot or cold as desired.

Ingredients to Consider on Specific Diets

Gluten & Casein Free .... Yes
Phenol Free .... Yes (if you use parsley and avoid basil)
Low Oxalate Diet .... Yes (if you use basil and avoid parsley)
Specific Carbohydrate Diet .... Yes
This recipe is also Soy free, Corn free and Rice free

Oral Motor Rating ☺ ☺ ☺ ☺

Beef Stew

Yields: 4 to 6 Servings

Ingredients

1 pound beef stew meat, cut in 1-inch cubes
1 tablespoon olive oil or coconut oil
3 cups beef broth 1 cup water
1/2 teaspoon sea salt
1/8 teaspoon pepper
2 small potatoes, peeled and cubed
1 cup carrots, diced
1 cup celery, chopped
1 small onion, chopped
1 bay leaf or 1 teaspoon dried parsley

> ***Bay Leaves***
> *Bay leaves are commonly added to soups to enhance flavor. They are a good source of vitamin A, and are helpful in treating many ailments of the liver, kidney and stomach.*

Directions

In a large soup pot with lid, heat oil and brown the beef. Add broth, water, salt and pepper. Heat and bring to a boil. Cover and simmer 2 1/2 hours, till beef is almost tender. Add vegetables and bay leaf or parsley. Cover and simmer for another 30 minutes. Adjust seasonings to taste and serve. NOTE: This may also be pureed in a blender until creamy and strained if desired.

Ingredients to Consider on Specific Diets

Gluten & Casein Free .... Yes
Phenol Free .... Yes (omit potatoes)
Low Oxalate Diet .... No
Specific Carbohydrate Diet .... No

This recipe is also Soy free, Corn free and Rice free

Oral Motor Rating 😊 😊 😊

Hearty German Soup (Pressure Cooked)

Yields: 4 Servings

Ingredients
3 cups dry pinto beans or black eyed peas
4 cups water
1 tablespoon olive oil
1 pound chicken or beef sausage links
2 garlic cloves, minced
1 quart chicken stock, vegetable broth, or beef stock
2 cups sauerkraut, drained
1 teaspoon sea salt
1/4 teaspoon black pepper (optional)

> **Sauerkraut**
>
> *Sauerkraut is fermented cabbage. It is packed with vitamins and minerals that are created during the fermentation process. Sauerkraut boosts the immune system.*

Directions
Soak beans overnight or at least for 7 hours. Drain the water, and add it to pressure cooker with the beans and 4 cups of water. Cook for 20 minutes. In a soup pot, heat oil and sauté the sausage links until lightly brown. Let them cool down, chop into small bite- size pieces and return to the pot. Add the cooked beans and their liquid, garlic, and chicken stock and simmer for 15 minutes or until sausage is cooked. Salt and pepper to taste, and add the sauerkraut at the last minute and serve.

Ingredients to Consider on Specific Diets

Gluten & Casein Free ....Yes	Phenol Free ....Yes
Low Oxalate Diet ....Yes	Specific Carbohydrate Diet ....No

This recipe is also Soy free, Corn free and Rice free

Oral Motor Rating ☺ ☺ ☺ ☺

Chicken Rice Soup

Yields: 6 Servings

Ingredients
2 quarts chicken stock or vegetable broth
1 cup brown rice (preferred soaked for 7 hours)
1 1/2 cups cooked chicken meat
1 1/2 cups mixed vegetables, finely diced
1/2 cup water
1/2 teaspoon sea salt
1/2 teaspoon pepper

Vegetables
Carrots, celery, red pepper, string beans and cauliflower work in this recipe. Use your child's favorites.

Directions
Bring stock and rice to boil and skim off any foam rising on top. Reduce heat and cook for about 1 hour, till rice is tender. Add water to make a soup-like consistency. Add the diced chicken and your choice of vegetables. Cook for 5 to 10 minutes, until just tender. Season the soup to taste with salt and pepper and serve.

Ingredients to Consider on Specific Diets

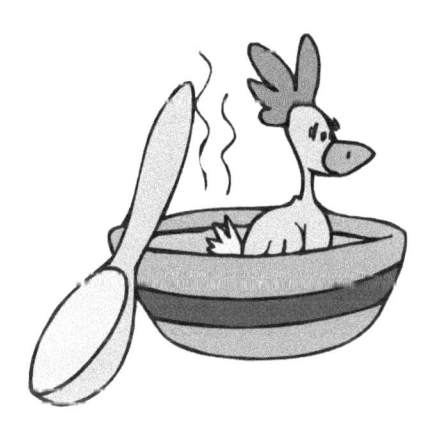

Gluten & Casein Free .... Yes	Phenol Free .... Yes
Low Oxalate Diet .... Yes	Specific Carbohydrate Diet .... No

This recipe is also Soy free and Corn free, but is not Rice free

Oral Motor Rating 😊 😊 😊

Mulligatawny Soup

Yields: 6 Servings

Ingredients

1/2 cup onion, chopped
2 tablespoons ghee, coconut oil, or olive oil
4 cups chicken stock or vegetable broth
2 pounds cooked chicken cut into bite-size pieces
2 medium tomatoes, chopped
1 large apple, coarsely chopped
1 large carrot, chopped
1 medium green pepper, cut into 1/2 inch pieces
1 teaspoon sea salt
1 teaspoon gluten-and casein-free curry powder
1 teaspoon lemon juice

> *Homemade Curry Powder Recipe*
> See the recipe in the "Homemade Specialties" section of Chapter 9.

Directions

In a Dutch Oven, or soup pot with lid, heat ghee or oil over medium heat. Add chopped onion and sauté for about two minutes. Remove from heat. Add broth, chicken, and all remaining ingredients. Heat to boiling, reduce heat. Cover and simmer about 10 minutes, or until carrots are tender. Garnish with parsley.

Ingredients to Consider on Specific Diets

Gluten & Casein Free .... Yes
Phenol Free .... Yes (moderate; most spices are moderate to high)
Low Oxalate Diet .... Yes
Specific Carbohydrate Diet .... Yes
This recipe is also Soy free, Corn free and Rice free
Oral Motor Rating ☺ ☺ ☺ ☺

Turkey or Chicken Soup

Yields: 6 to 8 Servings

Ingredients
2 pounds ground turkey or chicken
2 large onions, chopped
6 garlic cloves, minced
2 tablespoons olive oil or grape seed oil
1 quart water
1 quart chicken stock or vegetable broth
1 teaspoon sea salt
2 cups baby carrots cut in small pieces
1 package frozen or 1 bunch fresh kale
1/2 cup red peppers cut in small pieces

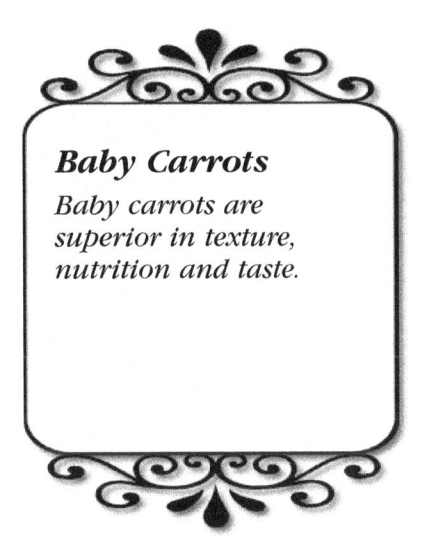

> ***Baby Carrots***
> *Baby carrots are superior in texture, nutrition and taste.*

Directions
In a large soup pot, heat oil and sauté garlic and onion until brown. Add water, salt, chicken broth, carrots, kale and red peppers. Simmer and cook for 30 minutes. Form ground meat into little "meatballs" about 1 to 2 inches round, and drop into soup. Cook for another 30 minutes and serve hot.

Ingredients to Consider on Specific Diets

Gluten & Casein Free .... Yes	Phenol Free .... Yes
Low Oxalate Diet .... Yes	Specific Carbohydrate Diet .... Yes

This recipe is also Soy free, Corn free and Rice free

Oral Motor Rating ☺ ☺ ☺ ☺

Two-Bean Chili Soup

Yields: 4 Servings

Ingredients
1 large onion, finely chopped
3 garlic cloves, minced
2 tablespoons olive oil
1 pound lean ground beef or buffalo
1 large green pepper, finely chopped
1 teaspoon sea salt
1/4 teaspoon black pepper ground (optional)
4 cups tomato juice
1 cup water 1 (15 ounce) can kidney beans, rinsed and drained
1 (15 ounce) can great northern beans, rinsed and drained

> **Beef**
> *If available, purchase organically grown beef. It is pesticide, hormone and antibiotic free. Beef is highly perishable, so it should always be kept at cold temperatures, either refrigerated or frozen.*

Directions
In a large soup pot, heat oil and sauté garlic and onion until brown. Add beef/buffalo, green pepper, salt and black pepper, and cook for 5 to 7 minutes. Add tomato juice, water and beans and simmer for 30 minutes and serve.

Ingredients to Consider on Specific Diets

Gluten & Casein Free ....Yes	Phenol Free ....Yes
Low Oxalate Diet........................Yes	Specific Carbohydrate Diet .... No

This recipe is also Soy free, Corn free and Rice free

Oral Motor Rating 😊 😊 😊 😊

SALADS
A daily need, nutrition must

Eating a salad every day offers numerous health benefits. It is one of the simplest and healthiest food habits that anyone can commit to. Salads are easy to make and they bring us a few steps closer to our recommended daily serving of fruit and vegetables.

Health Benefits of Eating Salad: Many studies have shown that many Americans don't get the recommended daily servings of fruit and vegetables. And eating a salad daily can bring you a few steps closer to that goal. **There are numerous health benefits provided when one eats salads.**

- **Eat salads for fiber:** Salads provide the body with a lot of fiber which in turn means lower cholesterol and less constipation. Furthermore, when you eat these green wonders, you feel fuller, eat less junk food, and maintain a healthier weight.

- **Vegetables and fruit in salads:** They are a rich source of many nutrients which contribute to our overall health. Green veggies provide the body with high levels of antioxidants (vitamin C and E, folic acid, lycopene, and beta-carotene) which lower our chances of developing many illnesses.

- **Salads good source of good fats:** Homemade salad dressings can be a source of consuming essential fatty acids when we incorporate safflower, sunflower, flax, hemp, BodyBio omega 6 to 3 Balanced Oil, and seeds into our salads.

- **Salads and raw food in diet:** Salads help add raw fruits and vegetables in the diet. They contain natural enzymes which help to properly digest food and prevent stressing the body. Sprouts, nuts and seeds can also be added for additional benefits since they are nutrient-dense foods.

- **Salads alkalize the body:** The basic health principal is to keep the body alkaline, because when the body becomes too acidic, health problems arise quickly. Certain foods cause the body to become either alkaline or acidic (a healthy person may want to eat 60 percent alkalizing, to 40 percent acidic). Raw fruits and vegetables in salads help stabilize the acid/alkaline balance in the body.

- **Salads are a rich source of vitamins and minerals:** Americans do not get enough of the vitamins and minerals of which salads are a rich source.

Tips for Making a Healthy Salad

- Choose the high-in-folate and vitamin C-rich dark leafy greens instead of iceberg lettuce. Good choices are spinach, endive, and mixed "baby" greens containing multicolored lettuces and romaine.

- Choose vegetables from "all the colors of the rainbow," such as red radishes, peppers and tomatoes, green/red/orange peppers, cucumbers and broccoli, purple cabbage and orange carrots.

- Avoid veggies in marinades, dressings, sauces, or mayonnaise, which add fat, salt, and trans fats. Instead, add good fats from seeds and nuts into the salad.

- Add cooked beans as chickpeas, lentils or kidney beans to salads for extra protein. This will help to fill you up and will stay with you far longer than the veggies and greens alone. When adding beans from cans, rinse them well to remove any preservatives and extra salt content.

- Choose meats and fish such as chicken, turkey, beef or tofu but avoid breaded, fried protein.

- Avoid commercial or bottled dressings, as they may be made with trans-fat oils. Read the label as they may contain MSG, hydrolyzed vegetable proteins, or other similar unhealthy ingredients. (Ingredients listed as "natural flavors," often contain MSG.) Instead, opt for high-quality dressings found at health food stores and homemade dressings. You can also use beneficial oils such as BodyBio Balance Oil to make it healthy.

- Sprouted beans, lentils and legumes can also be added to salads. Nuts and seeds can be eaten raw or ground and added to salads directly or mixed in salad dressings before serving.

- Finely chopped salads are often appealing to children rather than large pieces of salad that are difficult to chew properly.

VEGETARIAN SALADS

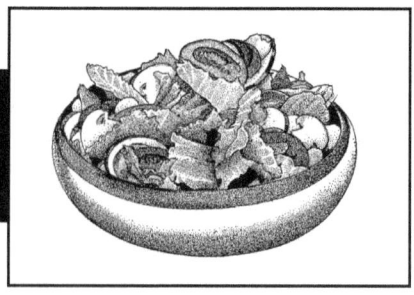

Spinach Pear or Guava Salad

Yields: 4 to 6 Servings

Ingredients
- 1 (16 oz) packet baby spinach
- 4 cups pear or guava, sliced
- 1/2 cup grape seed, sunflower, or rice bran oil
- 1/4 cup white wine vinegar or apple cider vinegar
- 1 teaspoon honey or maple syrup
- 1/4 teaspoon paprika (optional)
- 2 tablespoons sesame seeds (optional)

> **Sesame seeds**
> *Sesame seeds add a nutty taste and a delicate, almost invisible touch to recipes. They have a high oil content, and are used in breads, candies, main dishes, and as a garnish on pasta and vegetables.*

Directions
In a large bowl, toss together the spinach and sliced fruit. In a medium bowl, whisk together the oil, vinegar, honey, paprika and sesame seeds. Pour over the spinach and pear/guava, and toss to coat.

Ingredients to Consider on Specific Diets

Gluten & Casein Free .... Yes
Phenol Free .... Yes (moderate, use maple syrup avoid honey, spinach high)
Low Oxalate Diet .... No
Specific Carbohydrate Diet .... Yes (if you use honey)
This recipe is also Soy free, Corn free and Rice free (avoid rice branoil)

Oral Motor Rating 😊 😊 😊 😊

Tomato, Cucumber and Avocado Salad

Yields: 2 to 4 Servings

Ingredients
1 cup tomato, finely chopped
1 cup avocado, diced
1 cup cucumber, peeled and chopped
2 teaspoons lemon juice
1/2 teaspoon sea salt
1 tablespoon olive oil

> *Alkalizing Recipe*
>
> *This alkalizing recipe is very easy to make. To add essential oils, you can replace olive oil with 1 tablespoon of BodyBio Balance oil.*

Directions
In a large bowl, add the chopped tomato, cucumber and avocado. Mix them well. In a small bowl or cup, dissolve the salt in the lemon juice, add the olive oil, and pour over the salad.

Ingredients to Consider on Specific Diets

Gluten & Casein Free ....Yes	Phenol Free ....No
Low Oxalate Diet .... Yes	Specific Carbohydrate Diet .... Yes

This recipe is also Soy free, Corn free and Rice free

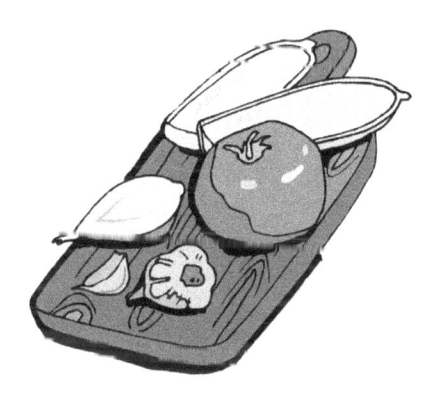

Oral Motor Rating 😊 😊 😊

CHAPTER 12: TASTY MEAL COMPANIONS

Bean Sprout Spinach Pine Nut Salad

Yields: 2 Servings

Ingredients
1/2 cup onions, finely chopped
1 tablespoon olive oil
1 cup bean sprouts
1/2 cup tomatoes, chopped
1 cup baby spinach leaves
1/2 cup pine nuts
Salt to taste

> *Recipe for Lentil Sprouts*
>
> *Soak lentils overnight and drain excess water. Lentils will sprout in two days; make sure to rinse them 2 to 3 times a day.*
>
> *It takes about 3 cups of dry lentils to make 5 cups of sprouts.*

Directions
In a pan, heat olive oil and sauté onion until light brown in color. Add bean sprouts and chopped tomatoes and sauté for another 2 to 3 minutes. Turn heat to simmer and let it cook for 10 minutes. Remove from heat and let it cool down a little bit. Place in a bowl and add baby spinach and pine nuts and mix them well. Serve warm or cold.

Ingredients to Consider on Specific Diets

Gluten & Casein Free	Yes
Phenol Free	Yes (moderate)
Low Oxalate Diet	Yes (moderate)
Specific Carbohydrate Diet	Yes

This recipe is also Soy free, Corn free and Rice free

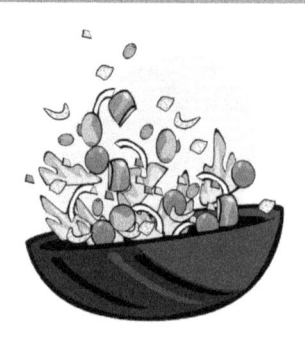

Oral Motor Rating ☺ ☺ ☺ ☺

Lentil Salad

Yields: 6 Servings

Ingredients

5 cups lentil sprouts, chopped
2 cups celery, minced
2 green onions with tops, minced
1 red pepper, chopped
3 tablespoons apple cider vinegar
2 teaspoons kelp granules (optional)

Dressing (Make ahead of time)
1 tablespoon raw sesame tahini
4 tablespoons olive oil
1/8 cup water

> ***Kelp Granules***
>
> *Kelp granules are a great source of iodine. Keep this shaker handy while cooking, dining, hiking or traveling. Sprinkle on the nutritional benefits of sea vegetables and skip the table salt.*

Directions

In a blender, make the dressing by adding tahini, olive oil, and water and blending until smooth. Mix the chopped/minced vegetables in a large bowl. Add apple cider vinegar and kelp granules, and pour dressing over it. Toss all until all mixed well and serve.

Ingredients to Consider on Specific Diets

Gluten & Casein Free ...... Yes	Phenol Free ...... Yes
Low Oxalate Diet ...... Yes	Specific Carbohydrate Diet ...... No

This recipe is also Soy free, Corn free and Rice free

Oral Motor Rating 😊 😊 😊 😊

Quinoa & Cilantro Salad with Lemon & Garlic

Yields: 4 to 6 Servings

Ingredients
2 cups quinoa, cooked
1 can black beans, chopped
1 medium red pepper, chopped
1/2 teaspoon sea salt
1/2 bunch cilantro, finely chopped
1/2 cup parsley or basil, minced

Dressing
2-3 garlic cloves, minced
1/4 cup freshly squeezed lemon juice
3 tablespoons BodyBio Balance Oil
1 teaspoon sea salt

Directions
Place the quinoa in a large bowl; add black beans, chopped red pepper, salt, and cilantro. Mix all well. In small bowl, combine garlic, lemon juice, oil, and sea salt. Pour over the salad and toss well. Serve at room temperature.

Directions for Quinoa

To yield 2 cups of cooked quinoa, take 1/2 cup uncooked quinoa and 1 cup water, and cook for 20 minutes.

Ingredients to Consider on Specific Diets

Gluten & Casein Free .... Yes
Phenol Free .... Yes (use parsley and avoid basil)
Low Oxalate Diet .... Yes (use basil and avoid parsley)
Specific Carbohydrate Diet .... No
This recipe is also Soy free, Corn free and Rice free
Oral Motor Rating 😊 😊 😊 😊

Broccoli Salad

Yields: 4 Servings

Ingredients
1 head broccoli, finely chopped
1 medium carrot, coarsely grated
1 small red onion, finely chopped

Dressing
1 egg or egg replacer
1 teaspoon dry mustard
1/2 teaspoon sea salt
2 tablespoons lemon juice 1 cup safflower oil
1 tablespoon hot water

> **Variation**
>
> *If your child is allergic to egg, and not soy, and is not currently on the SCD diet, use grape seed oil veganaise as a healthy alternate.*

Directions for Dressing
In a blender, make dressing by combining the egg, mustard, salt and lemon juice and blending well. With the blender still running, add the oil in a steady slow stream and blend until all oil is well mixed. Blend in hot water to stabilize. Serve immediately or refrigerate in a covered container and use within one week

Directions
In a large bowl, mix the vegetables and pour the dressing over all.
Toss and serve.

Ingredients to Consider on Specific Diets

Gluten & Casein Free	Yes
Phenol Free	Yes (moderate)
Low Oxalate Diet	Yes (moderate)
Specific Carbohydrate Diet	Yes

This recipe is also Soy free, Corn free and Rice free

Oral Motor Rating 😊 😊 😊 😊

Potato Salad

Yields: 6 to 8 Servings

Ingredients
6 to 8 medium sized potatoes
1 large onion, finely chopped
5 hard-boiled eggs

Dressing
1 cup SCD mayonnaise or grape seed oil veganaise
1 tablespoon apple cider vinegar
2 teaspoons mustard
1 teaspoon honey
1/2 teaspoon sea salt
1/4 teaspoon pepper
Paprika for garnish

> *Paprika*
>
> Paprika is a lovely red spice that is made from dried bell peppers. When red bell peppers are dried, they are ground into tiny particles, making paprika. It is added to soups and stews and sprinkled over the tops of meats as a seasoning.

Directions
Boil five eggs. Wash and peel potatoes. Boil in salted water until just tender; do not overcook. Drain, cool to room temperature and cut into small cubes. In a large bowl, combine potatoes, onions and 4 diced eggs (reserve one egg for garnish). In a small bowl, mix all dressing ingredients except paprika and mix well. Carefully stir this into potato mixture. Transfer to a bowl. Garnish top of salad with sliced egg and sprinkle with paprika. Cover and refrigerate for an hour and serve cold.

Ingredients to Consider on Specific Diets

Gluten & Casein Free ....Yes	Phenol Free..No
Low Oxalate Diet ....No	Specific Carbohydrate Diet .... No

This recipe is also Soy free, Corn free and Rice free

Oral Motor Rating :) :) :)

Three-Bean Salad

Yields: 4 Servings

Ingredients
- 1 cup navy beans, cooked or canned
- 1 cup pinto beans, cooked or canned
- 1 cup string beans, finely chopped
- 2 tablespoons sesame, sunflower, or safflower oil
- 1 tablespoon umeboshi paste, mixed with 1/4 water
- 1 tablespoon basil or parsley, freshly chopped

> **Umeboshi Paste**
>
> *Umeboshi paste is a tangy, salty condiment made from the pureed pulp of naturally processed, pickled umeboshi plums. It promotes healthy appetite and digestion. A small dab replaces both salt and butter in dishes. Ideal for making sushi, dips, sauces, salad dressing, and for seasoning vegetables.*

Directions
Combine all the three beans in large bowl. Add sesame oil, umeboshi paste, and fresh basil. Toss them till mixed and serve.

Ingredients to Consider on Specific Diets

Gluten & Casein Free .... Yes	Phenol Free .... Yes
Low Oxalate Diet .... Yes	Specific Carbohydrate Diet .... No

This recipe is also Soy free, Corn free and Rice free

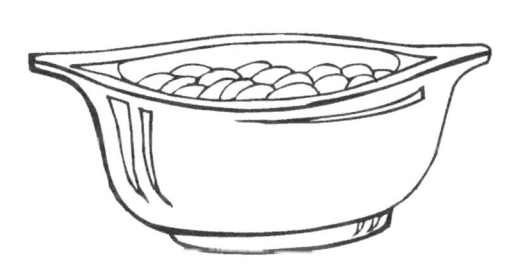

Oral Motor Rating 😊 😊 😊

CHAPTER 12: TASTY MEAL COMPANIONS

Cucumber Pressed Salad

Yields: 3 Servings

Ingredients
2 small "pickle" cucumbers, finely chopped
1 small onion, finely chopped
1 sheet toasted nori
1/3 bunch parsley or basil
1/2 teaspoon sea salt
1 teaspoon umeboshi paste
2 cups napa cabbage, thinly sliced
4 radish tops (green)

The Japanese Pickle/Salad Press*
It will allow you to make delicious quick pickles. Just place lightly salted vegetables into the bucket, lock the lid, and press. The pressure and salt will cause the juices to seep from the veggies and form mild brine. Press anywhere from three hours to three days. Then drain off the brine (save for a great soup stock) and enjoy.

Directions
Combine all ingredients in a salad press. Press all together for minimum of three days.

Ingredients to Consider on Specific Diets

Gluten & Casein Free .... Yes
Phenol Free .... No
Low Oxalate Diet .... Yes (use basil and parsley)
Specific Carbohydrate Diet .... Yes
This recipe is also Soy free, Corn free and Rice free

Oral Motor Rating :) :) :) :)

* Japanese pickle presses are available in Oriental shops or on such websites as http://www.kushistore.com (see "Kitchenware" in this website's catalog section).

Bok Choy Pressed Salad

Yields: 2 to 4 Servings

Ingredients
2 cups bok choy or napa cabbage, thinly sliced
1 onion, chopped
1/2 cup carrots, grated
1/4 teaspoon sea salt
1 tablespoon apple cider vinegar
1 tablespoon shiso powder

> **Shiso**
> *Shiso is a flavorful herb that deserves a place beside basil and cilantro in every culinary herb garden.*

Directions
Combine all ingredients well and place in salad press for one hour. This salad can be served warm or cold as desired.

Ingredients to Consider on Specific Diets

Gluten & Casein Free .... Yes	Phenol Free .... Yes
Low Oxalate Diet .... Yes	Specific Carbohydrate Diet .... Yes

This recipe is also Soy free, Corn free and Rice free

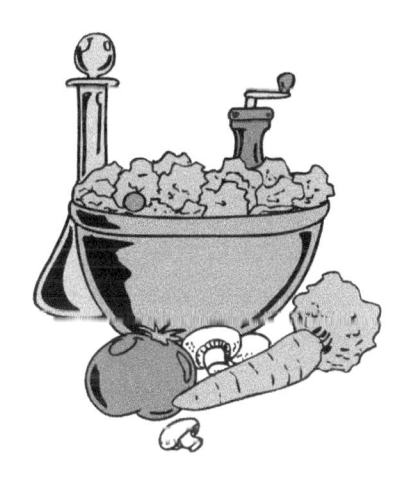

Oral Motor Rating ☺ ☺ ☺ ☺

Tempeh Salad

Yields: 4 to 6 Servings

Ingredients
8 ounces tempeh (plain or vegetable)
3 tablespoons olive oil
2 teaspoons lemon juice
2 garlic cloves, minced
1/2 cup carrots, grated
1 large stalk celery, minced
1 small onion, finely chopped
1 cup mixed vegetables
   (diced green peppers, scallions, dill,
   cucumber pickles)
Pinch of salt to taste

Tempeh
Tempeh is made by a natural culturing and controlled fermentation process that binds soybeans into a cake. It is also a good filing for a healthy sandwich.

Directions
Cut tempeh in small pieces and steam for 15 minutes. Cool a bit and then add chopped vegetables, oil, lemon, garlic and toss together. Serve at room temperature.

Ingredients to Consider on Specific Diets

Gluten & Casein Free .... Yes	Phenol Free .... Yes
Low Oxalate Diet .... Yes	Specific Carbohydrate Diet .... No

This recipe is also Corn free and Rice free

Oral Motor Rating 😊 😊 😊

NON-VEGETARIAN SALADS

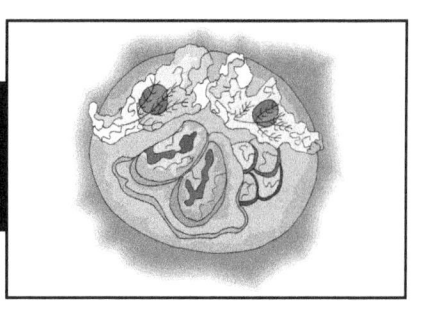

Hard-Boiled Egg Salad

Yields: 1 to 2 Servings

Ingredients
2 eggs, hard boiled
1 tablespoon olive oil
Salt and pepper to taste

Directions
Coarsely chop hard-boiled eggs, add olive oil, and salt and pepper to taste.

Ingredients to Consider on Specific Diets

Gluten & Casein Free .... Yes	Phenol Free .... Yes
Low Oxalate Diet .... Yes	Specific Carbohydrate Diet .... Yes

This recipe is also Soy free, Corn free and Rice free

Oral Motor Rating :) :)

Hamburger Salad

Yields: 4 Servings

Ingredients
1 pound ground beef or buffalo
1 teaspoon olive oil
3 garlic cloves, chopped fine
1 red onion, sliced
1 cup grape seed oil, veganaise or SCD mayonnaise
1 teaspoon sea salt
1/2 cup finely chopped walnuts

> ### Lean Organic Beef
> *Lean, organic beef is a very good source of protein as well as vitamins B12 and B6. (Children with ASD can often be deficient in both of these vitamins.)*

Directions
In an iron skillet, heat oil and add garlic and onions and cook for several minutes until onions start to look slightly transparent. Then add ground beef and cook until browned. Allow to sit for several minutes, and then drain off excess liquid. Add mayonnaise or Veganaise and walnuts. This salad can be served over cooked vegetables of your child's choice.

Ingredients to Consider on Specific Diets

Gluten & Casein Free ....Yes	Phenol Free ....Yes
Low Oxalate Diet ....Yes	Specific Carbohydrate Diet .... Yes

This recipe is also Soy free, Corn free and Rice free

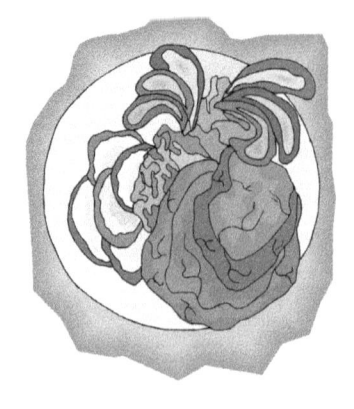

Oral Motor Rating 😊 😊 😊

Turkey Salad

Yields: 4 Servings

Ingredients
2 cups cooked turkey, chopped into bite-sized pieces
1 small red onion, finely chopped
1 celery stalk, finely chopped
1/2 cup red bell pepper, finely chopped
1 teaspoon sea salt

Dressing
1/4 cup raw organic apple cider vinegar
1/4 cup lemon juice, freshly squeezed
3 tablespoons olive oil
1 tablespoon Dijon mustard
1 teaspoon ground black pepper (optional)
1 teaspoon dried rosemary
1/2 teaspoon sea salt

> *Turkey*
>
> *Turkey is a very good source of protein as well as the trace mineral, selenium, which is of fundamental importance to human health. It is an essential component of several major metabolic pathways and immune function.*

Directions
Cook the turkey on low to medium heat in a covered pan, allowing it to cook in its own juices. After turkey is cooked, set aside and let it cool down. In a medium-size mixing bowl, mix the turkey with the vegetables, and pour dressing over all. Refrigerate several hours to marinate flavors. Serve over a bed of mixed greens.

Ingredients to Consider on Specific Diets

Gluten & Casein Free	Yes
Phenol Free	No
Low Oxalate Diet	Yes
Specific Carbohydrate Diet	Yes

This recipe is also Soy free, Corn free and Rice free

Oral Motor Rating 🙂 🙂 🙂

Ham and Fresh Asparagus Salad

Yields: 4 to 6 Servings

Ingredients
6 ham slices (1/4 inch thick)
12 large or 18 small stalks of fresh asparagus
1/2 cup lettuce
1/8 teaspoon black pepper
1/8 teaspoon garlic powder
1 teaspoon onion powder
2 tablespoons lemon juice
3 tablespoons BodyBio Balance Oil (flax/sunflower seed oil)
1/2 teaspoon sea salt

Directions
Blanch asparagus in boiling water for 1 to 2 minutes and let it cool down. Cut ham into small cubes. Add other ingredients in a bowl, mix and serve.

Ingredients to Consider on Specific Diets

Gluten & Casein Free .... Yes	Phenol Free .... Yes
Low Oxalate Diet .... Yes	Specific Carbohydrate Diet .... Yes

This recipe is also Soy free, Corn free and Rice free

Oral Motor Rating 😊 😊 😊

Chapter Thirteen

Delicious Accompaniments

Sauces, Dips, Dressings and Condiments

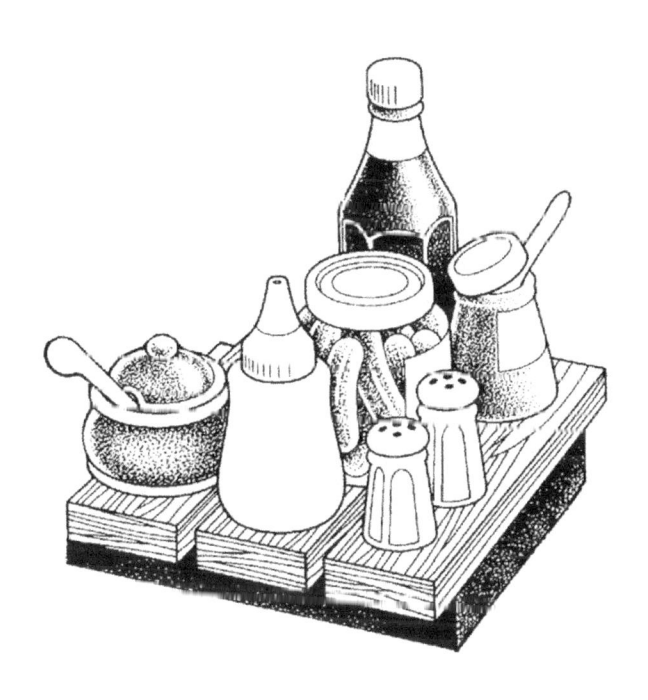

DELICIOUS ACCOMPANIMENTS
TABLE OF CONTENTS

SAUCES, DIPS, DRESSING and CONDIMENTS RECIPES

BBQ Sauce	317
Sweet Mustard Sauce	318
Homemade Ketchup	319
Ginger Scallion Dipping Sauce	320
Easy Cranberry Sauce	321
Italian Pesto	322
Zucchini Hummus	323
White Bean Hummus Dip	324
Spicy Thai Almond Sauce	325
Gingery Carrot Sauce	326
Ranch Dip or Dressing	327
Mango Salsa	328
Avocado Dip	329

BBQ Sauce

Ingredients
2 pounds ripe tomatoes
1 cup celery, chopped
1/2 cup green pepper, chopped
1 large onion, chopped
3 garlic cloves, chopped
1/4 cup honey
1/4 cup vinegar
1 tablespoon lemon juice
1 tablespoon paprika
1 teaspoon dry mustard
1 teaspoon sea salt
1/4 teaspoon cayenne pepper

Cayenne Pepper
Cayenne pepper is often used as a table condiment. The trick to using this spice is to use it with care and add gradually.

Directions
Core and cut tomatoes in chunks and cook on medium heat until soft. Pass through thin strainer to remove seeds and skin. Return the puree to the pot. Add remaining ingredients. Bring to a boil on medium heat, stirring often. Simmer for about 2 to 2 1/2 hours until thickened and of the consistency that you want. Remove from heat and cool. Smooth in blender, then return the puree to the pot and bring back to a boil (slowly). Store in a mason jar in refrigerator.

Ingredients to Consider on Specific Diets

Gluten & Casein Free ....Yes	Phenol Free ....No
Low Oxalate Diet ....No	Specific Carbohydrate Diet ....Yes

This recipe is also Soy free, Corn free and Rice free

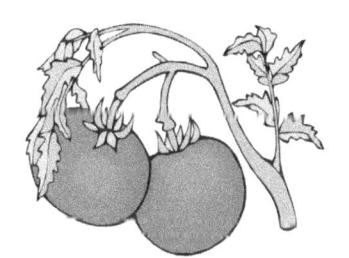

Oral Motor Rating 😊

Sweet Mustard Sauce

Ingredients
1/4 cup honey
1/4 cup plain mustard
1/4 cup sunflower or safflower oil
3/4 teaspoon apple cider vinegar
Pinch red pepper, optional
1 teaspoon garlic powder

Apple Cider Vinegar
Apple cider vinegar is made by the fermentation of apple cider. Apple cider vinegar contains numerous nutrients essential for children and it is also helpful in fighting fungal and bacterial infections.

Directions
Add all ingredients in a large bowl, and mix with a whisk, so all are blended together. Store in a Mason jar and refrigerate.

Ingredients to Consider on Specific Diets

Gluten & Casein Free .... Yes
Phenol Free .... No (mustard is very high)
Low Oxalate Diet .... Yes
Specific Carbohydrate Diet .... Yes
This recipe is also Soy free, Corn free and Rice free

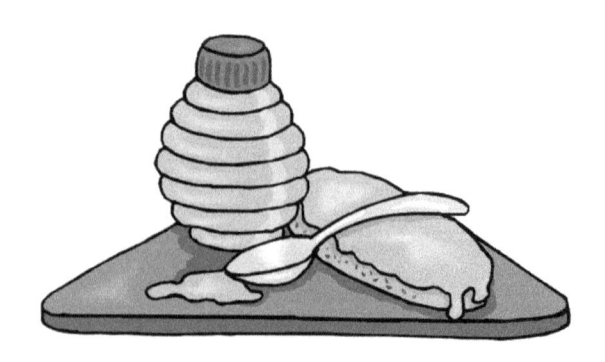

Oral Motor Rating 😊 😊 😊 😊

Homemade Ketchup

Ingredients
6 cups tomato juice (one large 48-oz. can)
1/2 cup white distilled vinegar
2 1/2 tablespoons honey or maple syrup

> *Ketchup*
>
> *Ketchup is an excellent example of a condiment that was formerly fermented, and thus health-promoting, whose benefits were lost with large scale canning methods and reliance on sugar for preservation.*

Directions
Simmer tomato juice and vinegar in a saucepan on low flame until it thickens, then add honey, cool, and refrigerate. Note: This homemade version of ketchup is easy to make and not loaded with artificial colorings and preservatives like commercial ketchup. To add the color, red vegetables can also be added, and as per your child's preference, more honey can be added. This ketchup can be refrigerated up to a week. The ingredients selected In recipe does fall into high in some diets; however keeping in mind the proportion of ketchup that will be used each day, this recipe is shown be compliant for each diet. After all, all kids want Ketchup!

Ingredients to Consider on Specific Diets

Gluten & Casein Free	Yes
Phenol Free	No
Low Oxalate Diet	Yes
Specific Carbohydrate Diet	Yes

This recipe is also Soy free, Corn free and Rice free

Oral Motor Rating 🙂

Ginger Scallion Dipping Sauce

Ingredients
1/2 cup brown rice vinegar
1 scallion, minced
1 teaspoon tamari
1 teaspoon cilantro, fresh minced
1 garlic clove, minced
1/2 teaspoon dark sesame oil
1/2 teaspoon ginger, minced
1/4 teaspoon red pepper flakes (or to taste)

> **Tamari**
> *Tamari is made from the salty fermented paste derived from soy beans, called miso. People with gluten intolerance should read labels on tamari soy sauce carefully to ensure that it is true tamari, fermented without any gluten.*

Directions
Combine all ingredients in a glass jar and shake to blend completely. Sauce will keep for several days stored in a tightly covered jar in the refrigerator.

Ingredients to Consider on Specific Diets

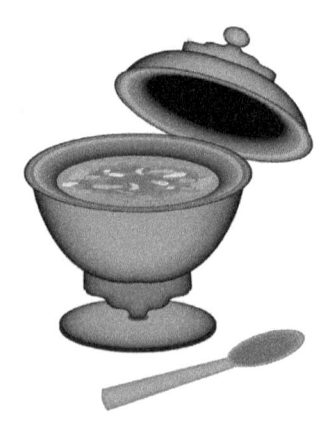

Gluten & Casein Free	Yes
Low Oxalate Diet	No
Phenol Free	No
Specific Carbohydrate Diet	No

This recipe is also Soy free, Corn free, but is not Rice free

Oral Motor Rating

Easy Cranberry Sauce

Ingredients
1 pound cranberries, fresh or frozen (4 cups)
1 cup water
1 cup honey

Directions
Rinse cranberries with cool water, and remove any stems or blemished berries. Over medium heat, bring water and honey to boiling in a saucepan and cook for 5 minutes, stirring occasionally. Add cranberries heat to boiling again, and cook about 5 minutes longer, still stirring occasionally until cranberries begin to pop. Pour sauce into bowl or container. Refrigerate about 3 hours or until chilled.

Ingredients to Consider on Specific Diets

Gluten & Casein Free	Yes
Phenol Free	No
Low Oxalate Diet	Yes
Specific Carbohydrate Diet	Yes

This recipe is also Corn free, Soy free and Rice free

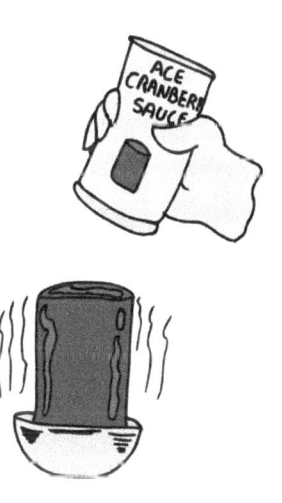

Oral Motor Rating 🙂

Italian Pesto

Ingredients
3 garlic cloves, finely chopped
2 cups fresh basil leaves, washed and dried
1/2 cup olive oil or grape seed oil
1/4 cup casein-free parmesan cheese
1/2 cup pine nuts (optional)

Basil
The delicious taste and aroma of basil is the signature of Mediterranean cooking. It may also be brewed into tea that has the ability to relieve intestinal gas.

Directions
Put all ingredients in a food processor, and pulse for 30 seconds. Add more oil if you want it smoother like a paste.

Ingredients to Consider on Specific Diets

Gluten & Casein Free .... Yes
Phenol Free .... No
Low Oxalate Diet .... No
Specific Carbohydrate Diet .... Yes

This recipe is also Soy free, Corn free and Rice free

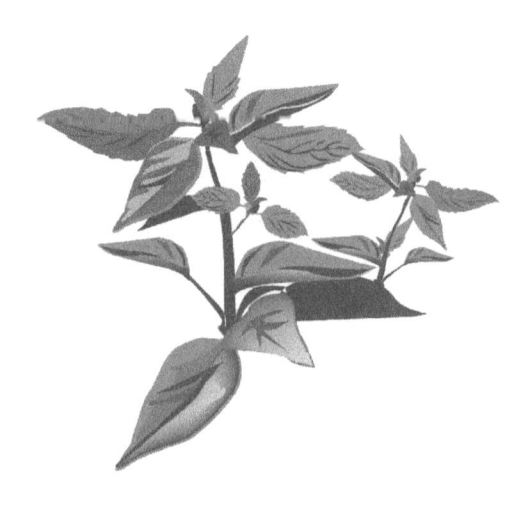

Oral Motor Rating 😊 😊

Zucchini Hummus

Ingredients
2 medium sized zucchini, peeled and chunked
1/2 cup raw tahini
1/2 cup fresh lime or lemon juice
1/3 cup olive oil, cold pressed
4 garlic cloves
1/4 cup parsley
1/4 teaspoon sea salt
1/2 tablespoon ground cumin (optional)

> **Variation to the Recipe**
>
> *Traditional hummus is made with chick peas. Using vegetables like zucchini is a great way to get more vegetables in your child's diet.*

Directions
In a high-speed blender, combine all ingredients. Blend until thick and smooth.

Ingredients to Consider on Specific Diets

Gluten & Casein Free................ Yes
Phenol Free............................ Yes (omit zucchini and substitute with butternut squash or chickpeas)
Low Oxalate Diet .... Yes
Specific Carbohydrate Diet .... Yes
This recipe is also Corn free, Rice free but is not Soy free

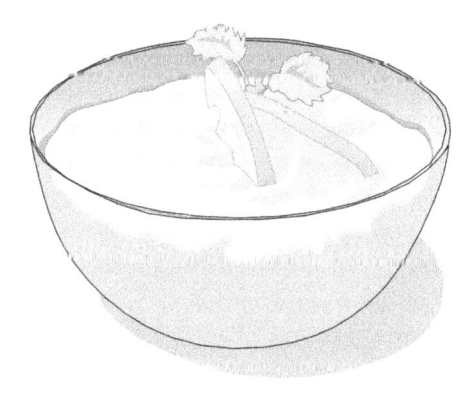

Oral Motor Rating 😊 😊

White Bean Hummus Dip

This dip, served with pita bread or chips, makes a nice appetizer for guests to nibble on as you prepare the evening's meal. The dip can be made up to three days ahead and stored in the refrigerator. Bring to room temperature before serving.

Ingredients
1/4 cup green onions, chopped
2 tablespoons lemon juice, fresh
2 tablespoons tahini (sesame-seed paste)
1/2 teaspoon oregano
1/4 teaspoon ground cumin (optional)
1/8 teaspoon sea salt
1/8 teaspoon black pepper
1 can cannellini, great northern, or navy beans, rinsed and drained
1 garlic clove, peeled

Directions
Combine all of the ingredients in a food processor, and process until the mixture is smooth.

Ingredients to Consider on Specific Diets

Gluten & Casein Free .... Yes
Phenol Free .... Yes
Low Oxalate Diet .... Yes
Specific Carbohydrate Diet .... Yes (if you use navy beans and avoid cannellini beans)

This recipe is also Soy free, Corn free and Rice free

Oral Motor Rating ☺ ☺

Spicy Thai Almond Sauce

Ingredients
1 1/2 cups raw almond butter
1/4 cup rice bran oil or grape seed oil
1 tablespoon apple cider vinegar
1 teaspoon cayenne powder
1 garlic clove, finely crushed

> ### Rice Bran Oil
> Rice bran oil is created using the hull of the rice grain. It is rich in antioxidants and several vitamins. It has mild flavor, so can be easily added in a salad dressing. When used as oil in baked goods, the rice bran oil provides a delicious nutty flavor.

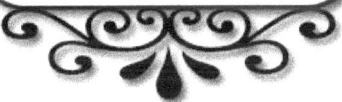

Directions
Add all ingredients and grind well. This can be a good dip to be used with fresh vegetables; also good on a crunchy green salad.

Ingredients to Consider on Specific Diets

Gluten & Casein Free .... Yes
Phenol Free .... No (almonds are very high)
Low Oxalate Diet .... No (almonds are very high)
Specific Carbohydrate Diet .... Yes

This recipe is also Soy free, Corn free, and Rice free (use grape seed oil)

Oral Motor Rating 🙂

Gingery Carrot Sauce

Ingredients
10 -15 small carrots, or
7 large carrots, chopped
1 large onion, diced
1 tablespoon coconut oil or ghee
1 celery stalk, chopped
1 small red pepper, chopped (optional)
2 garlic cloves, minced
1/2 teaspoon ginger, freshly grated or minced
2 cups water or stock
2 1/2 teaspoons sea salt

Ginger

Ginger is a spice which is used for cooking and is also consumed whole as a delicacy or medicine. It is the underground stem of the ginger plant.

Directions
Heat oil or ghee in a medium-size cooking pan and sauté carrots and onions until they are a little brown. Add celery, red pepper, garlic, and ginger and continue to sauté. Add water or stock and sea salt. Cover and simmer until carrots are cooked. Transfer all into blender and blend to get the sauce consistency you desire.

Note: This sauce can be used with gluten-free spaghetti or noodles.

Ingredients to Consider on Specific Diets

Gluten & Casein Free .... Yes	Phenol Free ....Yes
Low Oxalate Diet..Yes	Specific Carbohydrate Diet ....Yes

This recipe is also Soy free, Corn free and Rice free

Oral Motor Rating :)

HEALING AUTISM IN THE KITCHEN

Ranch Dip or Dressing

Ingredients
1 whole egg or egg replacer
1 teaspoon dry mustard
1/2 teaspoon sea salt
3 tablespoons lemon juice
2 teaspoons apple cider vinegar
2 tablespoons parsley flakes
2 teaspoons onion powder
1/2 teaspoon garlic powder
1 cup safflower or sunflower oil
1 tablespoon hot water

Mustard
Mustard is a plant in the cruciferous family and is rich in vitamin C. Mustard is used to add a piquant, pungent, spicy flavor to a variety of dishes. Mustard seeds can be ground to create dry powdered mustard.

Directions
In a blender, combine the egg, mustard, salt, lemon juice, vinegar, parsley flakes, onion and garlic powder, and blend well. With the blender still running, add the oil in a steady slow stream and blend until all oil is mixed well. Blend in hot water to stabilize. Serve immediately or refrigerate in a covered glass container and use within one week.

Ingredients to Consider on Specific Diets

Gluten & Casein Free	Yes	Phenol Free	Yes
Low Oxalate Diet	Yes	Specific Carbohydrate Diet	Yes

This recipe is also Soy free, Corn free and Rice free

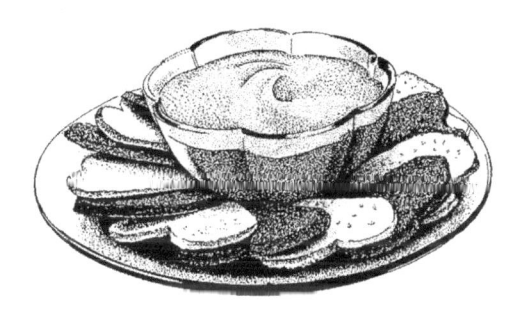

Oral Motor Rating 🙂 🙂

Mango Salsa

Ingredients
1 large ripe mango
1 large tomato, chopped
1 small onion, minced
2 tablespoons cilantro
3 tablespoons lime juice
1/4 teaspoon sea salt

> *Cilantro*
>
> *Cilantro is often sprinkled like parsley on cooked dishes or minced or puréed for use in sauces soups and curries. It can be used to flavor curries, soups, salsas, salads, burritos and even meat dishes.*

Directions
Peel and cube mango in small chunks. Mix in a small dish with tomato, onion and all other ingredients, and it's ready to eat.

Ingredients to Consider on Specific Diets

Gluten & Casein Free ....Yes	Phenol Free ....Yes
Low Oxalate Diet ....Yes	Specific Carbohydrate Diet ....Yes

This recipe is also Soy free, Corn free and Rice free

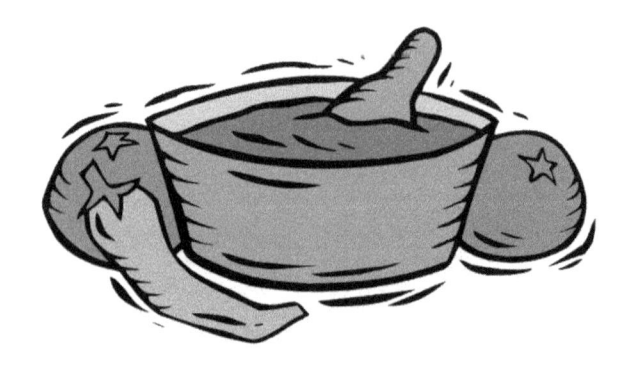

Oral Motor Rating 🙂 🙂

Avocado Dip

Ingredients
3 medium ripe avocados
1 small onion, finely chopped
1/4 teaspoon sea salt
Pepper to taste
2 garlic cloves, minced
1/2 teaspoon lemon juice
1 or 2 hard-boiled eggs (optional)

Avocado

Avocado is a fruit that has very high fat content — about 20 times more than any other fruit. Avocados are also a rich source of numerous minerals such as potassium, magnesium, iron, calcium and phosphorus.

Directions
Peel avocados, remove pits, and mash with a fork. Mix in one or two hard-boiled eggs and the finely chopped onion. Add salt, garlic, and pepper to taste. Sprinkle with lemon juice to prevent discoloration and add zing. Serve chilled.

Ingredients to Consider on Specific Diets

Gluten & Casein Free .... Yes
Phenol Free .... Yes (moderate to high)
Low Oxalate Diet ....   Yes
Specific Carbohydrate Diet .... Yes
This recipe is also Soy free, Corn free and Rice free

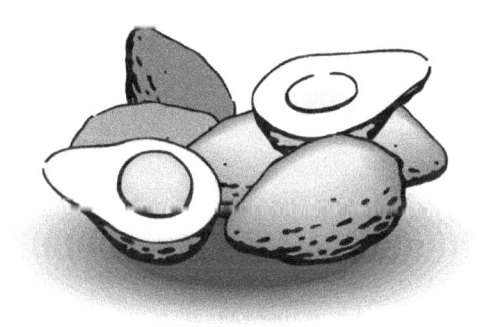

Oral Motor Rating :) :)

Notes:

CHAPTER FOURTEEN

Healthy Between-Meal Treats

Hunger-Satisfying Snacks

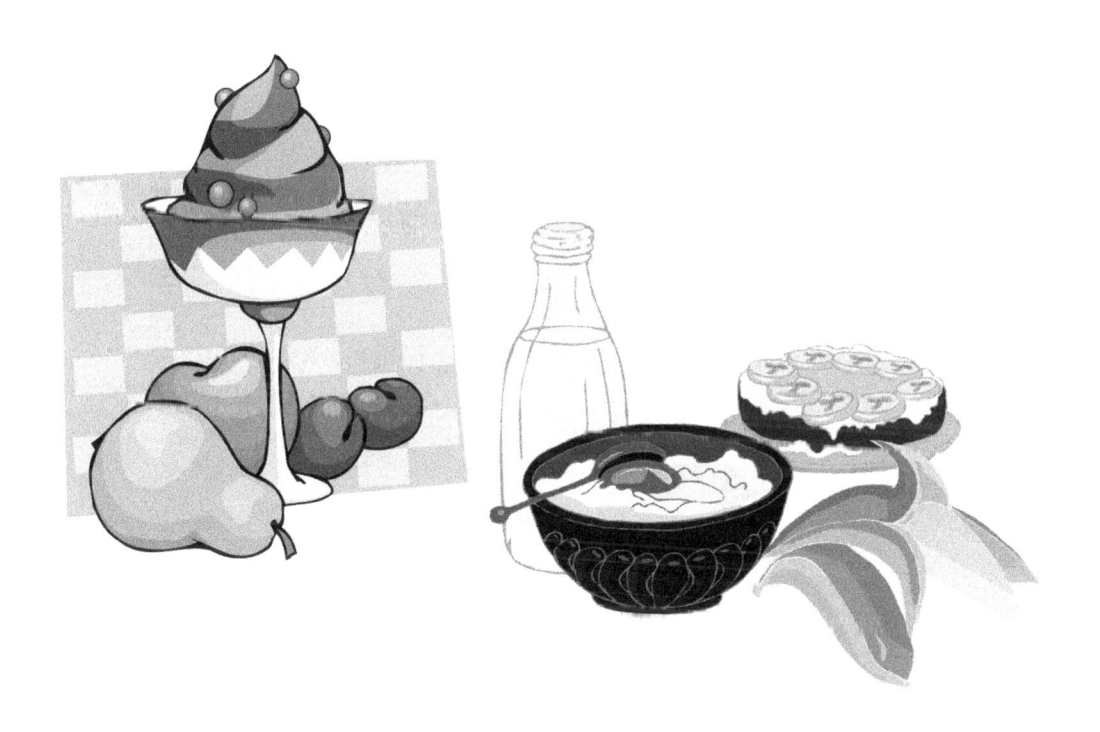

HEALTHY BETWEEN-MEAL TREATS
TABLE OF CONTENTS

SNACK RECIPES

Butternut Squash Crunch	333
Nut Butter Pudding	334
Crunchy Chickpea Bars	335
Buckwheat Crackers	336
Gluten-Free Chicken Nuggets	337
Pear Sauce	338
Nut "Ice Cream"	339
Rice Pudding	340
Flax and Sesame Seed Sticks	341
Spring Rolls	342
Quinoa Crackers	343
Sesame Finger Snacks	344
Graham Crackers	345

Butternut Squash Crunch

Yields: 4 to 6 Servings

This recipe comes out as a large loaf that you can cut into small desired size pieces.

Ingredients
1 large butternut squash, peeled and cut into small chunks
1/2 cup honey
1/2 cup almond milk
1 teaspoon ground cinnamon
1/4 teaspoon nutmeg, ground
1 teaspoon gluten- and casein-free vanilla extract
1/4 teaspoon sea salt
2 eggs, lightly beaten, or egg replacer

Topping Mixture:
2 tablespoons coconut or almond meal flour
3 tablespoons coconut butter

Directions
Preheat oven to 350º. Lightly grease a two-quart baking dish and set aside. Combine squash, honey, milk, cinnamon, nutmeg, vanilla, salt, and eggs in a large bowl and stir well. Prepare "crunch topping" by combining flour and butter in the bowl and mixing well. Spoon the squash mixture into the baking tray and crumble the topping over all. Bake for 25 minutes or until brown.

Ingredients to Consider on Specific Diets

Gluten & Casein Free .... Yes
Phenol Free .... No
Low Oxalate Diet .... No
Specific Carbohydrate Diet .... Yes
This recipe is also Soy free, Corn free and Rice free

Oral Motor Rating 😊 😊 😊

Nut Butter Pudding

Yields: 2 Servings

Ingredients
1 small banana, mashed
1/2 cup yogurt (SCD)
   (see recipe in Chapter 9)
1/2 cup almond butter, cashew
   or macadamia nut butter
1/4 teaspoon gluten-free vanilla extract
Pinch sea salt

> *Yogurt and pH*
>
> *When we make yogurt the pH falls to about 4.5 rather than 7.1-2 (as in fluid milk). The protein structure become less complex, causing less allergic reactions as compared to the casein found in same milk.*

Directions
Combine all ingredients in a blender. Blend until smooth, pour into serving dishes, and refrigerate. Serve cold.

Ingredients to Consider on Specific Diets

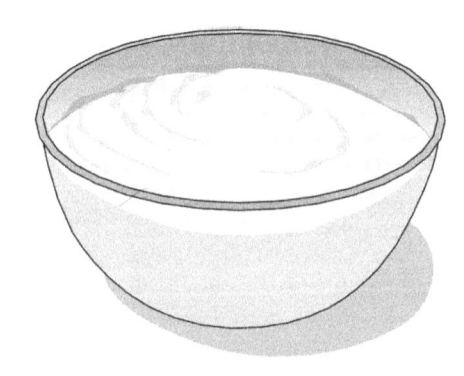

Gluten & Casein Free ....No
Phenol Free...Yes (If you use cashew or macadamia nut butter)
Low Oxalate Diet ....No
Specific Carbohydrate Diet ....Yes
This recipe is also Soy free, Corn free and Rice free

Oral Motor Rating 😊 😊

Crunchy Chickpea Bars

Yields: 4 Servings

Ingredients
2 cups chickpeas, cooked or canned
1/4 cup coconut or grape seed oil
1/2 cup honey or maple syrup
Pinch of salt

Chick Peas
Chick peas are perhaps better known as garbanzo beans. They are low on the glycemic index, and are a great staple for people with diabetes.

Directions
Preheat the oven to 350º. Mix chickpeas with melted oil, add honey and pour into a food processor and pulse 2 or 3 times. Spread the chickpea mixture on a lightly greased cookie sheet or one lined with parchment paper. Bake for 30-35 minutes, until browned and crisp. Cut in bars or bite-sized pieces.

Ingredients to Consider on Specific Diets

Gluten & Casein Free ....Yes	Phenol Free ....Yes (if you use maple syrup)
Low Oxalate Diet..Yes	Specific Carbohydrate Diet .... No

This recipe is also Soy free, Corn free and Rice free

Oral Motor Rating 😊 😊 😊 😊

Buckwheat Crackers

Yield: 24 Crackers

> ### *Buckwheat*
> *Buckwheat is also sold in whole or cracked form for use in breakfast cereals or to add texture to breads and other baked products. It has a distinctive nutty flavor quite pleasing in taste.*

Ingredients
1 1/2 cups buckwheat groats
1/2 cup flaxseed
1/4 cup coconut oil or olive oil
1 garlic clove, minced
2 tablespoons dried basil
(3x more if using fresh)
1 tablespoon dried oregano
(3x more if using fresh)
2 tablespoons dried parsley
(3x more if using fresh)
1 teaspoon sea salt
1 cup water

Directions
Soak the buckwheat grouts and flax seeds in water overnight. Drain off any remaining liquid. Combine grouts, flaxseeds, olive oil, garlic, and all the herbs in a blender and blend until batter is a thick consistency. Place the batter in a large bowl. Grease a cookie-baking sheet and spoon the batter into nice flat shapes about 1 1/2 inches round and about a third of an inch deep. Bake in the oven at 350º for 15 minutes on each side.

Ingredients to Consider on Specific Diets

Gluten & Casein Free ....Yes	Phenol Free ....No
Low Oxalate Diet ....Yes	Specific Carbohydrate Diet ......No

This recipe is also Soy free, Corn free and Rice free

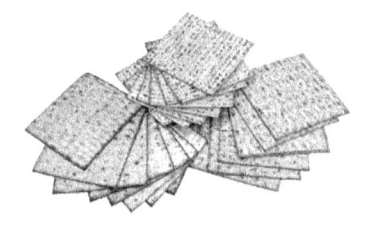

Oral Motor Rating 😊 😊 😊 😊

HEALING AUTISM IN THE KITCHEN

Gluten-Free Chicken Nuggets

Yields: 4 to 6 Servings

Ingredients
1 boneless, skinless chicken breast
1 1/2 cup coconut oil for frying
1 egg, beaten, or egg replacer
1 cup brown rice or almond flour
1 teaspoon sea salt
1 teaspoon garlic powder
1 teaspoon onion powder

Recipe Variation

If the child is egg intolerant, use melted ghee or Casein free milk or egg replacer. To make the nuggets crunchier, blend GF crackers/cereal in food processor or blender, and roll the nuggets in them before frying.

Directions
Heat oil in a pan. Slice chicken into bite size piece (slicing them thin enough to fry quickly). In a small bowl, beat egg. In another bowl, mix flour and seasonings. Dip nuggets in egg, coat with flour, and fry in oil until brown on all sides. Place on paper towel to drain excess oil.

Ingredients to Consider on Specific Diets

Gluten & Casein Free .... Yes
Phenol Free .... Yes (use brown rice flour)
Low Oxalate Diet........................ Yes (use brown rice flour)
Specific Carbohydrate Diet .... Yes (use almond flour)
This recipe is also Soy free, Corn free and Rice free (use almond flour)

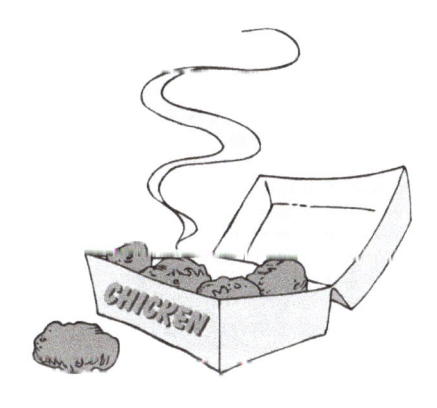

Oral Motor Rating 😊 😊 😊 😊

Pear Sauce

Yields: 3 to 4 Servings

Ingredients
4 small pears
1/2 cup water
2 tablespoon honey or maple syrup (optional)
Pinch cinnamon or nutmeg

Uses for Pear Sauce
This sauce can be used as a snack, spread like jam on top of breads, or mixed with other fruits to make desserts.

Directions
Peel and dice the pears. Place the fruit in a saucepan with water. Cover and cook on low to medium heat until fruit has cooked down and is soft. Add sweetener if necessary. Blend if a smoother texture is desired.

Ingredients to Consider on Specific Diets

Gluten & Casein Free .... Yes
Phenol Free .... Yes (omit honey)
Low Oxalate Diet .... Yes
Specific Carbohydrate Diet .... Yes (if you use honey)
This recipe is also Soy free, Corn free and Rice free

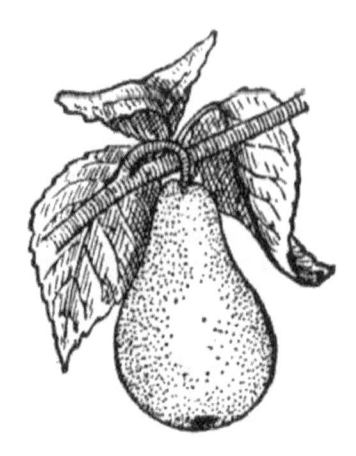

Oral Motor Rating :) :)

Nut "Ice Cream"

Yields: 3 Servings

Ingredients
2 SCD vanilla beans*
3 cups cashews or almonds
3 cups water
1 1/2 cups honey

*Or use 1/2 teaspoon pure vanilla extract, which is also SCD legal.

> ***Recipe Variation***
> *In this Nut "Ice cream," the texture and flavor makes cashews a great choice. Instead of cashews, others nuts can be substituted as well.*

Directions
Slice open the vanilla beans and scrape soft inside into blender (or substitute with pure vanilla extract). Add nuts, water, and sweetener. Blend on high until smooth. Place blender or mixture in freezer for 45 to 60 minutes to chill. Pour the mixture into an ice cream maker and freeze. Note: It's best to make homemade ice cream and serve it immediately. If you freeze it, it often freezes solid or icy.

Ingredients to Consider on Specific Diets

Gluten & Casein Free   Yes
Phenol Free .... No
Low Oxalate Diet .... No
Specific Carbohydrate Diet .... Yes
This recipe is also Soy free, Corn free and Rice free

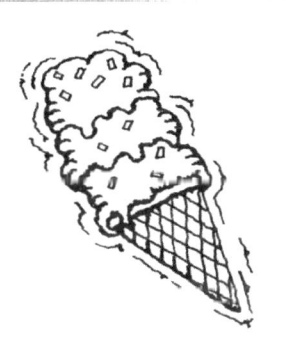

Oral Motor Rating :)

Rice Pudding

Yields: 6 to 8 Servings

Ingredients

1 cup sweet rice or short grain brown rice (previously soaked*)
3 cups water
1/4 teaspoon sea salt
2 tablespoons honey or maple syrup
1 1/2 cups coconut milk
1/4 teaspoon cinnamon or nutmeg
2 teaspoons gluten-free vanilla

> ### Rice and Digestion
> *To make the rice more digestible, soak rice 8 to 12 hours. Also, a spoonful of young coconut kefir or milk kefir to the soaking water helps "pre-digest" the grain/rice making it even more digestible.*

Directions

Bring 3 cups of water and rice to a boil in a large two-quart saucepan, cover and leave at lowest heat untouched for 45 minutes. Stir in the salt and honey. Remove the pot from the heat and add rice or almond milk, cinnamon or nutmeg, and the vanilla. *Soak rice 8 to 12 hours to remove the enzyme inhibitors. Adding a spoonful of young coconut kefir or milk kefir to the soaking water helps "pre-digest" the grain/rice, making it even more digestible.

Ingredients to Consider on Specific Diets

Gluten & Casein Free ....Yes
Low Oxalate Diet...Yes
Phenol Free ....Yes (if you use maple syrup)
Specific Carbohydrate Diet .... No

This recipe is also Soy free, and Corn free but is not Rice free

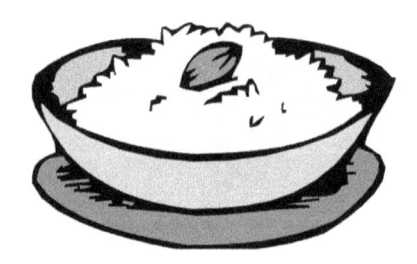

Oral Motor Rating 😊 😊

340 HEALING AUTISM IN THE KITCHEN

Flax and Sesame Seed Sticks

Yields: 4 to 6 Sticks

Ingredients
1 cup brown rice flour
1/4 cup ground flax seed
1 teaspoon garlic powder
1/4 cup sesame seeds
1/2 teaspoon baking powder (aluminum free)
1/2 teaspoon xanthan gum
1/2 cup warm water

> ### *Flax Seeds*
> *The warm, earthy and subtly nutty flavor of flaxseeds containing an abundance of omega-3 fatty acids, makes them an increasingly popular addition to the diet. Whether ground or whole, flax seeds add fiber to diet, along with other health benefits.*

Directions
In a bowl, mix all dry ingredients, and then add enough water and make dough. Make small balls of dough, and then roll them by hand to make long sticks. Deep fry in as much olive oil as needed, or bake them at 300º for 20 minutes.

Ingredients to Consider on Specific Diets

Gluten & Casein Free	Yes	Phenol Free	Yes
Low Oxalate Diet	Yes	Specific Carbohydrate Diet	No

This recipe is also Soy free and Corn free, but is not Rice free.

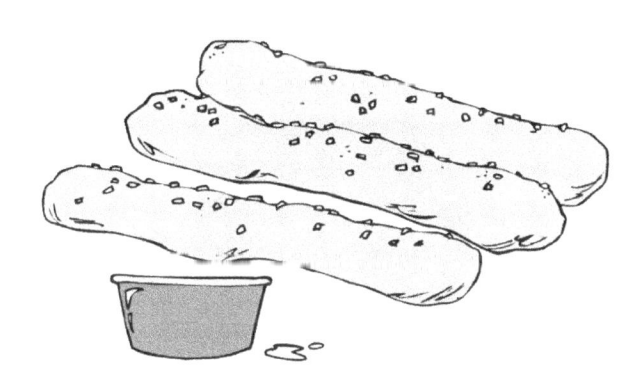

Oral Motor Rating 😊 😊 😊 😊

Spring Rolls

Yields: 12 to 14 Rolls

Ingredients
1 pound ground pork
1/2 head cabbage, thinly sliced
4-6 carrots, grated
1 onion, diced
1-2 garlic cloves, minced
1 teaspoon sea salt
1/2 teaspoon pepper (optional)
1/2 cup olive oil or coconut oil
12-ounce package round rice paper wrappers (about 30 wraps)

> ### *Rice Paper*
> *Rice paper is paper made from the pith of the rice plant, or from a variety of other plants including mulberry and hemp. They are used to make dumplings, spring rolls, and similar foods. The more rice in the blend of fibers used to make the paper, the more transparent it will be.*

Directions
Toss filling ingredients together and brown in a skillet or wok until thoroughly cooked. Dip wrapper quickly into the boiling water pan just to soften. Spoon 2 or 3 tablespoons of filling into the wrap, roll one side edge of wrap over filling, tuck in top and bottom ends, and continue rolling. Crisp the rolls by deep frying in a skillet. Drain on paper towels and serve.

Ingredients to Consider on Specific Diets

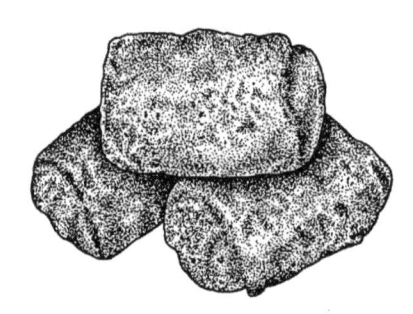

Gluten & Casein Free ....Yes	Phenol Free ....Yes
Low Oxalate Diet ....Yes	Specific Carbohydrate Diet ....No

This recipe is also Soy free, and Corn free, but is not Rice free

Oral Motor Rating 😊 😊 😊 😊

Quinoa Crackers

Yields: 8 Crackers

Ingredients
1 cup quinoa flour
1/2 cup rice flour
2 teaspoons baking powder(aluminum free)
1 teaspoon xanthan gum
1/2 teaspoon sea salt
2 tablespoons sunflower or safflower oil
1/2 cup water

> **Quinoa crackers**
> *Quinoa crackers are a healthy and nutritious snack that can be enjoyed with healthy dips and dressings or simply use a mayonnaise (like grape seed oil Veganaise).*

Directions
Preheat oven to 325º. Mix all the dry ingredients together, make a well in the middle, and add oil and water. Mix by hand; adding water as necessary till you have a dough-like consistency. Then roll out thin (1/8th of an inch) between two sheets of parchment paper or wax paper, cut into desired shapes and place on lightly greased cookie sheets. Prick each cracker several times with a fork and bake for 20 minutes.

Ingredients to Consider on Specific Diets

Gluten & Casein Free ....Yes	Phenol Free ....Yes
Low Oxalate Diet ....Yes	Specific Carbohydrate Diet ....No

This recipe is also Soy free and Corn free, but is not Rice free

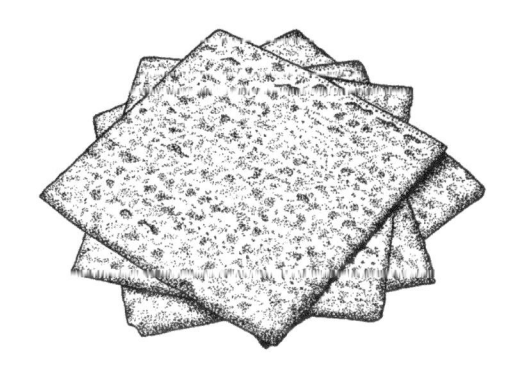

Oral Motor Rating 😊 😊 😊 😊

CHAPTER 14: HEALTHY BETWEEN-MEAL TREATS

Sesame Finger Sticks

Yields: 6 Sticks

Ingredients
1 cup quinoa or rice flour
2 teaspoons baking powder
1 teaspoon sea salt
1/2 cup coconut or olive oil
1/2 cup sesame seeds
1 tablespoon honey (optional)
2 teaspoons xanthan gum
1 cup water

Sesame Seeds

Sesame seeds contain a high source of calcium for the body. Children on the casein free diets can be deficient in calcium.

Directions
In a large bowl, mix all the dry ingredients. Add water and honey, and mix till you have workable dough. Roll small pieces of dough into two-inch oval shapes or logs approximately 3/4 inch thick, and roll in sesame seeds. Place on lightly greased baking sheets. Bake for 15 minutes at 350º until golden brown.

Ingredients to Consider on Specific Diets

Gluten & Casein Free ....Yes	Phenol Free............Yes (omit honey)
Low Oxalate Diet ....Yes	Specific Carbohydrate Diet ....No

This recipe is also Soy free and Corn free, but is not Rice free

Oral Motor Rating ☺ ☺ ☺ ☺

Graham Crackers

Yields: 32 Crackers

Ingredients
1 cup brown rice flour
3/4 cup almond or rice flour
1 1/2 teaspoon baking powder (aluminum free)
1/2 teaspoon xanthan gum (optional)
1/2 teaspoon cinnamon
1/2 teaspoon sea salt
1/2 cup honey
6 tablespoons almond butter or cashew nut butter
1/2 teaspoon gluten- and casein-free vanilla
1 cup water

> *Recipe Variation*
>
> This recipe is neither too salty nor too sweet. It can be easily modified to be more sweet or salty, based on the preference of the child.

Directions
Preheat oven to 400º. Combine flours, baking powder, xanthan gum, cinnamon, and salt. Set aside. In a large bowl, blend honey, butter, and vanilla. Add flour mixture and water alternately to mixing bowl, using just enough water to hold the batter in a soft ball. Then roll out thin (1/8th of an inch) between two sheets of parchment paper or waxed paper, cut into desired shapes, and place on cookie sheets. Prick each cracker several times with a fork and bake for 20 minutes or until lightly browned. Note: You can also cut the crackers into animal shapes for added fun.

Ingredients to Consider on Specific Diets

Gluten & Casein Free	Yes
Phenol Free	No
Low Oxalate Diet	No
Specific Carbohydrate Diet	No

This recipe is also Soy free and Corn free, but is not Rice free

Oral Motor Rating 😀 😀 😀 😀

Notes:

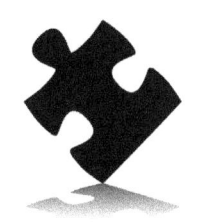

Chapter Fifteen

Sweets 'n' Treats

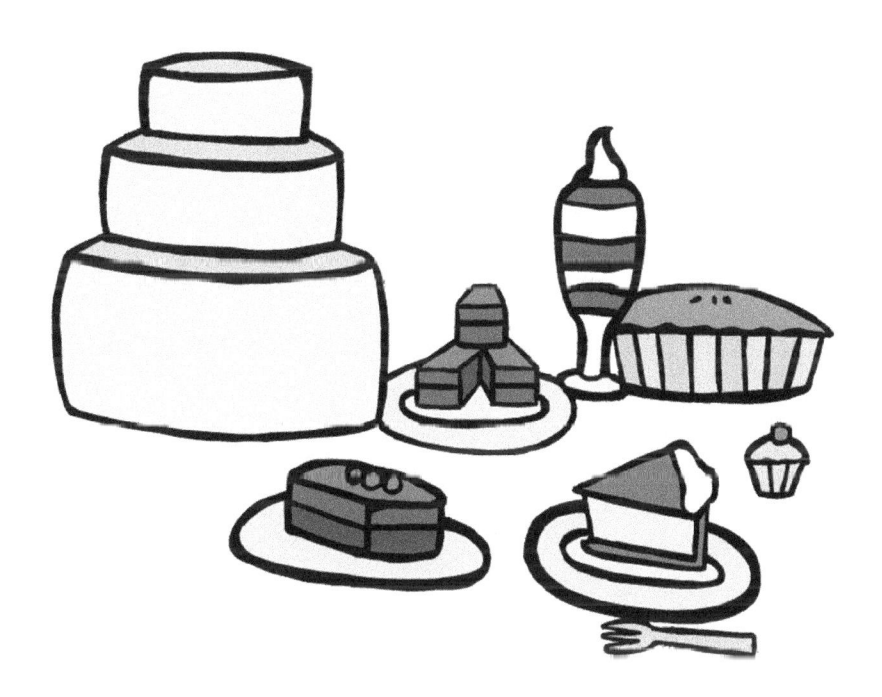

Satisfying the Sweet Tooth

The desire for sweets is notorious! Fighting this, especially with children with developmental delays, is a no-win situation. When given a choice over healthy food options, children naturally gravitate towards sweets, once it is introduced into the diet. This gave us an idea to develop healthy dessert recipes. Children love sweets, so give them something they can still benefit from nutritionally.

Sweets 'n' Treats
Table of Contents

COOKIES

Chocolate Chip Cookies	351
Pumpkin Cookies	352
Coconut Mango Cookies	353
Coconut Cookies	354
Crispy Walnut Crackers or Cookies	355
Gingersnap Cookies	356

PIES

Rolled Double Pie Crust	357
French Apple Pie	358
Pumpkin Pie	359
Peach Pie	360
Blueberry Pie	361

CAKES

Carrot Coconut Cake	362
Honey Cake	363
Apple Pudding Cake	364
Flourless Lemon and Almond Cake	365

BROWNIES AND BISCOTTI

No-Bake Lentil (Mung Dal) Blondie	366
Brown-Brown Brownies	367
Almond Butter Brownies	368
Chocolate Biscotti	369

MISCELLANEOUS DESSERTS

Apple Gelatin Dessert 370
Grape Dessert Delight 371
Baked Apples 372
Apple-Coconut Crisp 373
Donut Holes..374
Banana Nut Pudding..375
Coconut Macaroons 376
Banana Coconut Ice Cream 377

COOKIES

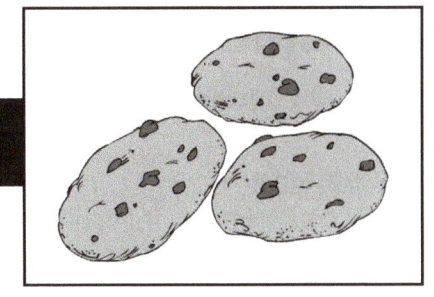

Chocolate Chip Cookies

Yields: 24 Cookies

Ingredients
1 1/2 cups rice flour
1/2 cup tapioca flour
1/2 cup potato starch
1 teaspoon baking soda
2 teaspoons xanthan gum
1 teaspoon sea salt
2 eggs or egg replacer
1 cup coconut oil
1 cup honey or maple syrup
1 tablespoon gluten- and casein-free vanilla
1 cup gluten- and casein-free chocolate chips
1 cup walnuts (optional), finely chopped

> ### Recipe Variation
> GFCF cookie mixes sometimes have a lot of sugar and can contain egg in the ingredients. This recipe can be used instead. Eggs can be substituted with egg replacer.

Directions
Preheat oven to 350º. Combine flours, potato starch, baking soda, xanthan gum and salt in a large bowl and set aside. In a small bowl, add eggs, oil, honey, and vanilla, and with a hand-held mixer, blend until smooth. Add this mixture to dry ingredients and mix well. Stir in chocolate chips and nuts (if desired). Drop tablespoonfuls on an ungreased cookie sheet spaced about half an inch apart. Bake for 8 to 10 minutes. Remove cookies from cookie sheet onto a wire rack or on paper towels to cool. Chocolate Chip Cookie Bars: Press cookie dough into a 9x13-inch baking pan. Bake at 350º for 25 to 30 minutes. Cool and cut into bars.

Ingredients to Consider on Specific Diets

Gluten & Casein Free ....Yes	Phenol Free ....Yes (if you use maple syrup)
Low Oxalate Diet...Yes	Specific Carbohydrate Diet .... No

This recipe is also Soy free and Corn free but is not Rice free

Oral Motor Rating 😊 😊 😊 😊

Pumpkin Cookies

Yields: 36 Cookies

Ingredients
2 1/2 cups almond or coconut flour
2 teaspoons baking soda
1 teaspoon xanthan gum (optional)
1 teaspoon cinnamon or nutmeg
1/2 teaspoon sea salt
1/2 cup coconut or grape seed oil
1 1/2 cups of honey
1 egg or egg replacer
1 cup canned pumpkin
1 teaspoon gluten- and casein-free vanilla
1/2 cup raisins or dried cranberries (optional)
1/4 cup gluten- and casein-free chocolate chips

> *Nutmeg*
> *Nutmeg is used in a variety of cuisines, and the essential oil of the seed has medicinal applications. Nutmeg is believed to aid digestion and relieve nausea.*

Directions
Preheat oven to 350º. In a small bowl, combine flour, baking soda, xanthan gum (optional), cinnamon or nutmeg, and salt. Mix well and set aside. In a large mixing bowl, using a hand-held mixer, beat oil and sweetener until light and fluffy. Stir in pumpkin and vanilla and beat till smooth. Fold in dry ingredients by hand, then stir in raisins or chocolate chips. Drop by tablespoonfuls onto a greased baking sheet. Bake 15 to 18 minutes.

Ingredients to Consider on Specific Diets

Gluten & Casein Free .... Yes
Phenol Free .... .No
Low Oxalate Diet .... Yes (if you use coconut flour)
Specific Carbohydrate Diet .... Yes
This recipe is also Soy free, Corn free and Rice free

Oral Motor Rating 😊 😊 😊 😊

Coconut Mango Cookies

Yields: 12 Cookies

Ingredients
1 egg or egg replacer
1/2 cup honey
1/4 teaspoon sea salt
1/2 cup almond flour
1 1/2 cups coconut, grated
1/2 cup walnuts, finely chopped
1/2 cup mango (dried fruit), chopped

> ***Mango***
> *Mango, also called "The King of Fruit," is a nutritious, not to mention delicious, fruit.*

Directions
Preheat oven to 350º. Using an electric mixer, blend the egg, honey, and salt together. Add flour to mixture and mix until well blended. Add coconut, walnuts and mango pieces and mix until thoroughly combined. Drop by tablespoonfuls on an oiled or parchment-covered baking sheet and bake for 10-12 minutes.

Ingredients to Consider on Specific Diets

Gluten & Casein Free......................Yes
Phenol Free ....No
Low Oxalate Diet.............................No
Specific Carbohydrate Diet ....Yes

This recipe is also Soy free, Corn free and Rice free (use almond flour)

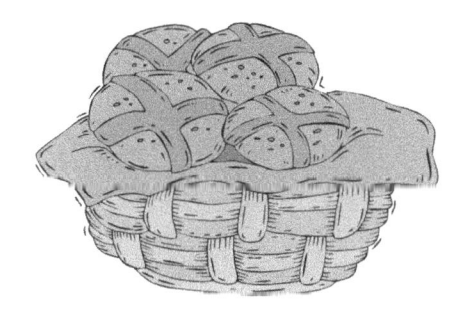

Oral Motor Rating ☺ ☺ ☺ ☺

Coconut Cookies

Yields: 6 Cookies

Ingredients

1 egg or egg replacer
1/2 cup honey or maple syrup
1/4 teaspoon sea salt
1/2 cup coconut flour
1 1/2 cup coconut, shredded, unsweetened
1 1/2 cup chopped dried fruit, (optional)

> *Coconut Shreds*
>
> *When baking, be careful. If a recipe calls for unsweetened shredded coconut and a sweet variety is used, the result will be far sweeter than desired. Shredded coconut is a better choice for batter for cakes, brownies, and other baked goods than coconut flour.*

Directions

In mixer, blend egg, honey, and salt. Add coconut flour; mix until well blended. Add coconut (and dried fruit if desired); mix well. Refrigerate batter for an hour or more. Shape into about two dozen slightly flattened balls on an oiled or parchment-lined cookie sheet. Bake 10 to 12 minutes at 350°.

Ingredients to Consider on Specific Diets

Gluten & Casein Free .... Yes
Phenol Free .... Yes (if you use maple syrup as sweetner)
Low Oxalate Diet .... Yes
Specific Carbohydrate Diet .... Yes
This recipe is also Soy free, Corn free and Rice free

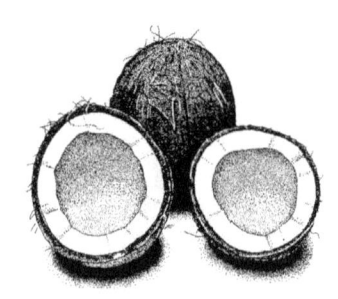

Oral Motor Rating 😊 😊 😊 😊

Crispy Walnut Crackers or Cookies

Yields: 12 Cookies

In the recipe you can use walnuts or any other nut, it should be toasted, finely ground and then measured for the recipe.

Ingredients
3/4 cup white rice flour
1/4 cup potato starch
1 1/2 teaspoons xanthan gum
1 teaspoon baking powder (aluminum free)
1/2 teaspoon sea salt
1/3 cup walnuts
4 tablespoons coconut butter or ghee
1/2 cup hempseed milk
2 teaspoons olive oil

Directions
In a mixing bowl, combine the rice flour, potato starch, xanthan gum, baking powder, salt and nuts. In a small saucepan, melt coconut butter and cool slightly. Add to flour mixture along with the milk. Using fingertips, work the dough, adding a teaspoon of warm water at a time (up to 1 1/2 tablespoons), until dough can be pressed into a ball. Allow dough to rest, covered, in a warm place for 15 minutes.

Preheat oven to 350º. Coat the bottom of a baking sheet with vegetable oil.

Set dough on center of sheet and press and roll dough until it reaches the edges of the pan. Trim edges. Brush with olive oil, and cut into squares. Prick with a fork, and sprinkle with kosher salt. Bake for 15 minutes. Turn pan to allow even baking and bake ten minutes more, or until tops are brown. Remove and cool, then store in an airtight container. Crackers keep for five days and may be frozen.

Note: The last step can be modified, and dough can be made in small balls and pressed to make cookies and baked on a baking sheet for 20 minutes at 350º.

Ingredients to Consider on Specific Diets

Gluten & Casein Free	Yes	Phenol Free	Yes
Low Oxalate Diet	Yes	Specific Carbohydrate Diet	No

This recipe is also Soy free, Corn free, but is not Rice free

Oral Motor Rating 😊 😊 😊 😊

Gingersnap Cookies

Yields: 24 Cookies

Ingredients
1 cup rice flour
1 cup quinoa flour
1 teaspoon cinnamon
1 teaspoon xanthan gum
1/2 teaspoon sea salt
1 teaspoon baking soda
1 teaspoon ground cloves
1 teaspoon ginger
1 cup honey
1 egg or egg replacer
1 cup coconut butter

> **Cloves**
> *Cloves are renowned for providing their uniquely warm, sweet and aromatic taste to gingerbread and pumpkin pie, but they can also make a wonderful addition to split pea and bean soups, baked beans and chili.*

Directions
Preheat oven to 350º. In a large mixing bowl, combine the first eight (dry) ingredients. In a small bowl, cream xylitol or honey, egg and coconut butter with hand-held mixer, and then add to dry ingredients. Blend all together with hand-held mixer to make a batter. Spoon out the batter into small shapes on a cookie sheet, keeping them at least 2 inches apart. Bake for 15 minutes.

Ingredients to Consider on Specific Diets

Gluten & Casein Free ....Yes	Phenol Free ....No
Low Oxalate Diet ....Yes	Specific Carbohydrate Diet ......No

This recipe is also Soy free and Corn free

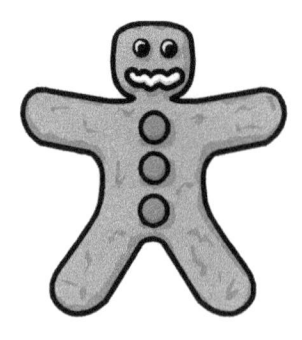

Oral Motor Rating 😊 😊 😊 😊

PIES

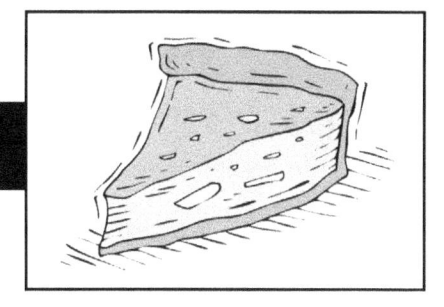

Rolled Double Pie Crust

Ingredients
1 cup brown rice flour
1/2 cup tapioca flour
1/2 cup almond flour
1 1/2 teaspoon xanthan gum
1/2 teaspoon baking soda
1/2 teaspoon sea salt
1/2 teaspoon honey or maple syrup
4 tablespoons coconut butter
1 egg or egg replacer
1 tablespoon gluten-free vinegar
4 tablespoons ice water

> **Tapioca**
> *Tapioca is a flavorless, colorless, odorless starch extracted from the root of the cassava plant. It is a staple food in some regions and is used worldwide as a thickening agent in foods. Tapioca is gluten free, and nearly protein free.*

Directions
Preheat oven to 350º. In medium mixing bowl, combine all dry ingredients. Cut coconut butter into the flour mixture using a pastry cutter. In a small bowl, beat egg using a fork; add honey, vinegar and ice water and stir into flour mixture. Knead to form two balls (it is better to be a little too moist than too dry). Cover with plastic wrap and refrigerate for one hour for easier handling.

Roll out bottom crust between sheets of wax paper or plastic wrap. Remove the top paper and transfer pastry into pie pan. Pour filling into crust. Roll out top crust between two fresh sheets of paper or plastic wrap and place over filling. Trim edges leaving 1/2-inch; fold under bottom crust to seal. Flute edges with fingers.

Bake as directed for filling used. For a one-crust pie: Roll out bottom crust, place in pie pan, and prick the bottom of the crust with a fork. Bake in a 400º oven for 10 to 15 minutes, or until lightly browned. Cool before filling.

Ingredients to Consider on Specific Diets

Gluten & Casein Free ....Yes	Phenol Free..........................Yes (omit honey)
Low Oxalate Diet ....Yes	Specific Carbohydrate Diet .... No

This recipe is also Soy free and Corn free

Oral Motor Rating ☺ ☺ ☺ ☺

French Apple Pie

Ingredients
5 cups pie apples, peeled, cored and sliced
1 teaspoon cinnamon, ground
3/4 cup honey or maple syrup
1/2 cup almond or hemp seed milk
2 tablespoons walnuts, finely chopped
2 pie crusts (use pie crust recipe p.357)

Directions
Preheat oven to 400º. In a medium bowl, mix apples, cinnamon, sugar/honey, and milk together. Spread apple mixture in an unbaked pie shell. Add the walnut topping. Cover with top crust and crimp edges with fingers to seal. Cut slits in top. Bake for 10 minutes. Turn oven to 350º and continue cooking for 30 to 40 minutes or until crust is lightly brown.

Ingredients to Consider on Specific Diets

Gluten & Casein Free .... Yes
Phenol Free .... Yes (if you use hempseed milk and maple syrup)
Low Oxalate Diet .... Yes (if you uses hempseed milk)
Specific Carbohydrate Diet .... No
This recipe is also Soy free, Corn free and Rice free

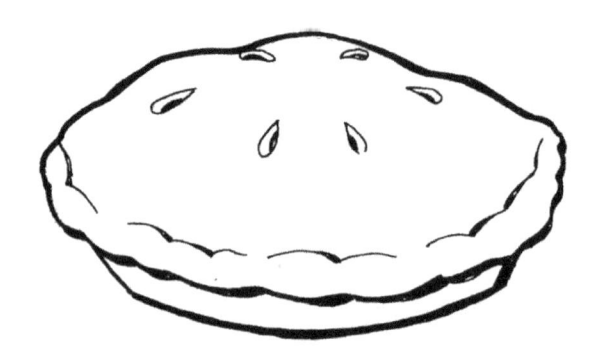

Oral Motor Rating 😊 😊 😊 😊

Pumpkin Pie

Ingredients
2 large eggs or egg replacer
15 ounces canned pumpkin
3/4 cup honey
1 tablespoon almond flour
1/2 teaspoon sea salt
1 teaspoon ground cinnamon or nutmeg
1 cup hot water
1/2 cup Dari Free powder
1 pie crust (use pie crust recipe p.357)

> ### *Dari Free*
> *DariFree is a fortified milk substitute. Creamy, mild, very pleasant flavored, very kid friendly, and rich in calcium is excellent for drinking and baking. It is made from potatoes. Many children with special needs cannot handle potatoes, so use with caution.*

Directions
Preheat oven to 425º. Line a deep-dish 9-inch pie pan with crust. In a medium bowl, beat eggs lightly. Stir in pumpkin, sugar, salt, cinnamon or nutmeg. Combine hot water, DariFree, and flour, and then add to the pumpkin mixture. Pour into pie shell. Bake for 15 minutes. Reduce heat to 350º and bake 60 minutes or until the center is soft set. Pie will set firmer after it cools (overnight in refrigerator is best).

Ingredients to Consider on Specific Diets

Gluten & Casein Free	Yes
Phenol Free	No
Low Oxalate Diet	No
Specific Carbohydrate Diet	No

This recipe is also Soy free, Corn free and Rice free

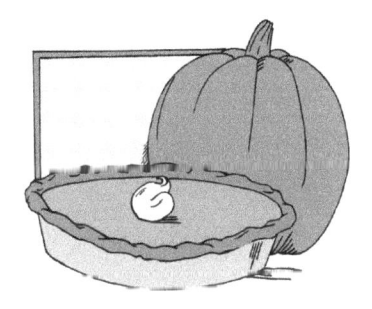

Oral Motor Rating 😊 😊

Peach Pie

Ingredients
5 cups peaches, peeled and sliced
3/4 cup honey
2 tablespoons coconut butter
1/4 teaspoon cinnamon
1/8 teaspoon sea salt
1/2 cup almond or hemp seed milk
1 double pie crust (use pie crust recipe p.357)

Peaches

Peaches and nectarines look very similar, but they can be told apart by their skin texture.

Peaches are fuzzy and dull, while nectarines are smooth and shiny.

Directions
Preheat oven to 400º. Combine sugar, coconut butter, cinnamon, and salt. Add peaches or pears and rice milk, toss gently, and spoon into unbaked pie shell. Top with second crust. Cut steam vents. Moisten edges and seal. Flute edges. Bake for 45 to 50 minutes.

Ingredients to Consider on Specific Diets

Gluten & Casein Free .... Yes
Phenol Free .... No
Low Oxalate Diet .... Yes (if you use hempseed milk)
Specific Carbohydrate Diet .... No
This recipe is also Soy free, Corn free and Rice free

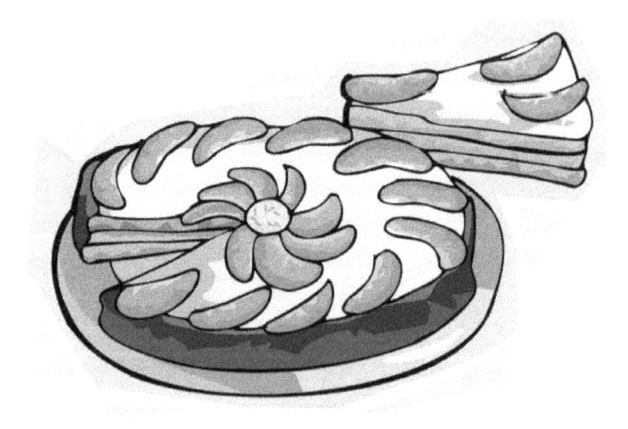

Oral Motor Rating ☺ ☺

Blueberry Pie

Ingredients
16 ounce package frozen blueberries, defrosted and drained
2/3 cup honey
2 tablespoons coconut butter
1/2 cup almond or hemp seed milk
1 tablespoon lemon juice
1/4 cup walnuts, finely chopped
1 double pie crust recipe (p.357)

Blueberries
Blueberries are among the fruits with the highest antioxidant activity. Blueberries are a very high phenol food, so use with caution.

Directions
Preheat oven to 425º. Mix sugar/honey and coconut butter together in a medium bowl. Stir in blueberries till well coated. Add milk, to make a good consistency. Pour blueberry mixture into an unbaked pie crust. Sprinkle with lemon juice. Cover with top crust and crimp edges with fingers to seal. Cut one or two 1-inch slits in the top. Bake for 45 minutes.

Ingredients to Consider on Specific Diets

Gluten & Casein Free .... Yes
Phenol Free .... No
Low Oxalate Diet .... Yes (if avoid blueberries and substituted with low oxalate fruits)
Specific Carbohydrate Diet .... No

This recipe is also Soy free, Corn free and Rice free

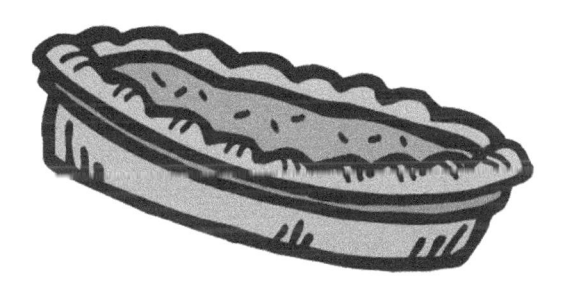

Oral Motor Rating 😊 😊 😊

CAKES

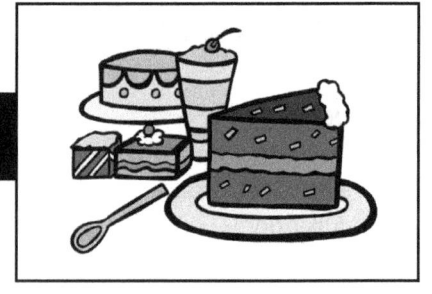

Carrot Coconut Cake

Ingredients
1 cup carrots, grated raw
3/4 cup coconut flakes
3/4 cup honey or maple sryup
1 teaspoon gluten-free vanilla
6 eggs or egg replacer
1 cup cashews or almonds, ground

> **Coconut Flakes**
> *Most air-dried shredded and flaked coconut products found in conventional supermarkets have additives to preserve them. However, freeze-dried coconut flakes have a very sweet taste and contain no preservatives or chemical additives.*

Directions
In a large bowl, blend the carrots, coconut, honey, and vanilla. Separate eggs. Beat the egg yolks to a creamy consistency. Fold them into the carrot-coconut mixture and let it sit in the refrigerator for one hour, or until the moisture has been absorbed. Add the ground cashews/almonds and blend.

Preheat oven to 400º. Grease and lightly flour two 9-inch cake pans or baking pans. Beat the egg whites until stiff. Fold them into the carrot-coconut mixture and pour into baking pan(s). Bake for 10 minutes, and then reduce the temperature to 350º and bake for an additional 20 to 30 minutes, or until the cake shows signs of leaving the sides of the pan. Cool on a wire rack.

Ingredients to Consider on Specific Diets

Gluten & Casein Free .... Yes
Phenol Free .... Yes (if you use cashews ground and maple syrup as a sweetener)
Low Oxalate Diet .... Yes (moderate to high, as all nuts are high)
Specific Carbohydrate Diet .... Yes

This recipe is also Soy free, Corn free and Rice free

Oral Motor Rating 😊 😊

Honey Cake

Ingredients
2 cups honey
3 eggs or egg replacer
1/2 cup safflower or sunflower oil
3 cups hemp seed, almond, or sorghum flour
1 teaspoon cinnamon
2 teaspoons baking soda
1 teaspoon ginger powder
1 apple, grated (can also use pear)
2 cups walnuts, finely chopped
1 teaspoon sea salt
1 cup apple juice
3/4 cup gluten- and casein-free chocolate chips (optional)
1/2 cup raisins (optional)

Ginger powder has pungent flavor. Its aroma is subtle and spicy. Add ginger to dishes at the beginning of cooking for a milder flavor, and at the end if you would like a more pronounced effect.

Directions
Beat honey and eggs in blender on medium speed. Add oil, flour, cinnamon, baking soda, and ginger powder. Add the walnuts, apple, salt and juice. Blend at medium speed to make a batter. Add chocolate chips or raisins, if desired. Preheat oven to 350º. Line the bottoms of two 9-inch by 5-inch loaf pans with parchment paper, then grease and flour. Pour the batter and bake for 20 minutes. Reduce the heat to 325º and bake for an additional 40 minutes. Cool cakes on wire racks, then loosen with a knife and turn onto serving plate.

Ingredients to Consider on Specific Diets

Gluten & Casein Free .... Yes
Phenol Free .... No
Low Oxalate Diet .... Yes (if you use hempseed, or sorghum flour)
Specific Carbohydrate Diet .... No
This recipe is also Soy free, Corn free and Rice free

Oral Motor Rating 😊 😊 😊

Apple Pudding Cake

Ingredients

For Apple Filling
10 baking apples
1 cup water
2 teaspoons cinnamon or nutmeg
1 teaspoon ginger powder
1/4 cup honey
1/4 cup coconut butter or ghee

For Cake Batter
1 1/4 cups almond
1/2 teaspoon cinnamon or nutmeg
1 teaspoon baking soda
3 tablespoons coconut butter or ghee
3 tablespoons honey

Directions

Peel and slice apples, place in sauce pan, Add enough water to cover 1/4 of the apples. Cook over medium high heat until apples are very soft and mushy. Using a large spoon, drain excess liquid into a bowl and set it aside to use in cake batter. Add cinnamon or nutmeg, ginger, honey and coconut butter or ghee; stir and simmer while preparing cake mixture.

Preheat oven to 350º. Combine one cup of the flour, the cinnamon or nutmeg, and baking soda; blend with your hands until all lumps are gone. Add butter, honey and the reserved juice from the cooked apples. Mix well. Batter should be smooth and pourable. If it seems too thin, add the extra quarter cup of flour.

Pour the apple mixture in a greased baking dish, and then pour cake batter over the apples, moving apples around a bit so the batter seeps in all around them. Bake for 45minutes to an hour. A knife or toothpick should come out clean, yet this is not a firm cake. It will be soft and juicy. (It is very yummy!)

Ingredients to Consider on Specific Diets

Gluten & Casein Free .... Yes
Phenol Free .... No
Low Oxalate Diet .... No
Specific Carbohydrate Diet .... Yes (use almond flour)
This recipe is also Soy free, Corn free and Rice free
Oral Motor Rating 😊 😊

Flourless Lemon and Almond Cake

Ingredients
1 1/3 cups almonds, finely chopped
4 tablespoons honey
4 eggs
5 teaspoons grated lemon peel, packed
1/2 teaspoon cinnamon
Pinch sea salt

Directions
Preheat oven to 375º. Butter and flour a 9-inch-diameter cake pan with 1 1/2 inch-high sides. Line the bottom of pan with waxed paper.

In a food processor, finely grind almonds with 2 tablespoons of the honey. Separate eggs. Combine yolks with the other two tablespoons of honey, the lemon peel, cinnamon, and salt. Using an electric mixer, beat for about two minutes until thick and smooth. Stir in almond mixture. Using clean beaters, beat egg whites in large bowl until stiff and dry. Fold a large spoonful of whites into almond mixture. Gently fold in remaining whites.

Pour batter into pan. Bake until tester inserted into center comes out clean, about 35 minutes. Cool in pan on rack. Turn out onto platter. Remove waxed paper.

Ingredients to Consider on Specific Diets

Gluten & Casein Free	Yes
Phenol Free	No
Low Oxalate Diet	No
Specific Carbohydrate Diet	Yes

This recipe is also Soy free, Corn free and Rice free

Oral Motor Rating 🙂 🙂

BROWNIES & BISCOTTI

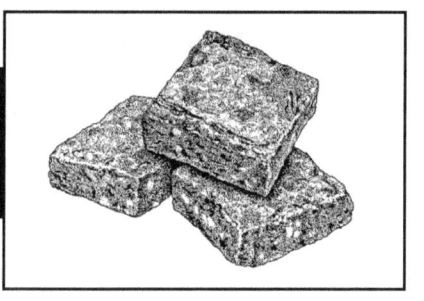

No-Bake Lentil (Mung Dal) Blondie

Yields: 12 Brownie Pieces

Ingredients
1 cup ghee or coconut butter
2 cups lentil (mung dal) flour
2 cups almond or hemp seed milk
1 cup of honey
1/4 teaspoon saffron (optional)
1 teaspoon cinnamon
4 drops gluten- and casein-free vanilla

Saffron

Saffron is the most expensive spice in the world, used to add flavor and color to recipes. It is a spice to be added one thread at a time. Just a thread or two can flavor and color an entire pot of rice. The flavor is distinctive and pungent.

Directions
In a heavy bottomed pan, heat the ghee or coconut butter and add the flour. Mix well, and stir till the flour is light brown in color. Reduce heat, and add milk a little at a time. Continue to cook over low heat, until all is mixed well. Over medium heat, add honey, saffron, cinnamon, and vanilla and cook for a minute. Let it cool down, and then spread the dough on flat surface. After it has cooled a little longer, cut into small pieces.

Ingredients to Consider on Specific Diets

Gluten & Casein Free................ Yes
Phenol Free.............................No
Low Oxalate Diet ....Yes (if you use hempseed milk)
Specific Carbohydrate Diet .... Yes (use almond milk)
This recipe is also Soy free, Corn free and Rice free

Oral Motor Rating 😊 😊

Brown-Brown Brownies

Yields: 12 Brownie Pieces

Ingredients
1/2 cup unsweetened cocoa
2 cups honey or maple syrup
2 cups coconut flour
1/2 cup ground flax seed
1/2 teaspoon sea salt
2 teaspoons baking soda
1 teaspoon xanthan gum (optional)
4 eggs or egg replacer
2/3 cup sunflower or safflower oil
1 teaspoon gluten- and casein-free vanilla
1 cup walnuts, finely chopped (optional)

Cocoa
Cocoa is the dried and fully fermented fatty seed from the cacao tree from which chocolate is made. "Cocoa" is referred to as the drink commonly known as hot chocolate.

Directions
Preheat oven to 350 F. In a large bowl, mix cocoa and sugar/honey with a wire whisk until thoroughly mixed. Stir in rice flour, ground flax seed, salt, baking soda, and xanthan, if desired. Add eggs (unbeaten), oil and vanilla. Stir with a large spoon only until blended. Spread into a greased and rice floured 13x9x2-inch baking pan. Sprinkle 1 cup nuts over batter (or 1/2 cup nuts over half the pan and leave the other half without for those who don't want nuts). Bake for 25-30 minutes. Cut into squares when cool.

Ingredients to Consider on Specific Diets

Gluten & Casein Free................ Yes
Phenol Free............................. Yes (if you use maple syrup as sweetner)
Low Oxalate Diet .... Yes
Specific Carbohydrate Diet .... No
This recipe is also Soy free, Corn free and Rice free

Oral Motor Rating 😊 😊

Almond Butter Brownies

Yields: 10-12 Brownie Pieces

Ingredients
1/2 cup almond butter or
cashew nut butter
4 tablespoons sunflower or safflower oil
1/2 cup honey
1 egg or egg replacer
1/2 teaspoon gluten- and casein-free vanilla
1 1/2 cups coconut flour
1/2 teaspoon sea salt
1/2 teaspoon baking soda

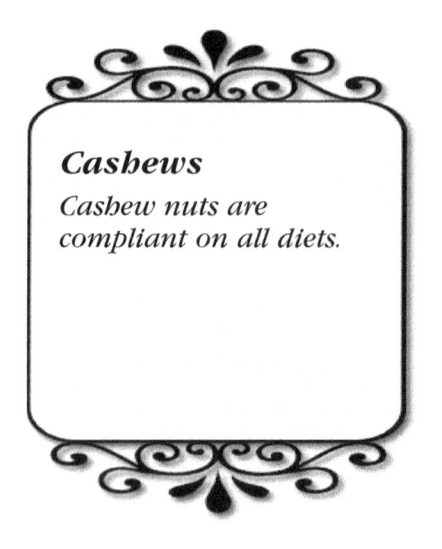

Cashews
Cashew nuts are compliant on all diets.

Directions
Mix by hand the butter, oil, honey, egg and vanilla. Blend in flour, salt and soda. Place in an 8-inch ungreased Pyrex pan. Bake at 350º for 35-40 minutes.

Ingredients to Consider on Specific Diets

Phenol Free............... No	Gluten & Casin Free ....Yes
Low Oxalate Diet .... No	Specific Carbohydrate Diet........Yes

This recipe is also Soy free, Corn free and Rice free

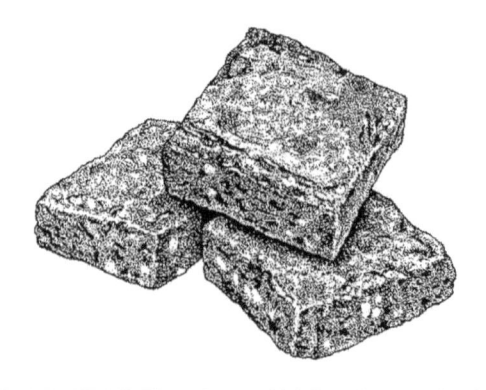

Oral Motor Rating ☺ ☺

Chocolate Biscotti

Yields: 6 Biscotti

Ingredients
6 eggs or egg replacer
1 1/4 cups safflower, sunflower oil, or coconut butter
1 1/2 cups honey or maple syrup
2 teaspoons gluten- and casein-free vanilla
5 cups coconut flour
1 cup gluten- and casein-free cocoa powder
1 teaspoon xanthan gum
2 teaspoons baking powder
1/2 teaspoon sea salt
1 1/2 teaspoon baking soda
1 cup walnuts, finely chopped Sugar for sprinkling on baked rolls

> **Gluten and Casein-free Biscotti**
>
> *Most GFCF Biscotti in health food stores are loaded with sugar and very costly. This simple recipe can be made at home.*

Directions

In a large bowl, combine eggs, oil, honey, and vanilla. Using hand held blender, blend at medium speed. In another bowl, stir together dry ingredients and then add to the creamed mixture. Stir in nuts, if desired and tolerated. Chill dough for an hour.

Preheat oven to 350º. Divide dough into 6 portions. Form each into tube-shaped rolls about 1 1/2 inch in diameter. Place rolls on greased baking sheet. Bake for 20 to 25 minutes.

While still warm, cut the rolls into half-inch slices on a slight diagonal. Lay the slices on a flat side, and sprinkle with sugar and toast in 275º oven for 25 minutes. Turn, sprinkle again and toast for additional 25 minutes.

Ingredients to Consider on Specific Diets

Gluten & Casein Free ....Yes	Phenol Free ....Yes (if you use maple syrup)
Low Oxalate Diet...Yes	Specific Carbohydrate Diet .... No

This recipe is also Soy free, Corn free and Rice free

Oral Motor Rating ☺ ☺ ☺ ☺

MISCELLANEOUS DESSERTS

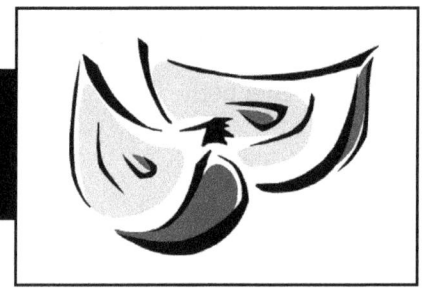

Apple Gelatin Dessert

Yields: 2 to 4 Servings

Ingredients
1/2 cup cold water
One package unflavored gelatin
2 cups apple juice

> **Gelatin**
>
> *Gelatin, or gelatine, is a substance derived from the processing of animal collagen. In the processed food industry, it is used as a thickener, a gelling agent, a stabilizer, and an emulsifier. It is used in foods as diverse as yogurt, pate, aspic, marshmallows and gummy candy, soups, salad dressings, and canned ham.*

Directions
Soften gelatin in the water, mix thoroughly, and set aside. Heat apple cider in a small saucepan for 3 or 4 minutes on a medium flame, and shut off. Add gelatin mixture to the hot apple cider and stir until the gelatin is completely dissolved. Transfer to a glass container and cover, storing in the refrigerator for at least one hour. Serve as a snack or dessert as you would gelatin.

Ingredients to Consider on Specific Diets

Gluten & Casein Free ....Yes	Phenol Free ....Yes
Low Oxalate Diet ....Yes	Specific Carbohydrate Diet ....Yes

This recipe is also Soy free, Corn free and Rice free

Oral Motor Rating 😊 😊 😊 😊

Grape Dessert Delight

Yields: 6 Servings

Ingredients
1/2 cup cold water
3 packages (3 tablespoons) unflavored gelatin
1 cup boiling water
One 12-ounce can frozen white grape juice (Welch's brand is legal)

> *100% white grape juice is more easily digested due to its carbohydrate, or natural sugar profile. Unlike other juices, 100% white grape juice has an even balance of fructose and glucose (two easy-to-digest natural sugars). The presence of sorbitol and unbalanced levels of fructose in other juices may lead to gas, intestinal discomfort, and even diarrhea.*

Directions
Let the gelatin soften in the cold water for approximately 1 minute. Bring a cup of water to a boil and then add the gelatin mixture to it, stirring for about 5 minutes until gelatin is completely dissolved. Add the undiluted frozen juice concentrate and stir until it is melted. Place mixture in a serving dish and chill overnight or until firm. Cut into squares and serve.

Ingredients to Consider on Specific Diets

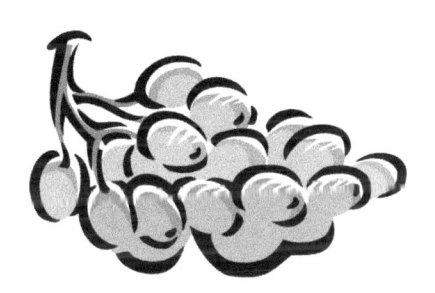

Gluten & Casein Free	Yes
Phenol Free	Yes (if use pear juice instead)
Low Oxalate Diet	Yes
Specific Carbohydrate Diet	Yes

This recipe is also Soy free, Corn free and Rice free

Oral Motor Rating 😊

Baked Apples

Yields: 4 to 6 Servings

Ingredients
2 pounds Granny Smith apples
1 teaspoon cinnamon
1/2 cup water

Granny Smith apples are light speckled and green in color, though some may have a pink blush. They are crisp, juicy, tart apples that are excellent for cooking, or eating out of hand. They also are favored for salads because the slices do not brown as quickly as other varieties.

Directions
Grease a 9 x 13-inch glass baking dish with coconut oil. Peel and core apples, and cut into one-inch pieces. In a bowl, combine the apples, cinnamon and water and then transfer the mixture to the baking dish. Bake at 425º for 45 minutes. Cool and serve.

Ingredients to Consider on Specific Diets

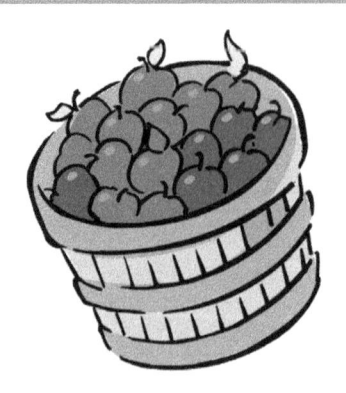

Gluten & Casein Free ....Yes	Phenol Free ....Yes
Low Oxalate Diet.........................Yes	Specific Carbohydrate Diet .... Yes

This recipe is also Soy free, Corn free and Rice free

Oral Motor Rating 😊 😊

Apple-Coconut Crisp

Yields: 4 to 6 Servings

Ingredients
6 baking apples
1/2 teaspoon ground nutmeg
   or gluten- and casein-free vanilla
3/4 cup honey
1 cup shredded coconut
1/4 cup walnuts or water chestnuts,
   finely chopped

> **Water Chestnuts**
>
> *Water chestnuts are used in a lot of dishes to add texture and flavor. Unlike many vegetables which soften as they are heated, water chestnuts stay firm, adding crunch to a recipe.*

Directions
Peel and slice baking apples. In a pot, combine apples and water. Bring to a boil, and let boil 15 minutes. Pour into a blender and puree. In a medium size bowl, mix nutmeg or vanilla extract and honey together in a medium bowl and then stir in apples and coconut. Spread apple mixture in a greased 8-inch square baking dish. Sprinkle top with nuts (as desired). Bake at 375º for 45 minutes.

Ingredients to Consider on Specific Diets

Gluten & Casein Free................ Yes
Phenol Free............................. No
Low Oxalate Diet .... Yes (omit walnuts)
Specific Carbohydrate Diet ...., Yes
This recipe is also Soy free, Corn free and Rice free

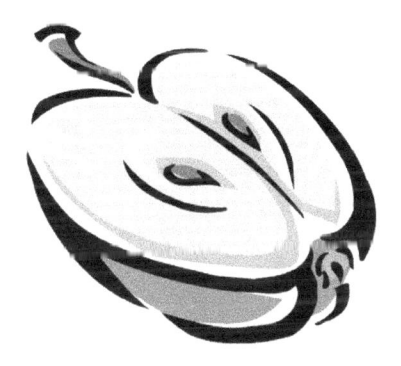

Oral Motor Rating ☺ ☺ ☺

CHAPTER 15: SWEETS 'N' TREATS 373

Donut Holes

Yields: 24 Donut Holes

Ingredients
1 1/2 cups almond flour
1/3 cup honey
2 tablespoons baking soda
1 1/2 tablespoons xanthan gum (optional)
1/2 teaspoon sea salt
1 egg or egg replacer
1/2 cup almond or coconut milk
1/4 teaspoon nutmeg
1/2 teaspoon gluten- and casein-free vanilla extract
6 tablespoons coconut, grape seed, sunflower, or safflower oil

Directions
In a large bowl, and add flour, honey or xylitol, baking soda, xanthan gum (optional) and salt. Mix well and set aside. In a small bowl, lightly beat the egg and milk, and stir in nutmeg or vanilla and oil. Add egg mixture to the dry ingredients and make dough. Roll out dough on well-floured surface and cut holes using the lid from the vegetable oil container. A cookie scoop also works very well for making donut holes. In a large frying pan, pour an inch of oil and heat to 375º. Fry the donuts a few at a time for about 1 to 1 1/2 minutes on each side until deep golden brown. Drain on paper towels.

Ingredients to Consider on Specific Diets

Gluten & Casein Free................. Yes
Phenol Free............................... No
Low Oxalate Diet .... No
Specific Carbohydrate Diet .... Yes (omit xanthan gum)
This recipe is also Soy free, Corn free and Rice free

Oral Motor Rating :) :) :)

Banana Nut Pudding

Yields: 2 Servings

Ingredients
1 medium ripe banana,
2 tablespoons almond or cashew butter
1/2 cup homemade SCD yogurt,
   or 1 cup almond or hemp seed milk

> *Note for parents:*
> In this recipe, cashew butter or almond butter can be used. The banana used in the recipe must be ripe with black spots on the skin.

Directions
In a small bowl, smash banana with fork until completely smooth. Mix in the nut butter, and then add the homemade yogurt or milk. Mix all until smooth. Refrigerate and serve cold.

Ingredients to Consider on Specific Diets

Gluten & Casein Free .... Yes
Phenol Free .... Yes (if you use cashew nut or peanut butter and hempseed milk)
Low Oxalate Diet .... No
Specific Carbohydrate Diet .... Yes
This recipe is also Soy free, Corn free and Rice free

Oral Motor Rating 🙂 🙂

Coconut Macaroons

Yields: 12 Macaroons

Ingredients
3 egg whites or egg replacer
1/3 cup honey or maple syrup
1/2 teaspoon sea salt
1 teaspoon gluten- and casein-free vanilla
1 1/4 cups shredded coconut

There are many different variations for this recipe. You can add chopped almonds to make almond coconut macaroons — a preferred choice of many children. To make the macaroons more crispy, sprinkle coconut flakes on top after baking. Keep in mind that will give the recipe an Oral Motor rating of 4.

Directions
Preheat oven to 300º. Using an electric mixer, whip eggs white until they form stiff peaks. Add honey, salt and vanilla and mix until well blended. Mix coconut into mixture. Spoon batter into cupcake papers in a muffin tin. Bake 25-30 minutes.

Ingredients to Consider on Specific Diets

Gluten & Casein Free .... Yes
Phenol Free .... Yes (avoid honey, use maple syrup)
Low Oxalate Diet .... Yes
Specific Carbohydrate Diet .... Yes
This recipe is also Soy free, Corn free and Rice free

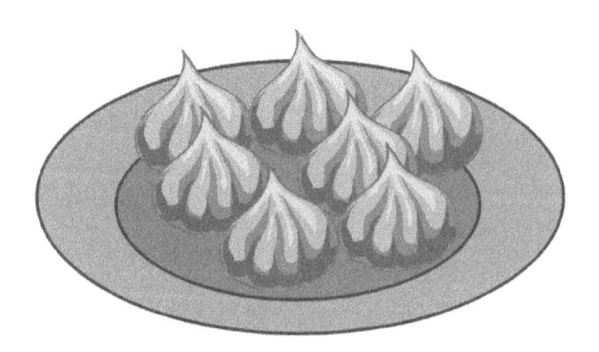

Oral Motor Rating 😊 😊 😊 😊

Banana Coconut Ice Cream

Yields: 4 to 6 Servings

Ingredients
2 cups coconut milk
2 ripe bananas
1/4 cup honey
2 eggs or egg replacer
1 cup SCD yogurt (optional)
1/2 cup walnuts or pecans, finely chopped

Pecans
Pecans have high fat content, which causes them to go rancid very easily. They must be stored well to make sure that they stay edible. Pecans are preferred as dessert nut, and appear in candies, pies, and cakes, as they provide a burst of rich and delicious buttery flavor.

Directions
In a bowl, blend all ingredients well and freeze in an ice cream maker.

Ingredients to Consider on Specific Diets

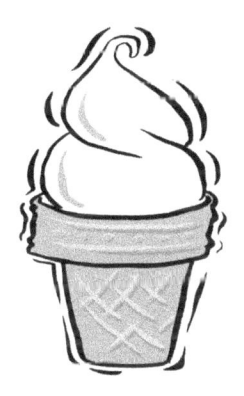

Gluten & Casein Free	Yes
Phenol Free	No
Low Oxalate Diet	No
Specific Carbohydrate Diet	Yes

This recipe is also Soy free, Corn free and Rice free

Oral Motor Rating 😊 😊

Notes:

Chapter Sixteen

Smoothies & Power Shakes

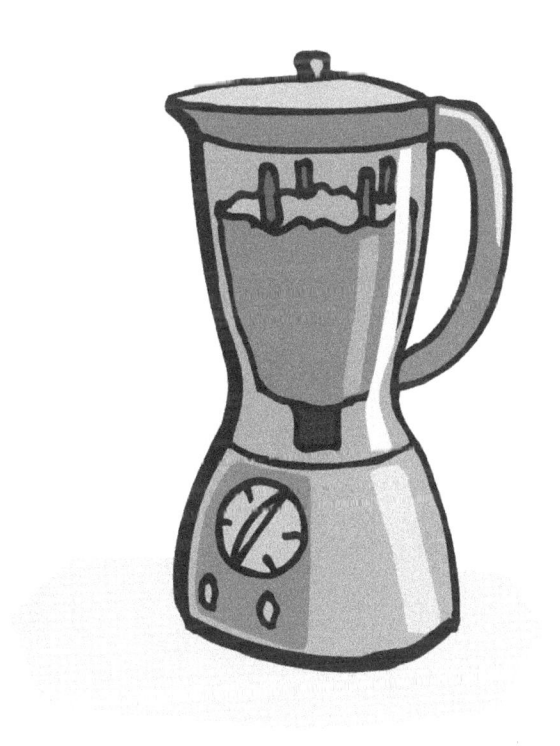

SMOOTHIES
TABLE OF CONTENTS

SMOOTHIE RECIPES

Blueberry and Banana Smoothie 381
Papaya Smoothie..382
Delicious Pear Smoothie 383
Banana Pineapple Shake 384
Coconut Protein Shake 385
Berry Kiwi Shake 386
Tropical Smoothie 387
Chocolate Shake..388
"Mmm Good" Mango Shake...389
Melon Shake...390
Vanilla Flavored Banana Smoothie 391
Eggnog Smoothie 392

Blueberry and Banana Smoothie

Yields: 2 Servings

Ingredients
1/4 cup seed cream
1 teaspoon cinnamon (optional)
2 cups nut milk
1/2 cup blueberries
1 banana
1 tablespoon honey

> **Nut Milk and Seed Cream**
>
> *Nut Milk and Seed Cream Recipes will be found in the "Homemade Specialties" area of Chapter 9.*

Directions
Grind the flax seeds along with cinnamon in a coffee grinder and set aside. Pour nut milk into your blender. Add all other ingredients and turn blender on low until the mixture is moving smoothly. Add seed cream and cinnamon powder. Then blend well on high for 2 minutes until creamy.

Ingredients to Consider on Specific Diets

Gluten & Casein Free	Yes
Phenol Free	No
Low Oxalate Diet	No
Specific Carbohydrate Diet	Yes

This recipe is also Soy free, Corn free and Rice free

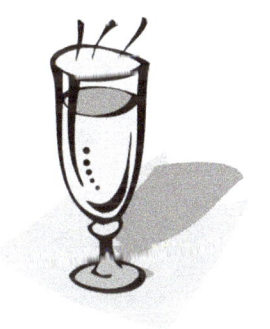

Oral Motor Rating 🙂 🙂

Papaya Smoothie

Yields: 2 Servings

Ingredients
1 cup almond or hemp seed milk
1 tablespoon honey or maple syrup
2 Papaya
1/4 cup seed cream or nut cream
1 tablespoon BodyBio Balance oil

Directions
Put all ingredients in a blender. Blend until all is well mixed, adding water to make the smoothie the consistency you desire.

Ingredients to Consider on Specific Diets

Gluten & Casein Free	Yes
Phenol Free	Yes (if you use hempseed milk, omit honey, and use seed creams)
Low Oxalate Diet	Yes (if you use hempseed milk and use seed creams)
Specific Carbohydrate Diet	Yes (if you use almond milk and honey as sweetner)

This recipe is also Soy free, Corn free and Rice free

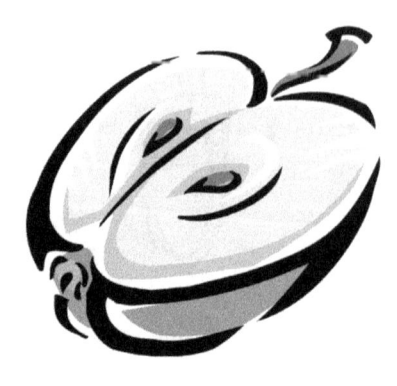

Oral Motor Rating 😊 😊 😊 😊

Delicious Pear Smoothie

Yields: 2 Servings

Ingredients
2 cups almond or hemp seed milk
1 pear, peeled, cored and cubed
1 tablespoon honey or maple syrup
2 tablespoons BodyBio Balance oil
1 tablespoon protein powder

> ### Protein Powders
> *Protein powders can be used based on the individual sensitivity and preference of your child. There are many options to choose from, including whey, soy bean, and egg.*

Directions
Put all ingredients in a blender and blend on medium speed for 30 seconds until smooth.

Ingredients to Consider on Specific Diets

Gluten & Casein Free	Yes
Phenol Free	Yes (if you use hempseed milk and omit honey)
Low Oxalate Diet	Yes (if you use hempseed milk)
Specific Carbohydrate Diet	Yes (if use almond milk and egg proteins powder)

This recipe is also Soy free, Corn free and Rice free

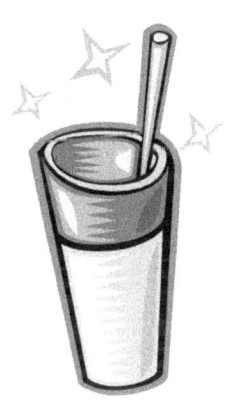

Oral Motor Rating :) :)

CHAPTER 16: SMOOTHIES

Banana Pineapple Shake

Yields: 2 Servings

Ingredients
1 cup almond, or hemp seed milk
1 medium banana
3 pineapple slices (fresh)
1 tablespoon honey or maple syrup
1/4 cup seed or nut cream
1 tablespoon BodyBio Balance oil

Pineapple

When buying pineapple, choose one that has gold-brown and firm skin. Avoid a pineapple whose skin is still green, as this will be unripe and very hard to slice.

Directions
Put all the ingredients in a blender. Blend for sixty seconds on medium speed or until mixture reaches desired consistency. Water can be added to make the smoothie the consistency you desire. Serve and enjoy.

Ingredients to Consider on Specific Diets

Gluten & Casein Free .... Yes
Phenol Free .... Yes (if you use hempseed milk, seed cream and omit honey)
Low Oxalate Diet .... Yes (if you use hempseed milk and seed cream)
Specific Carbohydrate Diet .... Yes (if you use almond milk)
This recipe is also Soy free, Corn free and Rice free

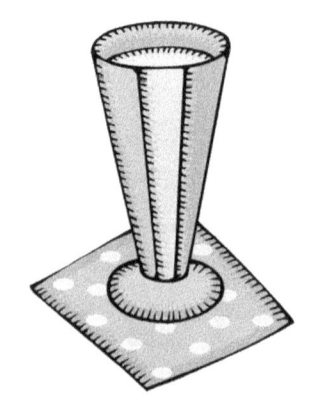

Oral Motor Rating ☺ ☺

Coconut Protein Shake

Yields: 2 Servings

Ingredients
1 cup coconut milk
1/2 cup organic coconut flakes
1 large ripe banana
1/4 cup almonds, finely chopped or
1 tablespoon almond butter
1 tablespoon honey
2 tablespoons BodyBio Balance oil

Directions
Put all of the above ingredients in a blender. Mix for 60 seconds on medium speed or until mixture reaches desired consistency. Serve and enjoy.

Ingredients to Consider on Specific Diets

Gluten & Casein Free .... Yes
Phenol Free .... No
Low Oxalate Diet .... No
Specific Carbohydrate Diet .... Yes
This recipe is also Soy free, Corn free and Rice free

Oral Motor Rating

Berry Kiwi Shake

Yields: 2 Servings

Ingredients
1/2 cup yogurt (SCD or coconut yogurt)
1/2 cup cranberry juice (unsweetened)
2 ripe kiwis (peeled and sliced)
2 tablespoons almond nut butter
2 tablespoons BodyBio Balance oil
1 tablespoon of honey

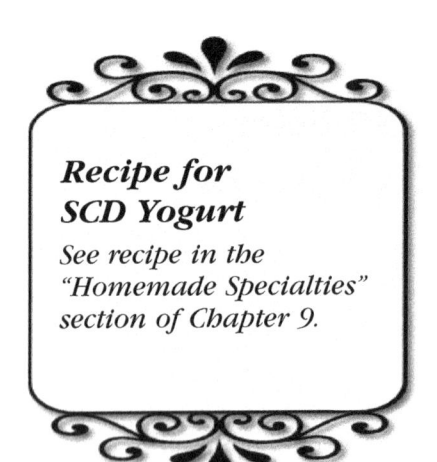

Recipe for SCD Yogurt
See recipe in the "Homemade Specialties" section of Chapter 9.

Directions
Put all of the above ingredients in a blender and mix for 30 seconds on medium speed or until mixture reaches desired consistency. Serve and enjoy.

Ingredients to Consider on Specific Diets

Gluten & Casein Free .... Yes (if you use coconut yogurt)
Phenol Free .... No
Low Oxalate Diet .... Yes (avoid kiwi and use orange instead)
Specific Carbohydrate Diet .... Yes

This recipe is also Soy free, Corn free and Rice free

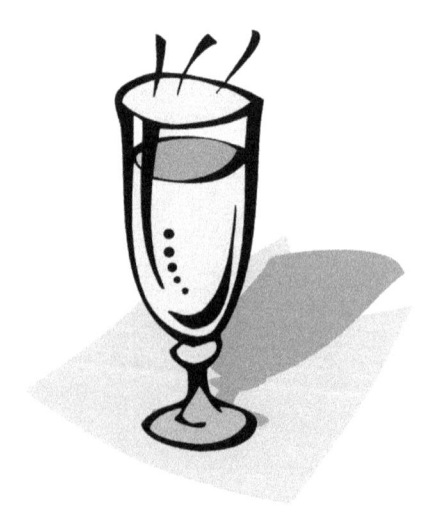

Oral Motor Rating 😊 😊

Tropical Smoothie

Yields: 3 Servings

Ingredients
2 cups unsweetened coconut milk
1 banana
1 mango, peeled and chopped
1 cup raw pineapple
1 tablespoon honey
2 tablespoons protein powder
2 tablespoons BodyBio Balance oil

Directions
Put all of the above ingredients in a blender. Mix for 30 seconds on medium speed or until mixture reaches desired consistency. Serve and enjoy.

Ingredients to Consider on Specific Diets

Gluten & Casein Free	Yes
Phenol Free	No
Low Oxalate Diet	Yes
Specific Carbohydrate Diet	Yes (if you use egg protein powder)

This recipe is also Soy free, Corn free and Rice free

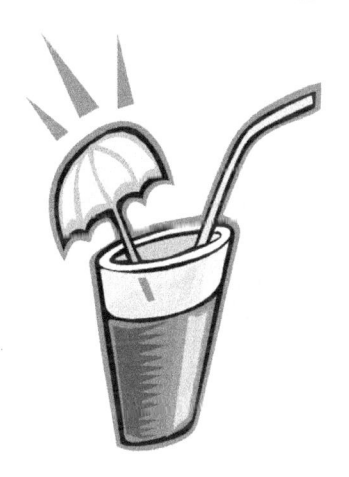

Oral Motor Rating 😊 😊

Chocolate Shake

Yields: 4 Servings

Ingredients
2 tablespoons seed or nut cream
2 cups almond milk or unsweetened coconut milk
2 bananas
1 tablespoon honey or maple syrup
2 tablespoons BodyBio Balance oil
2 tablespoons organic unsweetened cocoa powder
2 tablespoons Egg Protein Powder

> ### *Raw Honey*
> *Raw honey is the concentrated nectar of flowers that comes straight from the extractor. It is the only unheated, pure, unpasteurized, unprocessed honey. It is an alkaline-forming food and contains ingredients similar to those found in fruits, which become alkaline in the digestive system.*

Directions
Put all of the above ingredients in a blender. Mix for 45 seconds on medium speed or until mixture reaches desired consistency. Serve and enjoy.

Ingredients to Consider on Specific Diets

Gluten & Casein Free .... Yes
Phenol Free .... Yes (if you use coconut milk, seed cream and maple sryup as sweetner)
Low Oxalate Diet .... Yes (if you use coconut milk and seed cream)
Specific Carbohydrate Diet .... Yes (if you use honey)
This recipe is also Soy free, Corn free and Rice free

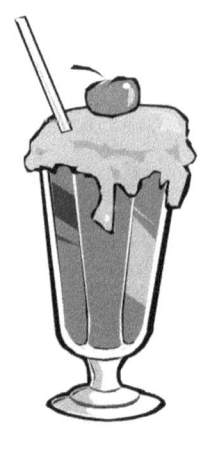

Oral Motor Rating 🙂 🙂

"Mmm Good" Mango Shake

Yields: 2 Servings

Ingredients
1 cup almond or hemp seed milk
1/2 cup pomegranate juice
1 ripe mango, peeled, cored and chopped
1 banana
2 tablespoons protein powder or
2 tablespoons seed or nut cream
1 tablespoon BodyBio Balance oil

Pomegranate juice

Use unsweetened pomegranate juice. Many people also enjoy its rich taste, making it a welcome beverage.

Directions
Put all of the above ingredients in a blender. Mix for 60 seconds on medium speed or until mixture reaches desired consistency. Serve and enjoy.

Ingredients to Consider on Specific Diets

Gluten & Casein Free .... Yes
Phenol Free .... Yes (if you use hempseed milk, seed creams and omit pomegranate juice)
Low Oxalate Diet .... Yes (if you use hempseed milk)
Specific Carbohydrate Diet ..... Yes (if you use almond milk)

This recipe is also Soy free, Corn free and Rice free

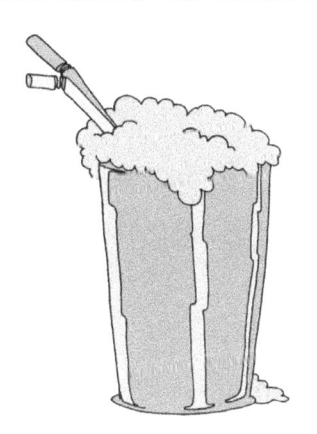

Oral Motor Rating 😊 😊

Melon Shake

Yields: 2 Servings

Ingredients
2 cups almond or hempseed milk
1/2 cantaloupe, peeled, seeded, and sliced
5 fresh strawberries
1 tablespoon honey or maple sryup
2 tablespoons protein powder, or
2 tablespoon seed or nut cream
1 tablespoon BodyBio Balance oil

Cantaloupe

Cantaloupe is a rich source of Vitamin C, beta-carotene and is loaded with potassium. It is filled with healing qualities that help control blood pressure and help fight against cancer.

Directions
Pour all ingredients in a blender. Mix for 60 seconds on medium speed or until mixture reaches desired consistency. Serve and enjoy.

Ingredients to Consider on Specific Diets

Gluten & Casein Free .... Yes
Phenol Free .... Yes (if you use hempseed milk, seed creams and omit honey)
Low Oxalate Diet .... Yes (if you use hempseed milk and seed creams)
Specific Carbohydrate Diet .... Yes (if you use almond milk and honey as sweetener)
This recipe is also Soy free, Corn free and Rice free

Oral Motor Rating ☺ ☺

Vanilla Flavored Banana Smoothie

Yields: 3 Servings

Ingredients
2 cups almond or hempseed milk
1 banana
1 tablespoon honey or maple sryup
2 tablespoons tahini, or any seed or nut butter
1 teaspoon gluten- and casein-free vanilla
2 tablespoons BodyBio Balance oil

> ### *Tahini*
> *Tahini is a paste of ground sesame seeds used in cooking. Tahini may be purchased in cans, jars, fresh or dehydrated. Tahini comes in two varieties; hulled and unhulled. It is sometimes used to replace peanut butter on bread.*

Directions
Pour all ingredients in a blender. Mix for 30 seconds on medium speed or until mixture reaches desired consistency. Serve and enjoy.

Ingredients to Consider on Specific Diets

Gluten & Casein Free .... Yes
Phenol Free .... Yes (if you use hempseed milk, omit honey and nut butter)
Low Oxalate Diet .... Yes (if you use hempseed milk and omit nut butter)
Specific Carbohydrate Diet .... Yes (if you use almond milk and honey as sweetener)
This recipe is also Soy free, Corn free and Rice free
Oral Motor Rating 😊 😊

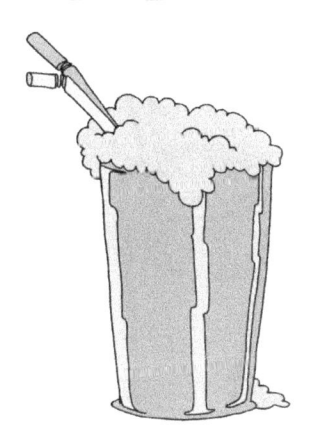

Eggnog Smoothie

Yields: 2 Servings

Ingredients
2 hard-boiled egg yolks
1 tablespoon honey or maple syrup
1 teaspoon gluten- and casein-free vanilla extract
1/8 teaspoon ground nutmeg (optional)
1/4 teaspoon cinnamon
1 cup almond or hempseed milk
1 tablespoon BodyBio Balance oil

Egg in the Recipe
This smoothie recipe uses only the yolks of hard boiled eggs. This makes the smoothie taste good and is well accepted by children.

Directions
Put all of the above ingredients in a blender. Mix for 30 seconds on a medium speed or until mixture reaches desired consistency. Serve and enjoy.

Ingredients to Consider on Specific Diets

Gluten & Casein Free .... Yes
Phenol Free .... Yes (if you use hempseed milk and omit honey)
Low Oxalate Diet .... Yes (if you use hempseed milk)
Specific Carbohydrate Diet .... Yes (if you use almond milk and honey as sweetener)
This recipe is also Soy free, Corn free and Rice free

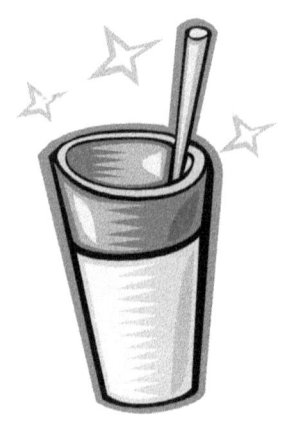

Oral Motor Rating ☺ ☺

Conversion Tables and Measurement Charts

Cooking Measurement Equivalents

16 tablespoons = 1 cup
12 tablespoons = 3/4 cup
10 tablespoons + 2 teaspoons = 2/3 cup
8 tablespoons = 1/2 cup
6 tablespoons = 3/8 cup
5 tablespoons + 1 teaspoon = 1/3 cup
4 tablespoons = 1/4 cup
2 tablespoons = 1/8 cup
2 tablespoons + 2 teaspoons = 1/6 cup
1 tablespoon = 1/16 cup
1 tablespoon = 3 teaspoons
2 cups = 1 pint
2 pints = 1 quart
48 teaspoons = 1 cup

Temperature* Fahrenheit / Celsius

32 / 0
212 / 100
250 / 120
275 / 140
300 / 150
325 / 160
350 / 180
375 / 190
400 / 200
425 / 220
450 / 230
475 / 240
500 / 260

All temperatures given in this book are Fahrenheit.

Liquids

1/4 teaspoon = 1 ml
1/2 teaspoon = 2 ml
1 teaspoon = 5 ml
1 tablespoon = 20 ml
1/4 cup = 60 ml
1/3 cup = 80 ml
1/2 cup = 125 ml
2/3 cup = 170 ml
3/4 cup = 190 ml
1 cup = 250 ml
1 quart = 1 liter

Weight

1 ounce = 30 grams
2 ounce = 60 grams
3 ounce = 90 grams
4 ounce = 125 grams
8 ounce = 225 grams
16 ounce = 500 grams

INDEX OF RECIPES

~ A ~

Alkaline Coleslaw	229
Almond and Coconut Pancakes	192
Almond Butter Brownies	368
Almond Coconut Granola	218
Apple Gelatin Dessert	370
Apple Pudding Cake	364
Apple Coconut Crisp	373
Applesauce Bread	189
Artichoke Pate Roll-Ups	245
Asparagus Soup	277
Avocado Dip	329
Avocado Meatloaf	264
Avocado Summer Soup	279

~ B ~

Baked Apples	372
Baked Butternut Squash	232
Baked Turkey Patties	250
Banana Bread	188
Banana Coconut Ice Cream	377
Banana Muffins	202
Banana Nut Pancakes	201
Banana Nut Pudding	375
Banana Pineapple Shake	384
Basil Veggie Stew	273

~ B ~

BBQ Sauce	317
Bean Sprout Spinach Pine Nut Salad	302
Beef Stew	291
Beefy Spinach with Mushrooms	247
Beet and Carrot Soup	289
Berry Kiwi Shake	386
Blueberry and Banana Smoothie	381
Blueberry Pie	361
Bok Choy Salad	309
Breakfast Spring Rolls	214
Broccoli Beef	260
Broccoli Salad	305
Brown Pear Muffins	206
Brown Rice Pancakes	194
Brown-Brown Brownies	367
Brussels Sprouts	227
Butternut Squash Crunch	333
Butternut Squash Soup	276

~ C ~

Carrot Coconut Cake	362
Carrot Cutlets	216
Carrot Pancakes	191
Cauliflower, Carrot and Celery Soup	280
Chicken Breasts Roasted in Fresh Garden Herbs	259
Chicken Chow Mein	265
Chicken Nuggets	257
Chicken Patties	253
Chicken Rice Soup	293
Chicken Teriyaki with Broccoli	255
Chocolate Biscotti	369
Chocolate Chip Cookies	351

~ C ~

Chocolate Shake 388
Chopped Meat Patty..199
Cinnamon Baby Carrots with Roasted Sesame Seeds........................234
Coconut Bread or Crackers 185
Coconut Chicken Broth 290
Coconut Cookies..354
Coconut Macaroons 376
Coconut Mango Cookies...353
Coconut Omelet...213
Coconut Protein Shake 385
Creamed Peas and Potatoes 240
Creamy Macaroni (Mac & Cheese) 242
Crispy Walnut Crackers or Cookies 355
Crunchy Chickpea Bars...335
Cucumber Pressed Salad..308
Curried Celery and Lima Bean Soup 282

~ D ~

Deep-Fried Shrimp 266
Delicious Pear Smoothie 383
Donut Holes..374
Dutch Style Red Cabbage 230

~ E ~

Easy Chicken Pancakes...200
Easy Cranberry Sauce 321
Easy English Pea Soup 281
Easy Gluten-Free Flatbread 184
Easy Pressure-Cooked Vegetables...239
Egg Bread...190

~ E ~

Egg Rolls 212
Eggnog Smoothie 392

~ F ~

Flax and Sesame Seed Sticks 341
Flourless Lemon and Almond Cake 365
French Apple Pie 358
French Onion Soup 288
French Toast 217
Fried Chicken Patties 197

~ G ~

Ginger Scallion Dipping Sauce 320
Gingersnap Cookies 356
Gingery Carrot Sauce 326
Gluten-Free Chicken Nuggets 337
Golden Pancakes or Waffles 196
Graham Crackers 345
Grape Dessert Delight 371

~ H ~

Ham and Fresh Asparagus Salad 314
Hamburger Salad 312
Hard-Boiled Egg Salad 311
Hash Brown Casserole 220
Hearty German Soup 292
Homemade Ketchup 319
Honey Cake 363
Hot Breakfast Porridge 215
Hummus-Stuffed Portobello Caps 243

~ I ~

Italian Pesto 322

~ J ~

Jam Muffins 205

~ L ~

Lentil Cauliflower and Parsley Pancakes 193
Lentil Salad 303

~ M ~

"Mmm Good" Mango Shake 389
Mango Salsa 328
Meat Loaf 248
Melon Shake 390
Mini Squash Muffins 207
Mulligatawny Soup 294

~ N ~

No-Bake Lentil (Mung Dal) Blondie 366
Nut "Ice Cream" 339
Nut Butter Pudding 334

~ O ~

Oriental Cabbage Soup 287

~ P ~

Papaya Smoothie	383
Peach Pie	360
Pear Sauce	338
Pizza Crust	226
Potato Celery Soup	272
Potato Salad	306
Pumpkin Cookies	352
Pumpkin Muffins	203
Pumpkin Pie	359
Pumpkinseed Fruit Bread	186

~ Q ~

Quick Black Bean Soup	284
Quick Chicken Vegetable Stir-Fry	261
Quick Creamy Cereal or Pudding	219
Quinoa & Cilantro Salad with Lemon & Garlic	304
Quinoa Crackers	343
Quinoa Pilaf	235

~ R ~

Ranch Dip or Dressing	327
Raw Buckwheat Crackers	336
Red Bell Peppers Stuffed With Millet	241
Red Lentil Soup	283
Red Pepper and Mushroom Soup	278
Rice Pudding	340
Roasted Mixed Vegetables	244
Roasted Potatoes with Garlic and Rosemary	238
Rolled Double Pie Crust	357

~ S ~

Salmon Patties 254
Sautéed Broccoli 228
Sautéed Kale with Garlic 231
Sautéed Snow Peas with Ginger and Onion 237
Sephardic Leek Soup 285
Sesame Chicken Wings 263
Sesame Finger Snacks 344
Simmered Greens 236
Soft Boiled Eggs 209
Soft Scrambled Eggs 210
Sorghum Bread 183
Spaghetti Carbonara 256
Spaghetti Squash 233
Spaghetti with Meat Sauce 262
Spicy Thai Almond Sauce 325
Spinach Pear or Guava Salad 300
Spinach Tofu or Chicken Curry 252
Split Pea Soup 286
Spring Rolls 342
Stuffed Acorn Squash 225
Sweet Mustard Sauce 318

~ T ~

Tandoori Chicken 267
Tempeh Salad 310
Three-Bean Salad 307
Tomato, Cucumber and Avocado Salad 301
Tropical Muffins 208
Tropical Smoothie 387
Turkey Burgers with Sweet Mustard Sauce 251
Turkey Meatballs 249

~ T ~

Turkey or Chicken Lettuce Wraps 258
Turkey or Chicken Soup 295
Turkey Salad 313
Two-Bean Chili Soup 296

~ V ~

Vanilla Flavored Banana Smoothie 391
Vegetable Cutlets or Pancakes 195
Vegetable Fried Rice 246
Very Very Green Smoothie 382

~ W ~

Water Chestnut Soup 274
Watercress Soup 275
White Bean Hummus Dip 324

~ Y ~

Yam Latkes 198

~ Z ~

Zucchini Bread 187
Zucchini Hummus 323
Zucchini Omelet 211

RESOURCES
FOR MORE INFORMATION ON
TOPICS DISCUSSED IN EACH CHAPTER

Chapter One Resources:

Nutrient and Nutrient-Dense Foods. *Dietary Guidelines for Americans 2005*, "Adequate Nutrients Within Calorie Needs" (www.health.gov/DietaryGuidelines)

Eating Habits of Children with Autism. Article in *Pediatric Nursing (May, 2000)* by Gail P. Williams, Nancy Dalrymple and Jamie Neal

Effects of Carbohydrates on Children with ASD. "Relationship of Dietary Intake to Gastrointestinal Symptoms in Children with Autistic Spectrum Disorders," by S. Levy, M. Souders, R. Ittenbach, E. Giarelli, A. Mulberg, J. Pinto-Martin. *Biological Psychiatry* (Volume 61, Issue 4, pages 492-497)

Proteins and Amino Acids:

- Food and Nutrition Board, National Academy of Sciences, "Dietary Reference Intakes for Energy, Carbohydrate, Fiber, Fat, Fatty Acids, Cholesterol, Protein, and Amino Acids" (Macronutrients) (2005)
- Lemon, PW. (1996). "Is increased dietary protein necessary or beneficial for individuals with a physically active lifestyle?" *Nutrition Review* 54:S169-S175

Fats and Essential Fatty Acids. *Know Your Fats: The Complete Primer for Understanding the Nutrition of Fats, Oils and Cholesterol* by Mary G. Enig, Ph.D. (Bethesda Press, 2000)

Vitamins:

- *Smart Medicine for a Healthier Child: A Practical A-to-Z Reference to Natural and Conventional Treatments* by Janet Zand and Rachel Walton (Avery, 1994, pages 50-51)
- *Advanced Nutrition and Human Metabolism*, Second edition, by Sareen S. Gropper, Jack L. Smith (West Publishing Company, pages 223-224)

Minerals:

- *Smart Medicine for a Healthier Child: A Practical A-to-Z Reference to Natural and Conventional Treatments* by Janet Zand and Rachel Walton (Avery, 1994, pages 52-53)
- *Advanced Nutrition and Human Metabolism*, Second edition, by Sareen S. Gropper, Jack L. Smith (West Publishing Company, pages 325-337)

Chapter Two Resources:

Guide to Food Selection. *Nourishing Traditions: The Cookbook that Challenges Politically Correct Nutrition and the Diet Dictocrats*, by Sally Fallon and Mary Enig (New Trends Publishing, Inc., pages 64-65)

Nuts and Seeds: Nutrient-Dense Food. Futers Nut Butters – www.futtersnutbutters.com

Guide to Edible Oils and Health:
- Omega Nutrition – www.omeganutrition.com/home.php
- Spectrum — A Passion for Healthy Oils – www.spectrumorganics.com

Sea Weeds: Health Treasure. *Aveline Kushi's Complete Guide to Macrobiotic Cooking: For Health, Harmony, and Peace*, by Aveline Kushi with Alex Jack (Warner Books)

Fermented Foods: Fruits and Vegetables. *Nourishing Traditions: The Cookbook that Challenges Politically Correct Nutrition and the Diet Dictocrats*, by Sally Fallon and Mary Enig (New Trends Publishing, Inc., pages 89-222)

Beans, Lentils and Legumes Guide and Health Benefits. *Aveline Kushi's Complete Guide to Macrobiotic Cooking: For Health, Harmony, and Peace*, by Aveline Kushi and Alex Jack (Warner Books, pages 248-253)

Chapter Three Resources:

Hidden Food Sources & Guide to Natural Sweeteners:
- *Nourishing Traditions: The Cookbook that Challenges Politically Correct Nutrition and the Diet Dictocrats*, by Sally Fallon and Mary Enig (New Trends Publishing, Inc., pages 536-537)
- *Aveline Kushi's Complete Guide to Macrobiotic Cooking: For Health, Harmony, and Peace*, by Aveline Kushi and Alex Jack (Warner Books, pages 320-321)

Chapter Five and Chapter Seven Resources:

Gluten and Casein-Free Diet (GFCF Diet) – www.gfcfdiet.com

Low Oxalate Diet – http://lowoxalate.info/

Phenol and Feingold (Additives) Free Diet. TACA Organization – http://GFCF-diet.TalkAboutCuringAutism.org. (Search for "Phenols, Salicylates & Additives")

Specific Carbohydrate Diet (SCD) – www.SCDiet.org.
- Breaking the Vicious Cycle – www.BreakingtheViciousCycle.info
- Recipes for the Specific Carbohydrate Diet – www.SCDrecipes.com
- The Healing Crow Organization — The Omen of Good Health, www.HealingCrow.com

Talk About Curing Autism Now (TACA) – www.TalkAboutCuringAutism.org (click GFCF DIET button)

Chapter Six Resources:

Raw Food Diet. Do a keyword search for "Raw Food Diet" to turn up several helpful articles on this About.com site: http://altmedicine.about.com

Food Rotation Diet. Food Allergy Organization – http://www.food-allergy.org/rotation.html

Food Elimination Diet. The Food Intolerant Consumer website – http://www.foodintol.com/eliminationdiet.asp

Food Sensitivity and Food Intolerance. The Food Intolerant Consumer website, www.foodintol.com/

Chapter Eight Resources:

Oral Motor Issues:

- *Improving Speech and Eating Skills in Children with Autism Spectrum Disorders — An Oral Motor Program for Home and School* by Maureen A. Flanagan (Autism Asperger Publishing Company)
- *Treating Eating Problems of Children W/ Autism Spectrum Disorders and Developmental Disabilities: Interventions for Professionals and Parents* by Keith E. Williams (Pro-Ed Publishing)

Additional Resources Meals (Breakfast, Lunch & Dinner):

- Eat Right/American Dietetic Association – www.eatright.org. (Click the MEDIA tab button for the 2/2/04 news release about the importance of breakfast.)
- Child Development Institute – www.childdevelopmentinfo.com. Many discussions about child and teen health and safety issues from leading experts and professional organizations. Search on this site for "nutrition" to turn up a number of pages relative to discussions in this book.
- *Pediatric Nutrition in Chronic Diseases and Developmental Disorders: Prevention, Assessment, and Treatment* by Shirley Walberg Ekvall and Valli K. Ekvall (Oxford University Press)